Manual of
Clinical Methods
Fourth Edition

Manual of
Clinical Methods

Fourth Edition

PS Shankar MD, FAMS, DSc(hc)

Emeritus Professor of Medicine
Medical Director, MR Medical College
Gulbarga

Oxford & IBH Publishing Co. Pvt. Ltd.

New Delhi

(A Unit of CBS Publishers & Distributors Pvt Ltd *)*

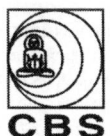

CBS

CBS Publishers & Distributors Pvt Ltd

New Delhi • Bengaluru • Chennai • Kochi • Kolkata • Mumbai
Bhopal • Bhubaneswar • Hyderabad • Jharkhand • Nagpur • Patna
• Pune • Uttarakhand • Dhaka (Bangladesh) • Kathmandu (Nepal)

Manual of
Clinical Methods
Fourth Edition

ISBN-13: 978-81-204-1687-1
ISBN-10: 81-204-1687-2

© 2005, 1992, 1987, 1976, PS Shankar
Reprint 2017, 2020

OXFORD & IBH
New Delhi
(A Unit of CBS Publishers & Distributors Pvt Ltd)

CBS Publishers & Distributors Pvt Ltd
204 FIE, Patparganj Industrial Area, Delhi 110 092
E-mail: delhi@cbspd.com, cbspubs@airtelmail.in

Ph: 4934 4934   Fax: 4934 4935   Website: www.cbspd.com
                                               e-mail: publishing@cbspd.com;
                                               publicity@cbspd.com

Branches

- **Bengaluru:** Seema House 2975, 17th Cross, K.R. Road,
  Banasankari 2nd Stage, Bengaluru 560 070, Karnataka, India
  Ph: +91-80-26771678/79   Fax: +91-80-26771680   e-mail: bangalore@cbspd.com
- **Chennai:** 7, Subbaraya Street, Shenoy Nagar, Chennai 600 030, Tamil Nadu, India
  Ph: +91-44-26260666, 26208620   Fax: +91-44-42032115   e-mail: chennai@cbspd.com
- **Kochi:** 42/1325, 1326, Power House Road, Opp KSEB, Kochi 682 018, Kerala
  Ph: +91-484-4059061-65   Fax: +91-484-4059065   e-mail: kochi@cbspd.com
- **Kolkata:** 6/B, Ground Floor, Rameswar Shaw Road, Kolkata-700014 (West Bengal), India
  Ph: +91-33-2289-1126, 2289-1127, 2289-1128   e-mail: kolkata@cbspd.com
- **Mumbai:** 83-C, Dr E Moses Road, Worli, Mumbai-400018, Maharashtra, India
  Ph: +91-22-24902340/41   Fax: +91-22-24902342   e-mail: mumbai@cbspd.com

Representatives

• Bhopal	0-8319310552	• Bhubaneswar	0-9911037372	• Hyderabad	0-9885175004
• Jharkhand	0-9811541605	• Nagpur	0-9421945513	• Patna	0-9334159340
• Pune	0-9623451994	• Uttarakhand	0-9716462459	• Dhaka	01912-003485
• Kathmandu (Nepal)	977-9818742655			(Bangladesh)	

Printed at Chaman Enterprises, Daryaganj, New Delhi, India

FOREWORD

I have great pleasure in writing this foreword to Dr. P.S. Shankar's book.

This book is designed to help in the training of undergraduate students in the subject of Clinical Medicine. Valuable practical hints have been given towards proper history-taking and recording of case notes. This is followed by general examination of the patient with elaborate details of the many points to be observed regarding posture, appearance, height, build, nutrition, skin and different parts of the body, head and face, trunk and limbs. The latter and the larger portion of the book deals with examination of various systems, digestive, respiratory, cardiovascular, nervous and locomotor. Considerable emphasis has been given to the methods of elicitation of clinical signs, their meaning and importance.

In the twenties and thirties, physical examination was the main and most important step in diagnosis. Ancillary aids were used only under special indications, and such aids were very few. Since then, biochemistry has evolved tremendously, giving a large number of laboratory tests yielding important information on the structure and function of organs and tissues. In the same period, a large number of very useful electro-medical appliances were made available to yield important information such as X-ray studies electrocardiograms, electroencephalograms and electromyograms. Teachers of the day in medicine, are keen to impart as much knowledge of these developments to their students, especially to the postgraduates, but to some extent to the undergraduates. As a result of all this, there is in evidence today, a greater faith in this ancillary data to the neglect of careful history taking and clinical examination. In this context, the publication of this 'Manual of Clinical Methods' is welcome. The importance of a careful examination, the way of carrying it out, and the information it yields, have been very well detailed in it. And the author has to be congratulated for the able way in which this has been done. This book will certainly contribute to a better moulding of the undergraduate students in their methods of clinical examination.

Bombay   Dr. R.V. Sathe
                                             M.D., F.R.C.P. (Lond)

PREFACE TO THE FOURTH EDITION

It is 30 years since the publication of first edition of Manual of Clinical Methods. During this period new diseases have been identified, new modalities of investigations and treatment have been formulated and medical education technology has witnessed significant changes. These significant advances have not replaced the good clinical history from the patient and elicitation of physical signs using the faculties of sight, hearing and touch. They form the basis of the diagnosis. Though actual methods of examination have not fundamentally changed, the interpretation of the clinical signs and the relative importance of some of them have changed, as methods of investigations and understanding of the pathophysiology of many diseases have improved significantly. Medical education technology has stressed the importance of problem-solving technique that rely on Evidence-based medicine.

The book has maintained the aims set out in the preface of the first edition. The book tries to help the student in the medical ward and outpatient to take a proper history, to make a careful examination of different systems and to evaluate the findings to arrive at a proper diagnosis. The emphasis is on developing clinical skills, as many diseases can be diagnosed by history and physical examination without recourse to expensive, highly sophisticated investigative methods.

All the chapters have been thoroughly revised in the light of advances in clinical science. New material has been added to the chapters on general examination and systemic examination. New diagrams and clinical photographs have been added. Attempts have been made to provide all information in a comprehensive manner.

Thanks are due to my wife Ambika without whose support and encouragement this book would not have been produced. I thank the publisher for giving all encouragement and support to revise this book and arrange for its publication.

January 01, 2005   P.S. Shankar

PREFACE TO THE FIRST EDITION

> *"To carefully observe the phenomena of life in all its phases, normal and perverted, to make perfect the most difficult of all arts, the art of observation, to call to aid the Science of experimentation, to cultivate the reasoning faculty so as to be able to know the true from the false-these are our methods"*
>
> *William Osler*

This book has been written for the medical students entering the clinical course. The scope of the book is described in the title 'Manual of Clinical Methods'. The diagnosis of various conditions can be made on the basis of a careful and accurate history and a methodical physical examination. The radiological and laboratory examinations, act as supplementary measures to the diagnosis. Those methods, however accurate, cannot replace the physical methods of examination. The time-honoured methods of inspection, palpation, percussion and auscultation using the sense of sight, touch and hearing, are employed to make accurate observations.

The aim of the book is to outline the principles and methods of history taking, and description of the standard methods, routinely adapted to elicit various physical signs. An attempt is made, to give an explanation of these methods on the findings in healthy people and in diseased states, in a comprehensive manner. The first two chapters deal with history taking, and the subsequent chapters cover general and systemic examinations of various systems. An attempt is made to give up-to-date methods of examination. The line diagrams and photographs used are to illustrate the methods employed to demonstrate the physical signs and some classic examples of the diseased states.

CONTENTS

ONE

INTRODUCTION

> *"Nature, in the production of disease, is uniform and consistent, so much so, that for the same disease in different persons the symptoms are for the most part the same; and the self same phenomena that you would observe in the sickness of a Socrates you would observe in the sickness of a simpleton"*
>
> *Thomas Sydenham (1624-1689)*

The patient (derived from Latin word, patiens, meaning sufferance) presents himself to his doctor for the relief of his ailment with which he is suffering. It is the duty of the physician to determine its cause (diagnosis). On the basis of it, he can treat the condition, and advise about the prognosis. The diagnosis can be arrived at by the application of two fundamental methods of examination: history taking (anamnesis, interrogation) and physical examination.

The history is obtained from an account of the complaints which the patient narrates. The complaints the patient speaks of are **symptoms**. These symptoms may be felt by the patient, as altered sensations (pain, cough, breathlessness) or as altered body function (frequency of micturition, constipation, diarrhoea). The objective changes as determined during the examination, are referred to as **signs**. These are further demonstrated by the classical methods of examination (inspection, palpation, percussion and auscultation) with the unaided senses and stethoscope and are referred to as 'physical signs'.

The clinical diagnosis is made on the following procedures:

1) History: Interrogation and recording of all symptoms of present illness, details of past illness, family history and personal history.

2) Physical examination: Elicitation of the signs of the disease by making a general and systemic examination.

3) Analysis of the salient features of the history and physical signs to arrive at a clinical diagnosis. The data logically interpreted based on experience and knowledge of the diseases.

The clinical diagnosis has to be substantiated by the routine laboratory investigations (examination of blood, urine, stools and sputum), and confirmed by special investigations using laboratory and imaging methods.

TWO

HISTORY TAKING

> "A doctor who cannot take a good history and a patient who cannot give one are in danger of giving and receiving bad treatment"
>
> *anonymous, quoted by Paul D White*

Record of Symptoms

The history is a record of the symptoms of the patient. History taking has been regarded as an art. It can be perfected by constant practice. When it is written in the form of a case-sheet, it should give the history in a comprehensive manner containing all the salient features.

Rapport with the Patient

The elicitation of a good history and physical signs, depends on a good rapport established between the doctor and the patient. The patient has to develop confidence in the doctor, so that he gives an accurate account of his ailments. Good bedside manners and courtesy extended by the doctor to the patient, helps to achieve this end. According to Perry, "In this era of high technology and managed care, as the practice of medicine has become so impersonal, more instrumental, and dehumanizing in its approach, the sense care and comfort the patient receives from the so-called *'laying on hands'* fosters the close rapport, trust and confidence so important to the privileged and sacred doctor-patient relationship. As it is said, no one cares how much you know, until they know how much you care".

Elicitation of History

After recording the preliminary data of the patient, the main complaints and relevant details of the current sickness are elicited and it is followed by a history taking of his past illness, and of his family.

While eliciting the history slowly and calmly, the patient must be allowed to relate his problems in his own way. He should not be distracted from his objective of narrating his ailment, unless a valid clarification is sought. He should be so prompted with queries then, that he gives answers related to the ailment. If he wanders off the subject, he should be gently steered back to the issue in question. History taking does not follow any rigid norms. An element of flexibility is needed as each case is different, and has to be treated as circumstances warrant.

The doctor must show genuine interest while listening to the patient's narration and give him a sympathetic hearing. There are patients who give a good account of their ailment, without having to be prompted. There are others who are inhibited and are unable to give a proper account of their ailments—the interrogator then must use tact, wit and charm to extract relevant information. The anxious patient may exaggerate his symptoms. The feelings of the patient must be respected, without a suggestion, even by facial expression that might upset the patient. While he should be encouraged to relate his tale of woe, he should be helped to stay with his story with greater relevance and significance.

The medical student, as also a doctor, should learn the regional language where he is studying or working. This will enable him to talk with the patient directly without the help of an interpreter. He must be aware of the local customs, habits and festivals as there are patients who tend to relate the beginning of their complaints to such festivals like that of Dasara, Diwali, a religious ceremony or fair, or a full moon or new moon day. History has to be written in the words of the patient (for example, swelling of the feet, or inability to use both lower limbs). Many patients are not aware of any medical terminology and may use vague terms. The terms like pain in the stomach, kidney pain, heart trouble, rheumatism, migraine or acidity are to be avoided. The questions should be simple and the terminology, must be readily understood by the patient. The patient may be asked to describe the discomfort he experiences.

Positive and Negative Symptoms

All efforts are to be made to get information from the patient,

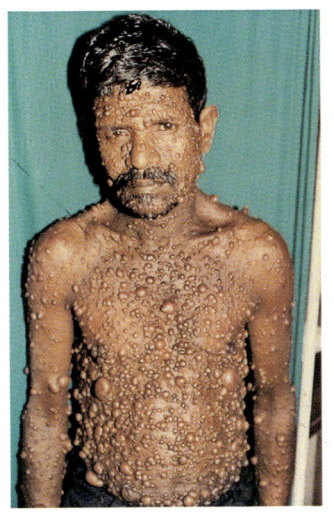

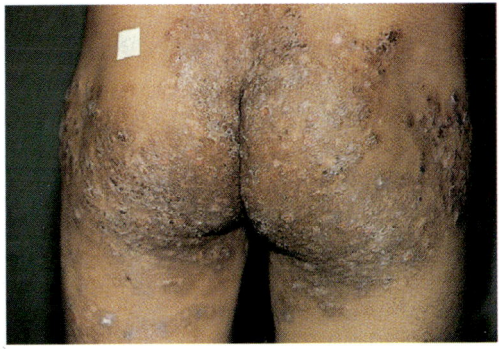

Taenia corporis

Neurofibromatosis

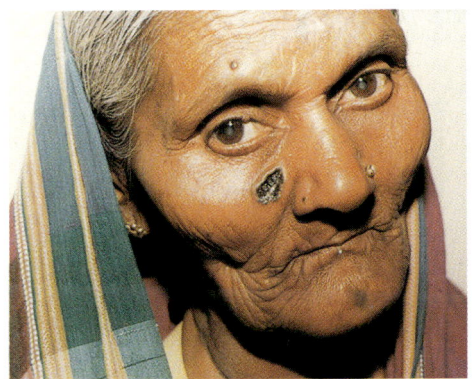

Basal cell carcinoma

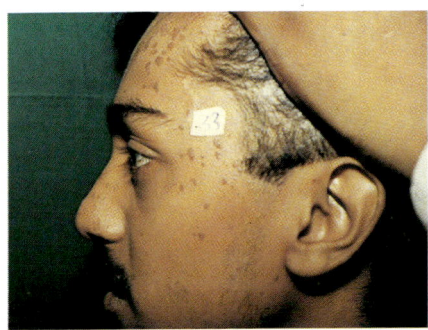

Verruca plana

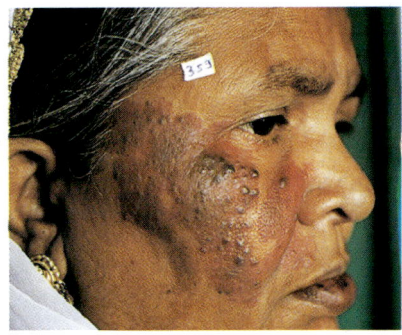

Port-wine stain

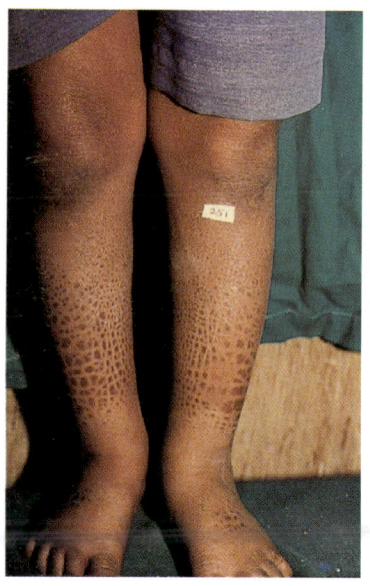

Icthyosis

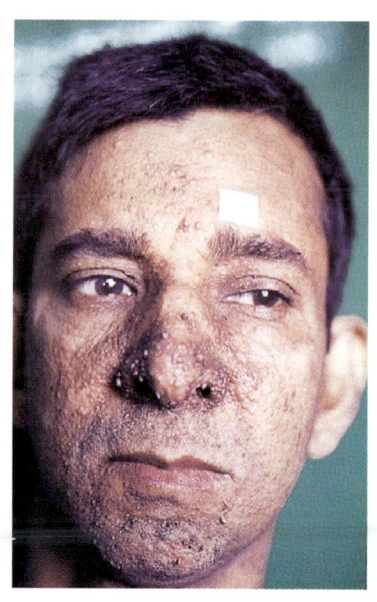

Adenoma sebaceum

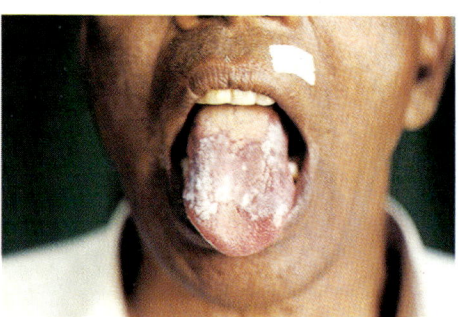

Oral candidiasis

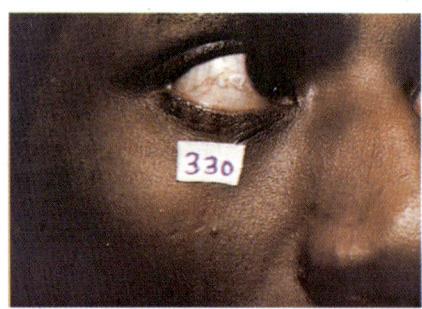

Bitot's spots

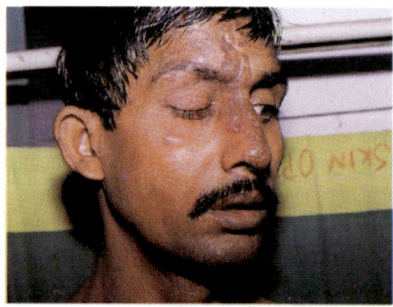

Herpes zoster ophthalmicus

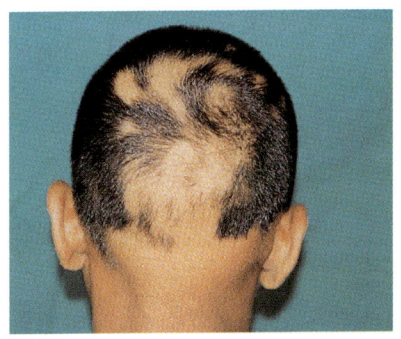

Alopecia aerata

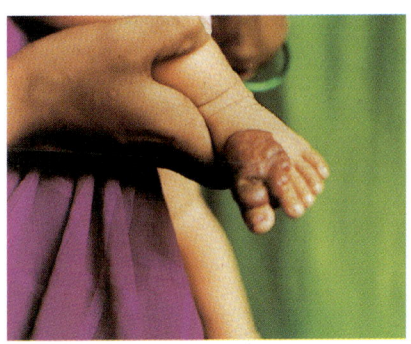

Capillary haemangioma

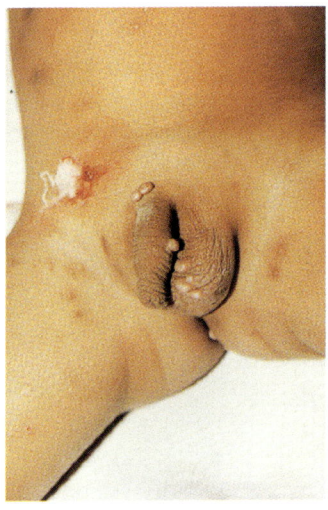

Molluscum contagiosum

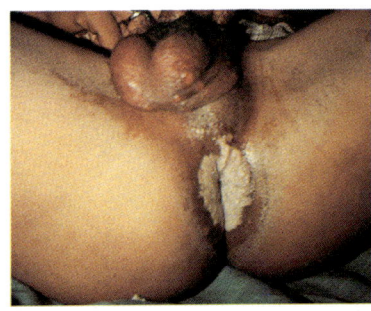

Condylomata lata-secondary syphilis

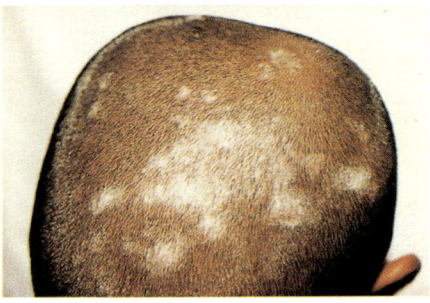

Taenia capitis

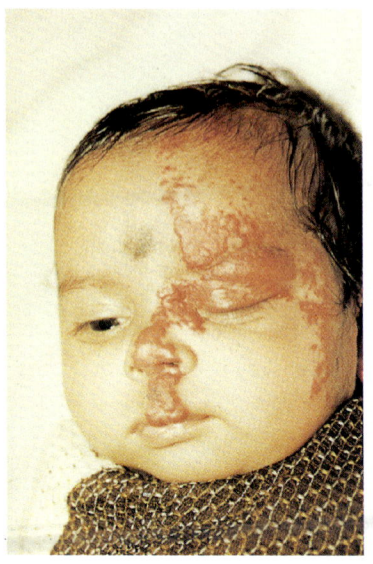

Haemangioma

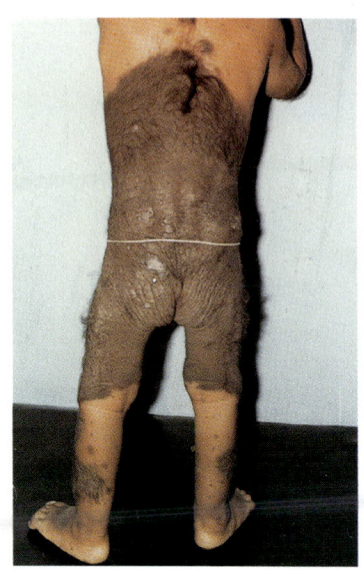

Bathing trunk naevus

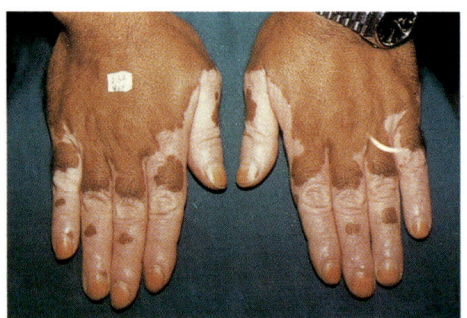

Vitiligo

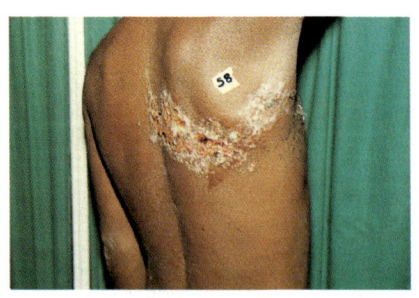

Herpes zoster

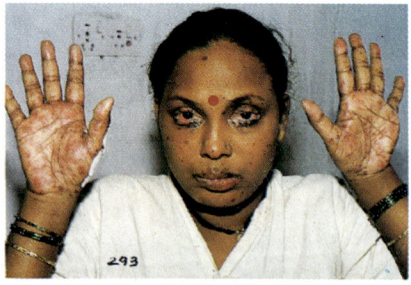

Stevens-Johnson syndrome

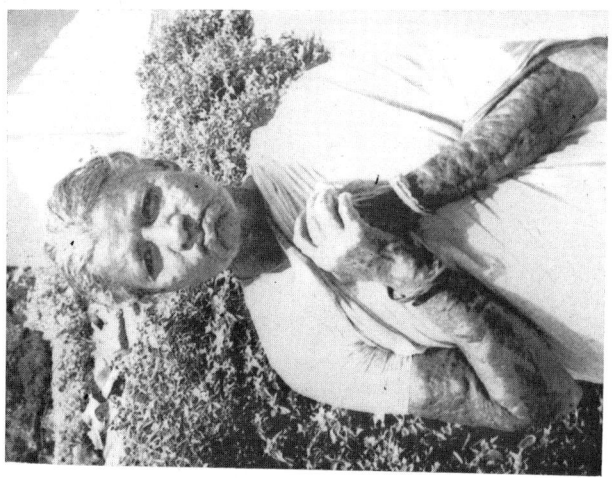

Nodular lepromatous leprosy

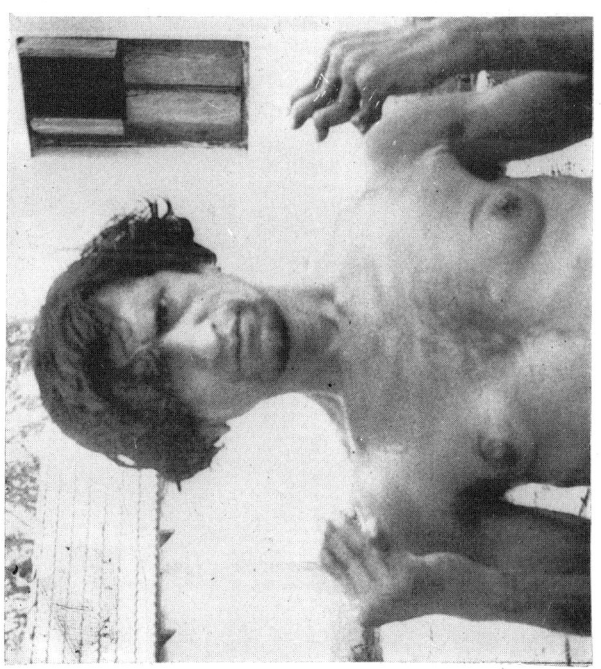

Lepromatous leprosy with bilateral Gynaecomastia
and claw hand deformity

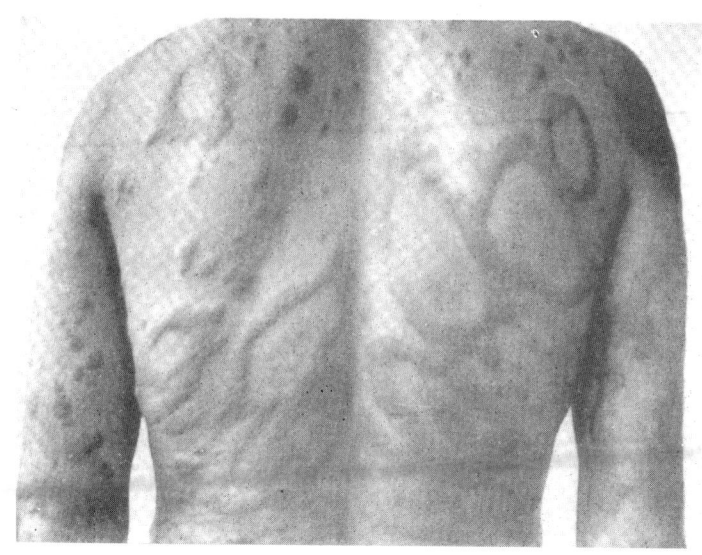

Ring shaped mid-borderline leprosy

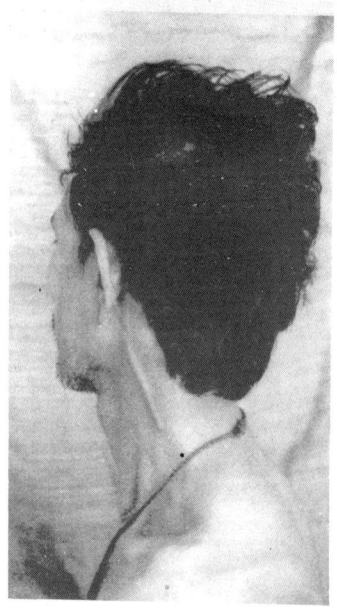

Thickened great auricular nerve in tubercular leprosy

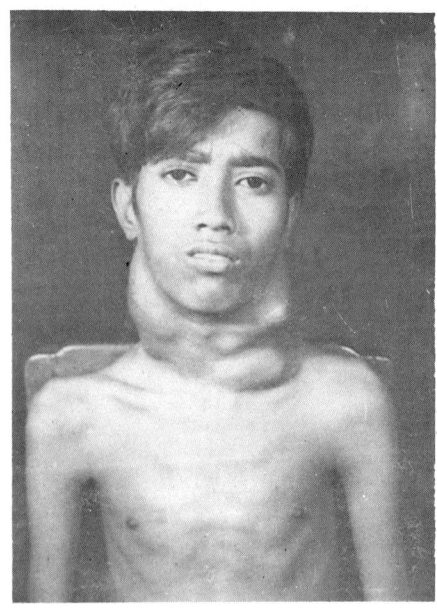

Cervical lymphadenopathy

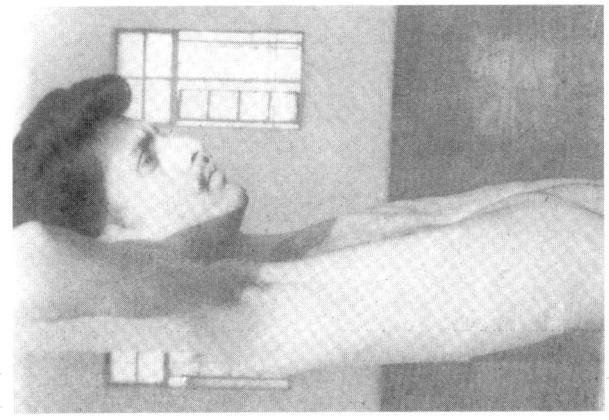

Flat chest with depressed sternum and costal cartilages

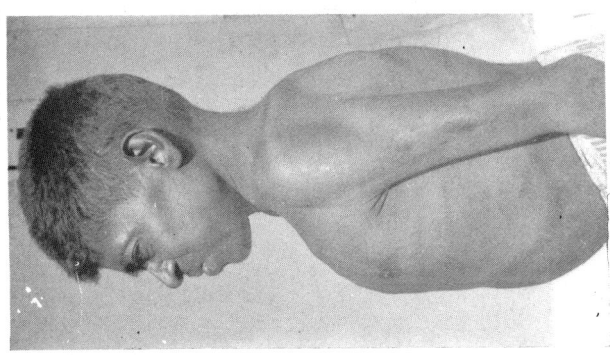

Chronic obstructive pulmonary disease demonstrating overinflated chest

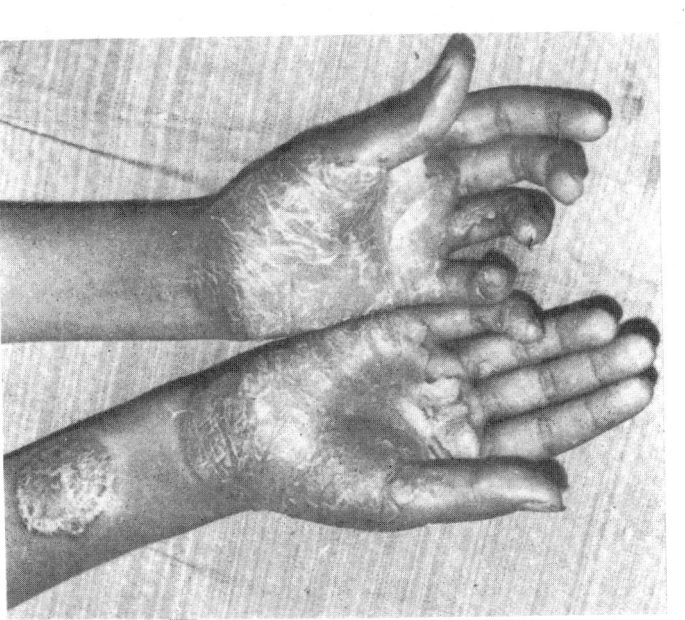

Psoriasis

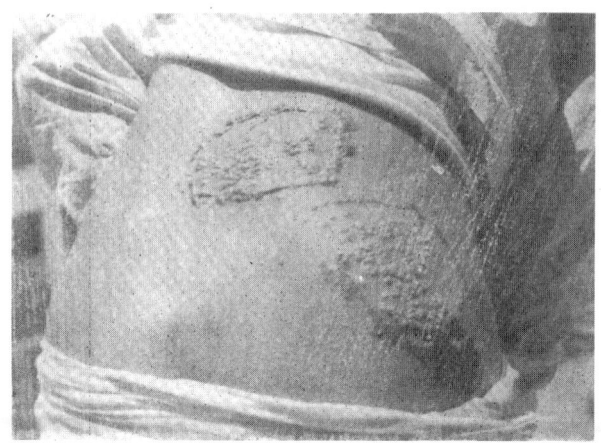

Herpes zoster

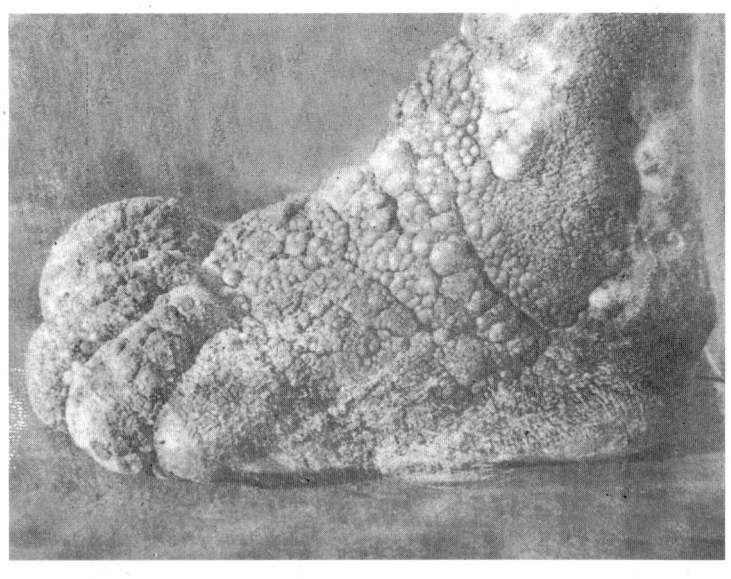

Elephantiasis nastras

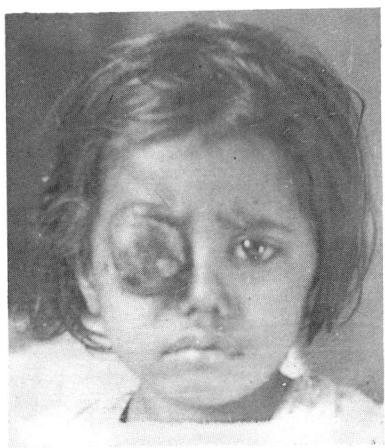

Retinoblastoma

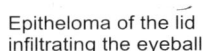

Epitheloma of the lid
infiltrating the eyeball

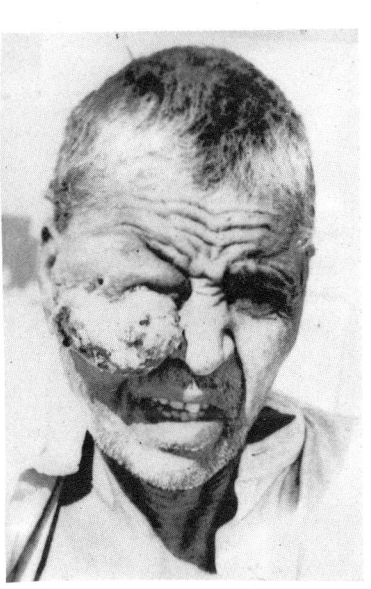

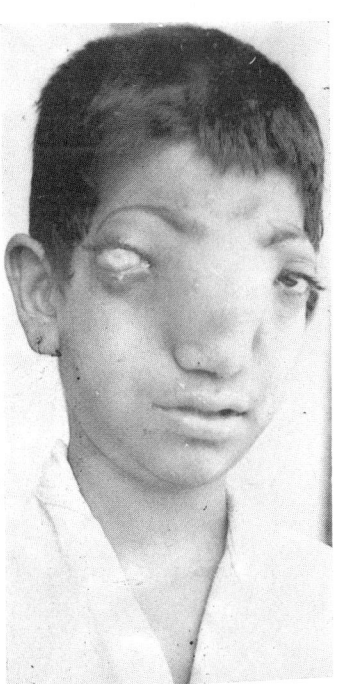

Ethamoidal carcinoma

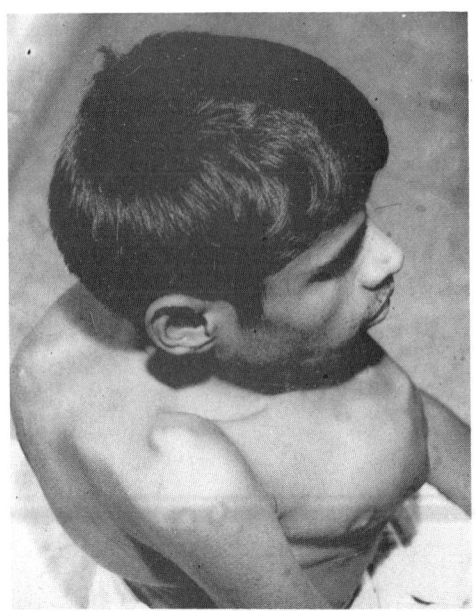

Kyphosis

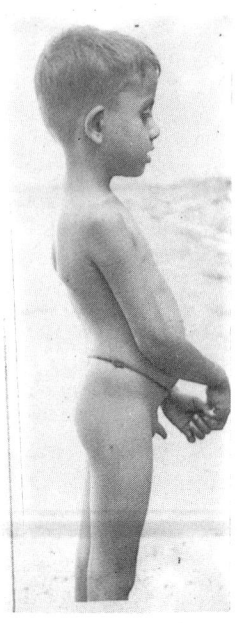

Lordosis

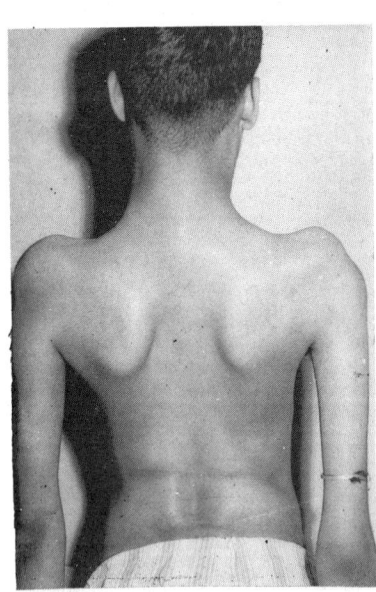

Winging of the scapulae from muscular dystrophy.

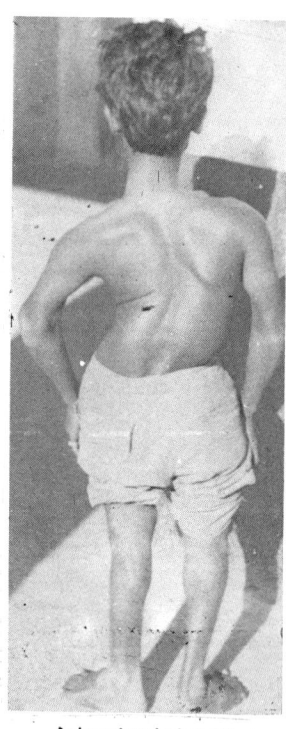

Achondroplasia with Kyphoscoliosis

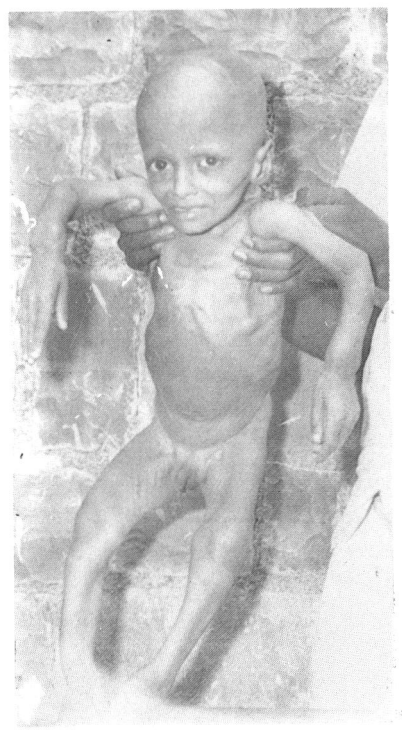

Rickets

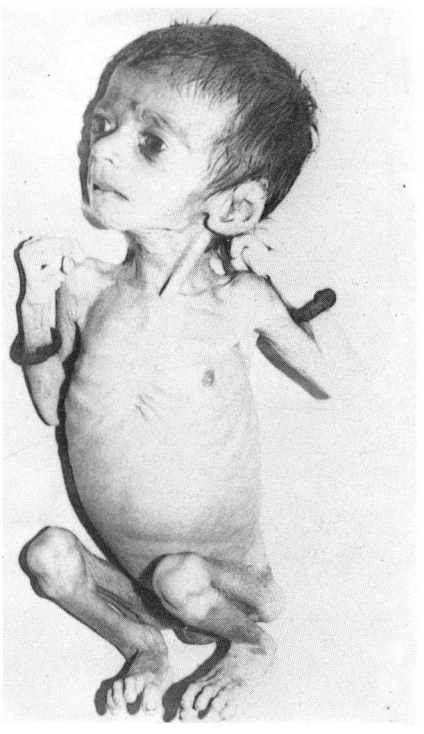

Marasmus

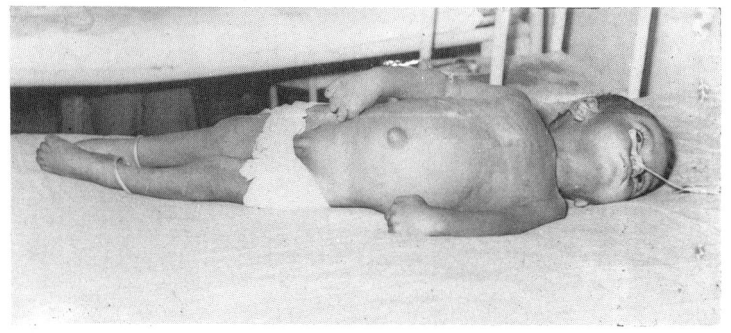

Decerebrate rigidity

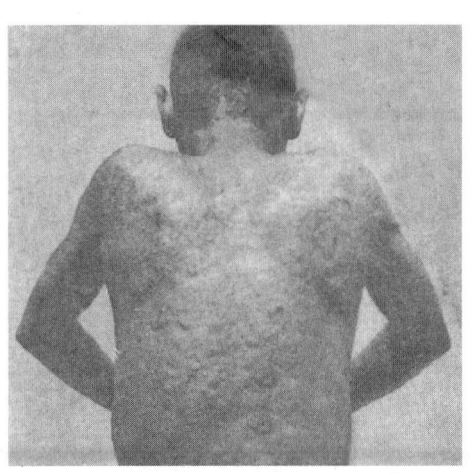

Atropho-dermo-vermicularis

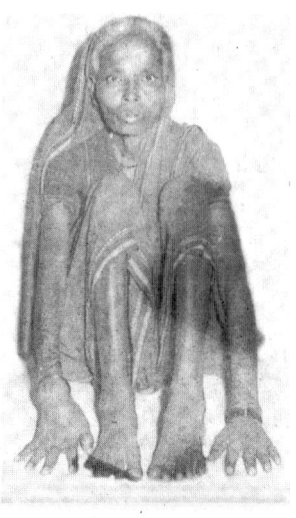

Pellagra

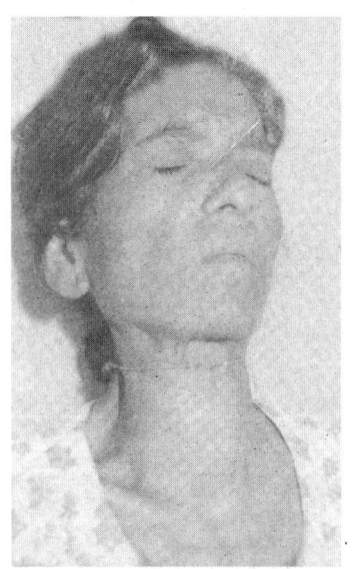

Acne keloidalis with goitre

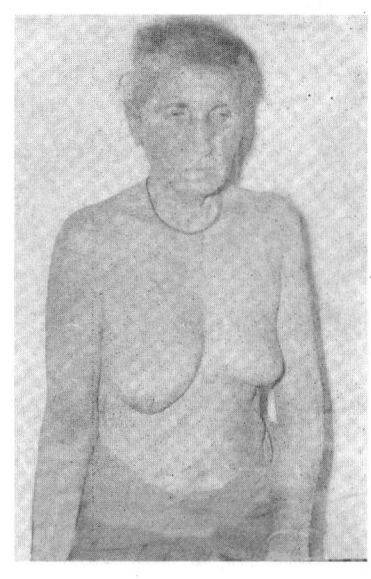

Vaccinia

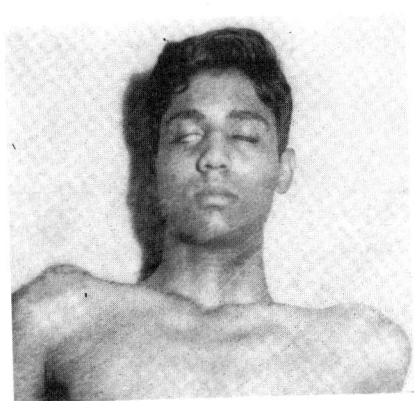

Facio-scapulo-humeral muscular dystrophy

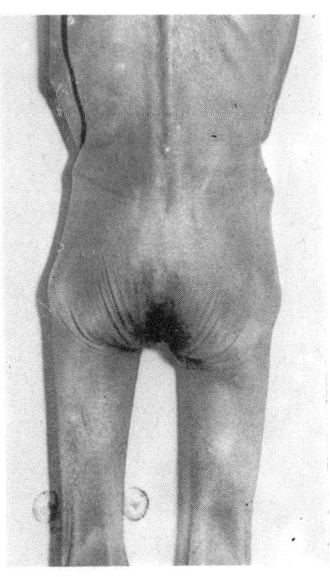

Wasting of gluteal muscles

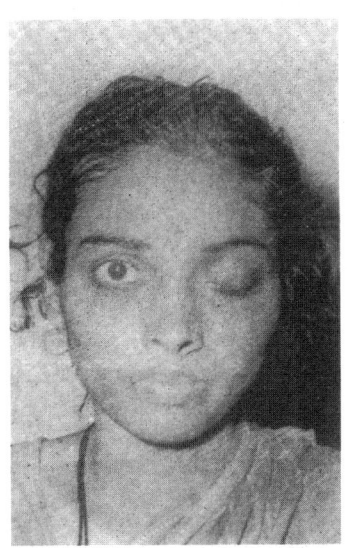

Left ptosis

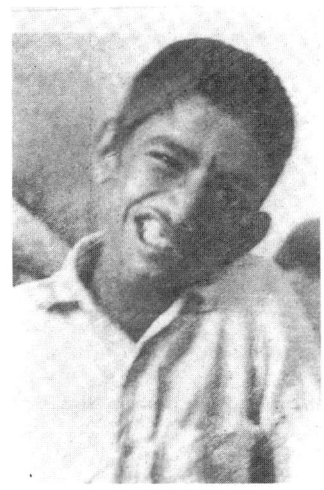

Left-sided facial palsy

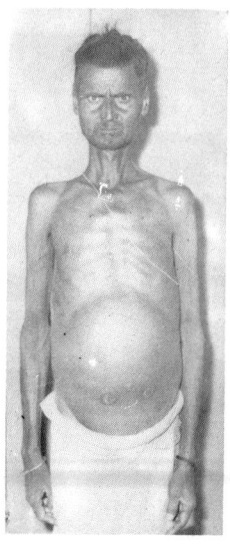

Pseudocyst of upper abdomen

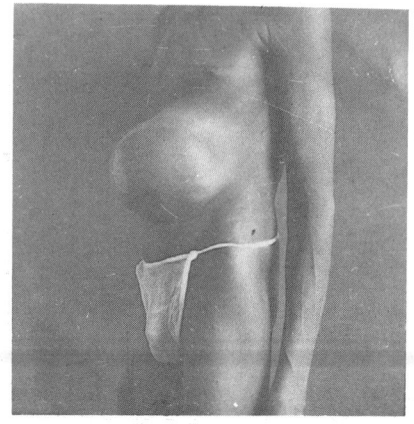

Fibrosarcoma

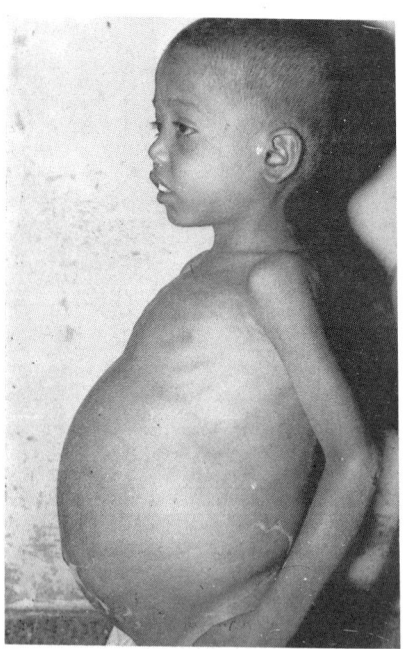

Ascites

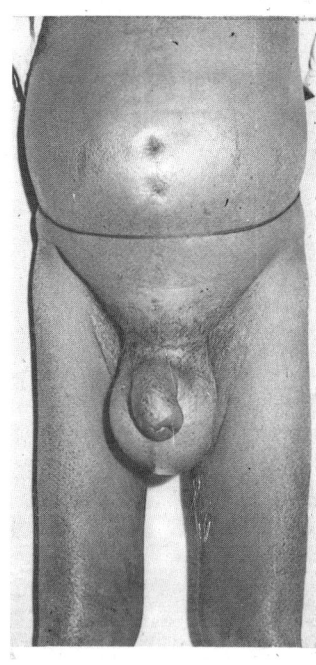

Anasarca

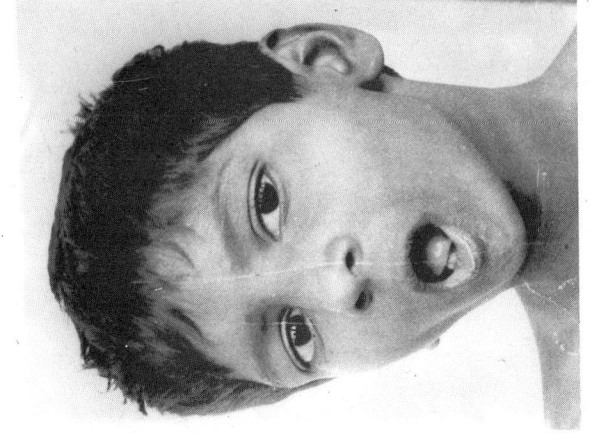

Face: Microglossia and micrognathia

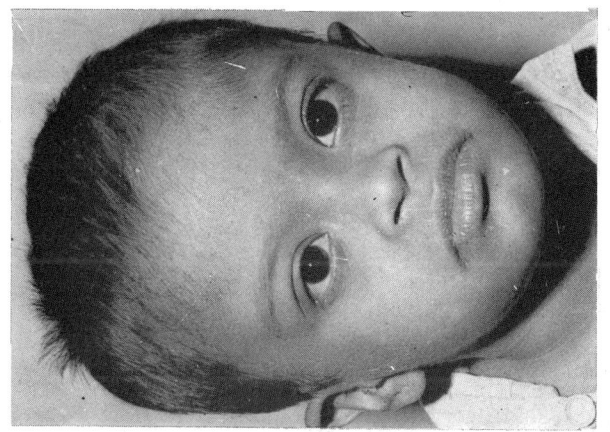

Hyperteleorism

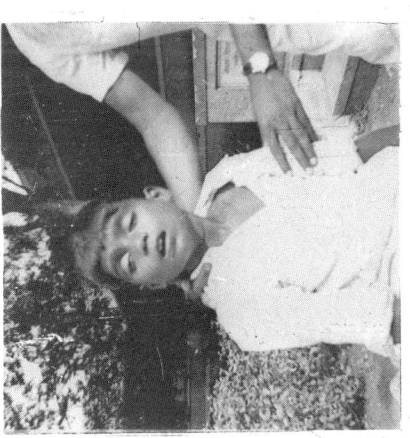

Bilateral ptosis

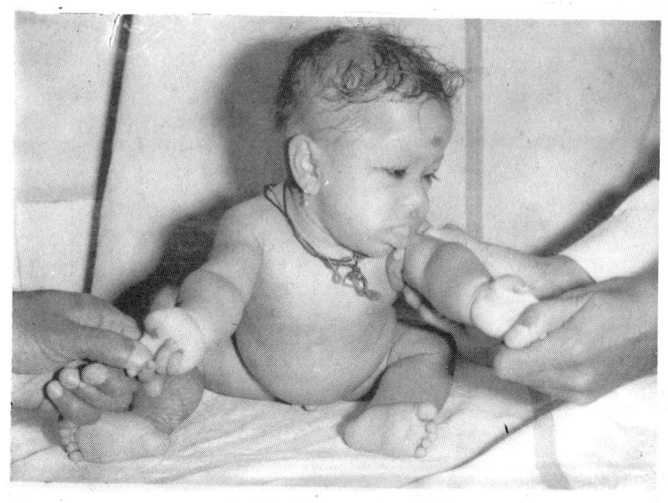

Cretin. Note hypertrophy of the muscles

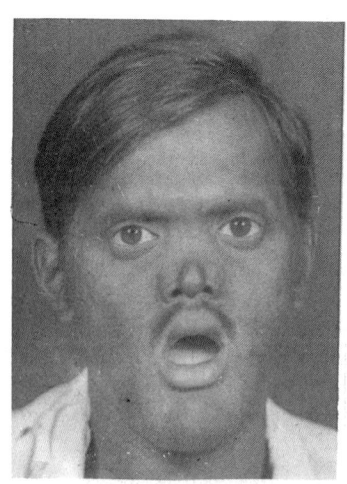

Endulous person-note depressed bridge and hide, deformed nose

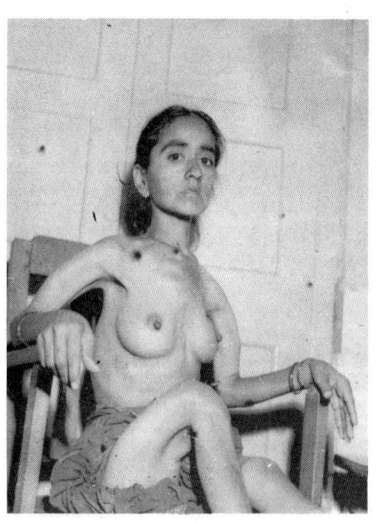

Osteogenesis imperfecta

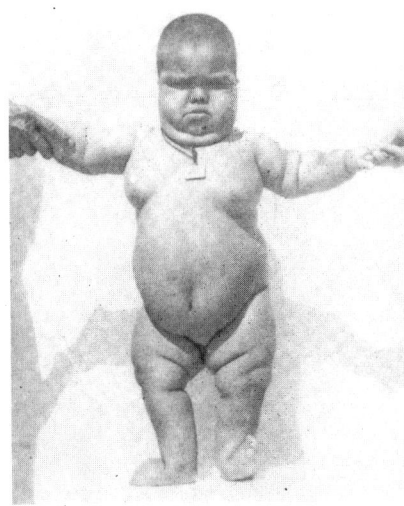

Dystrophia adiposogenitalis
Note talipes equinovarus
deformity

Cystic hygroma

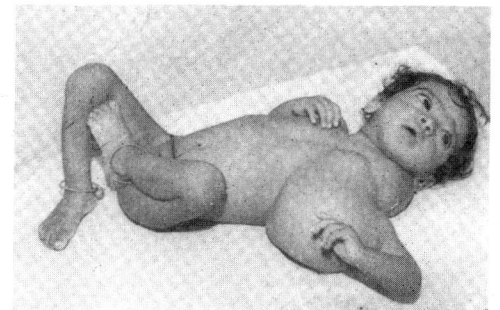

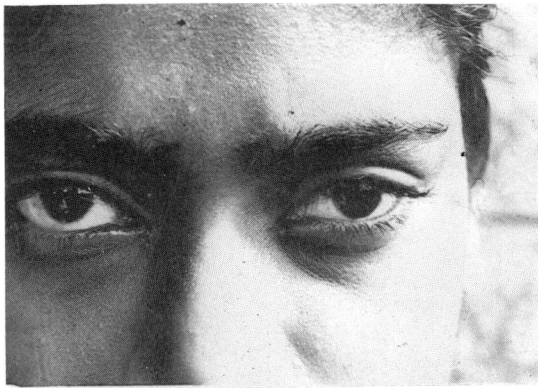

Face showing unequal palpebral fissure

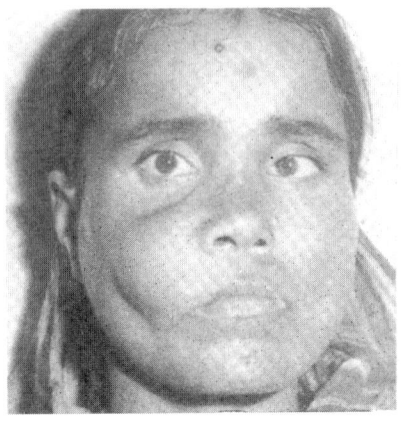

Cystic swelling of the maxilla

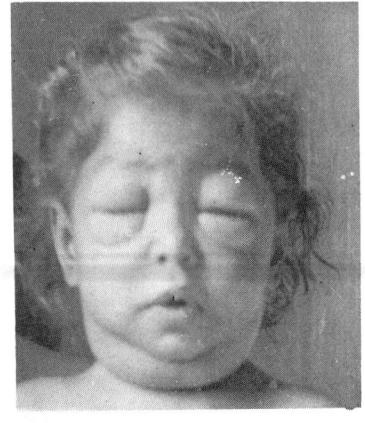

Acute nephritis-facies

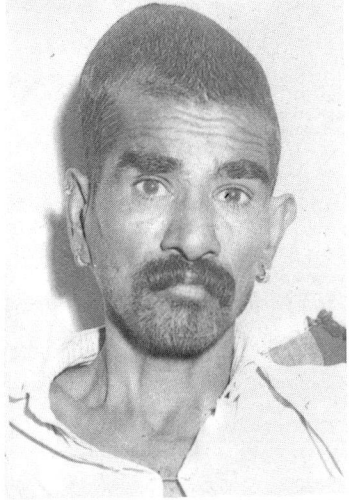

Tower skull

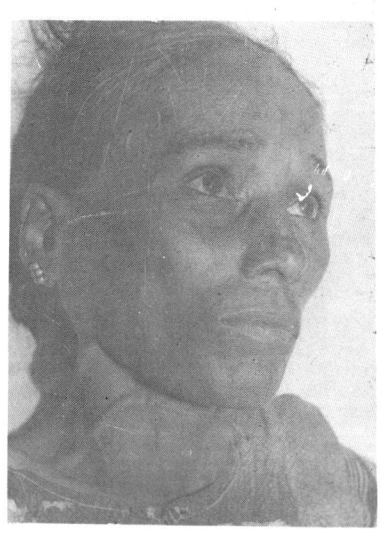

Prominent veins over
neck and forehead

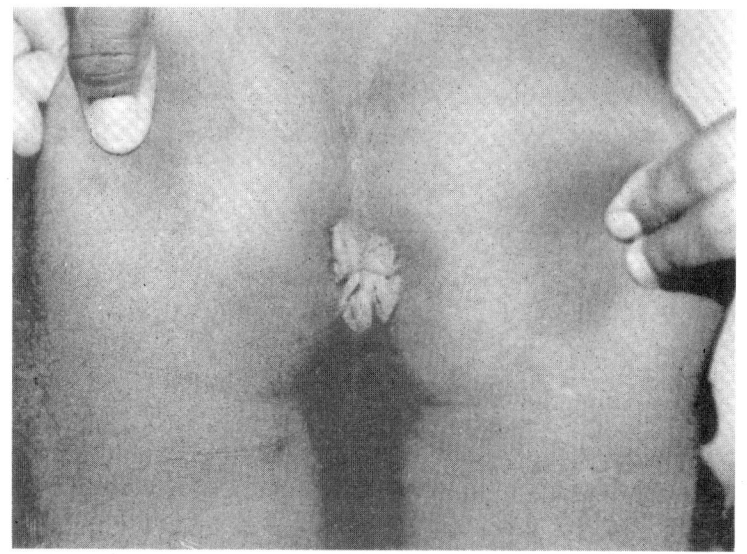

Anal condyloma

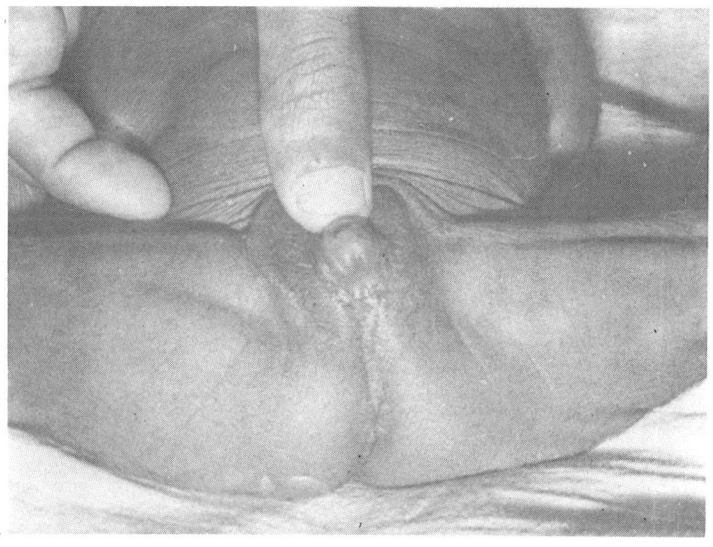

Hermaphroditism

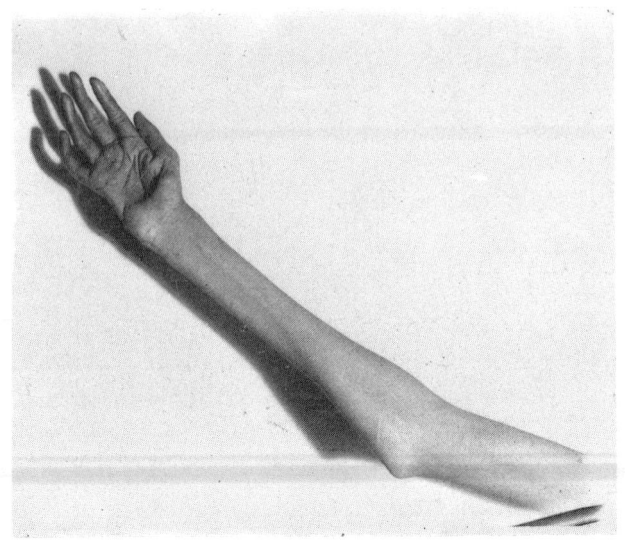

Gengrene of the hand

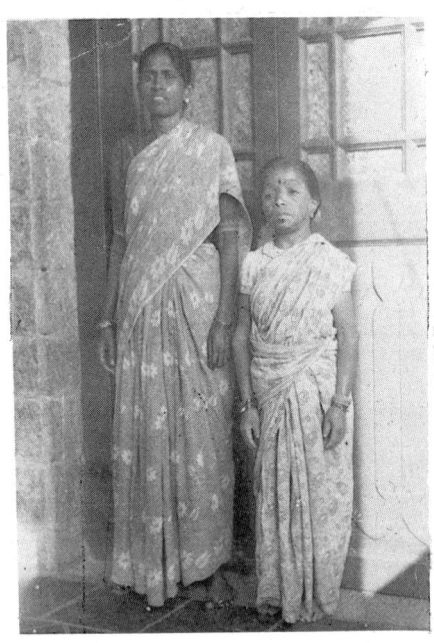

Hypothyroid dw with normal person
of same age

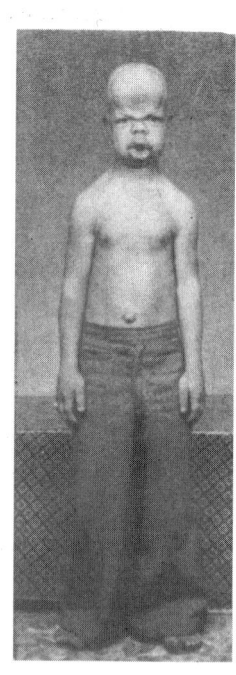

Gorgoylism

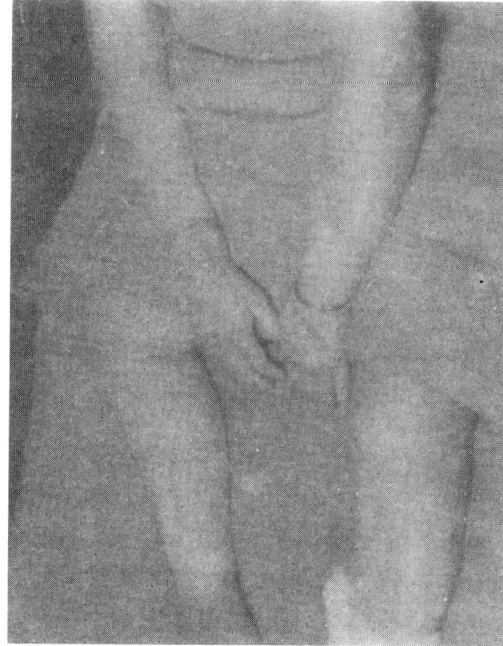

Pitting oedema

Bilateral Inguinal lymphadenopathy

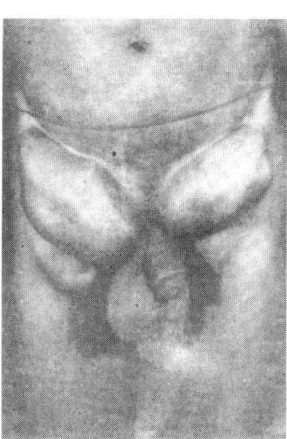

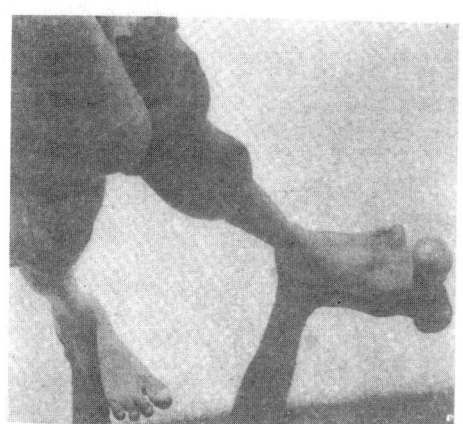

Hypertrophy of the great toe with maldevelopment
of other toes. Note fusiform swelling of the knee

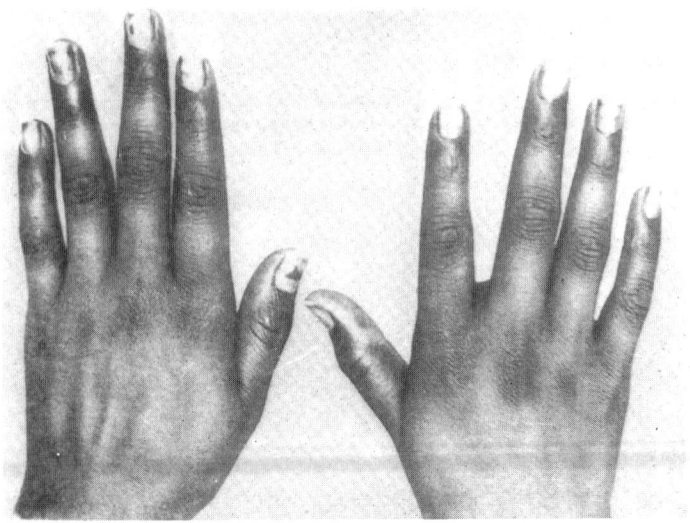

Knuckle pigmentation
in megaloblastic
anaemia

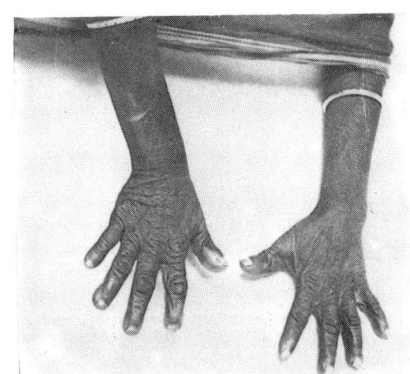

Skin of myxoedema patient

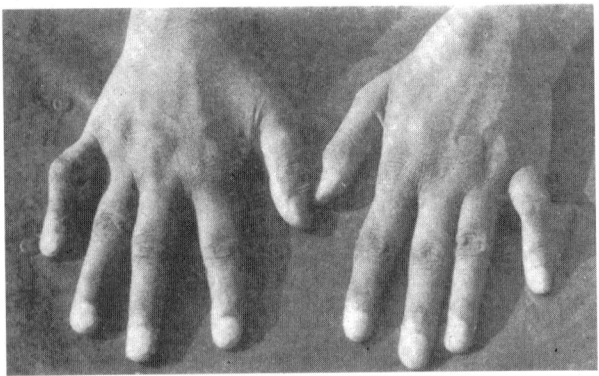

Koilonychia

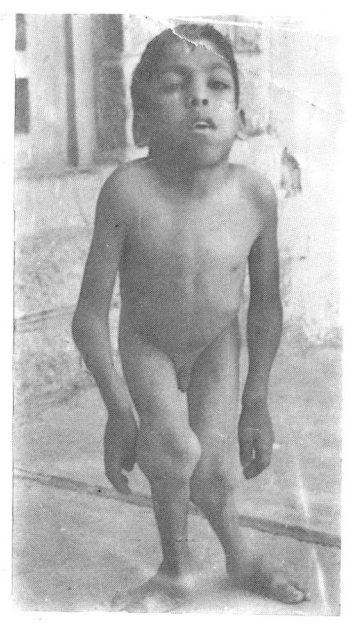

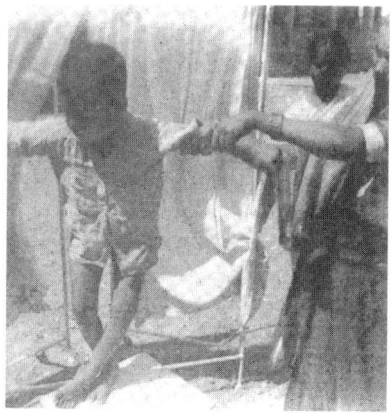

Cerebral diplegia

Morquio syndrome

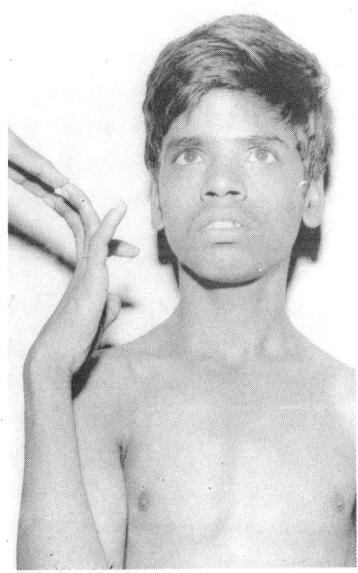

Ehler Danlos Syndrome
Hyperextensibility of the joint

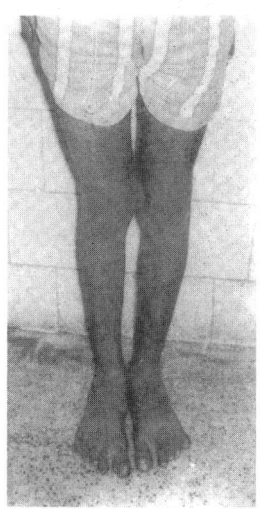

Knock Knee

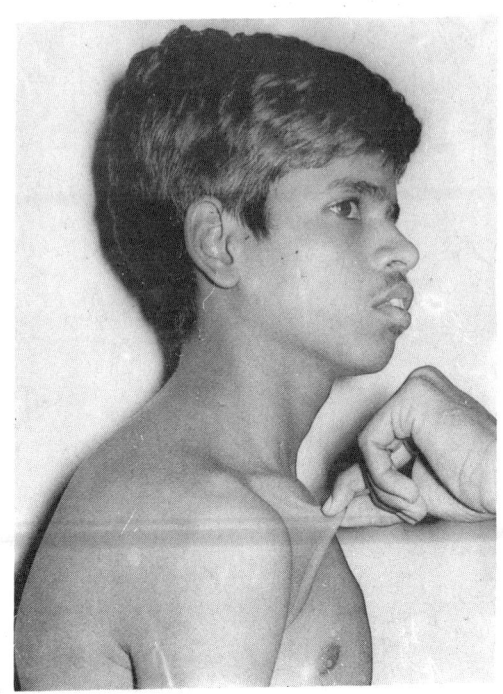

Ehler Danlos Syndrome
Hyperelastlcity of the skin

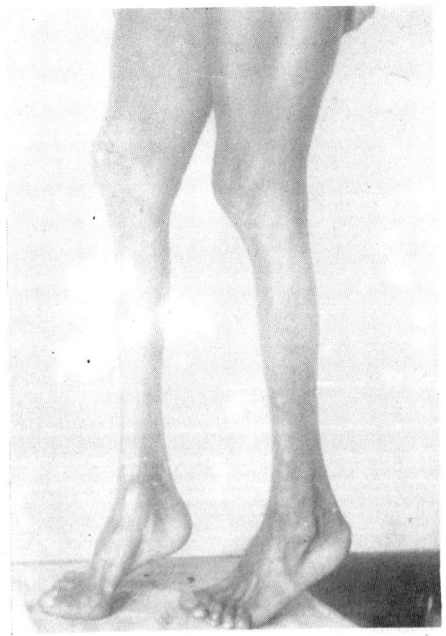

Peroneal muscular atrophy

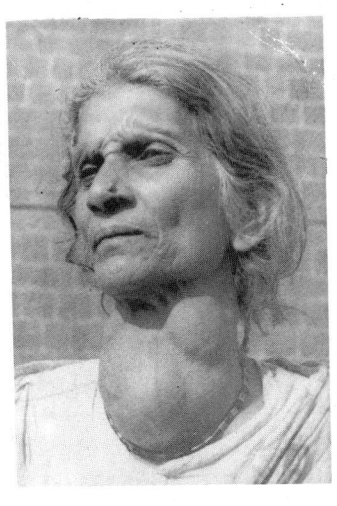

Multinodular goitre

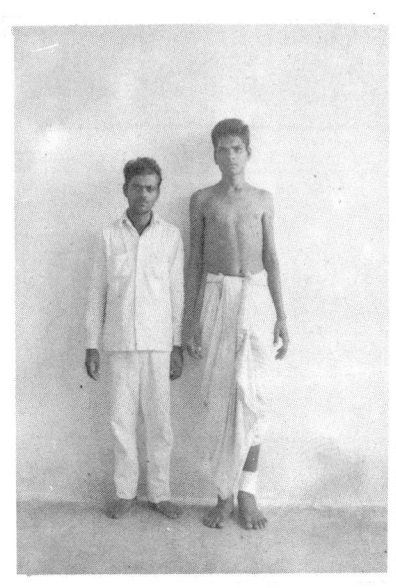

Gigantism

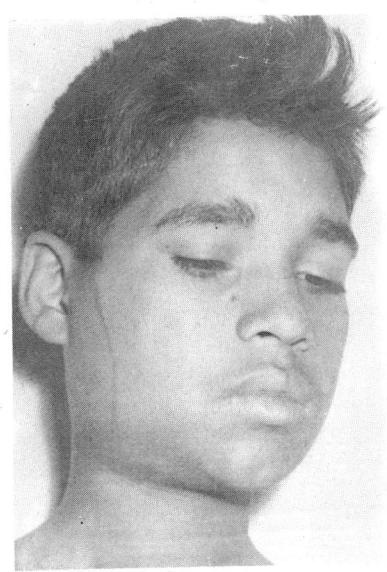

Parotid enlargement

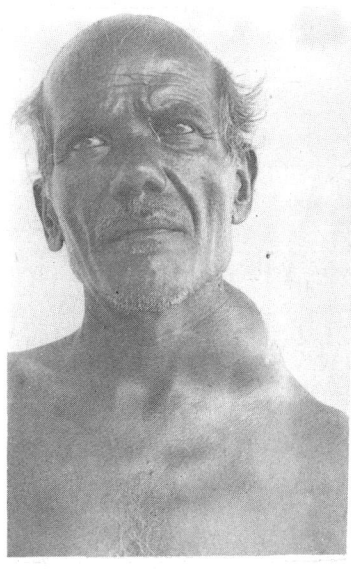

Abscess swelling in lateral side of neck

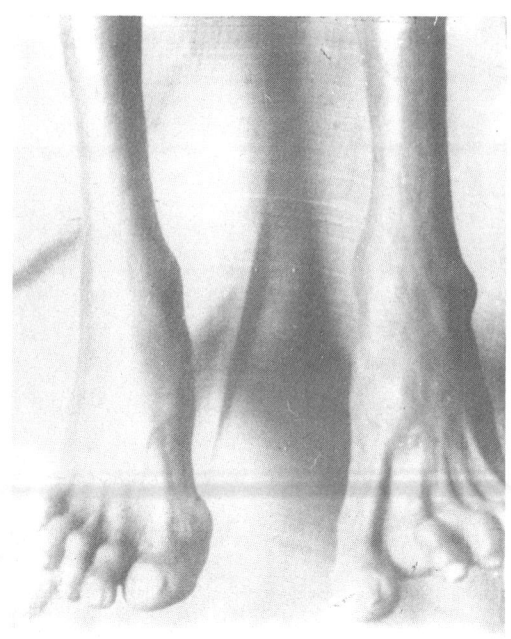

Intrinsic muscle wasting in feet

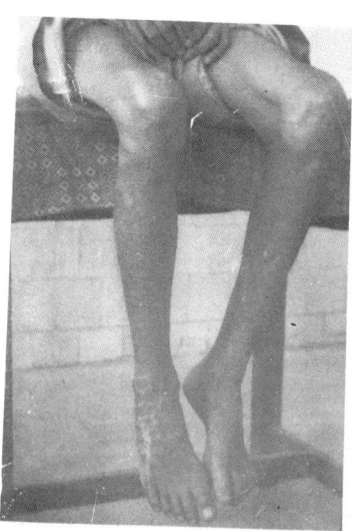

Bilateral Foot drop with
wasting of thigh muscles

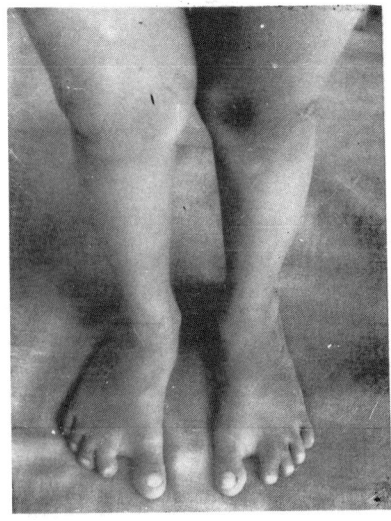

Down's syndrome: marked separation of great toe from second toe

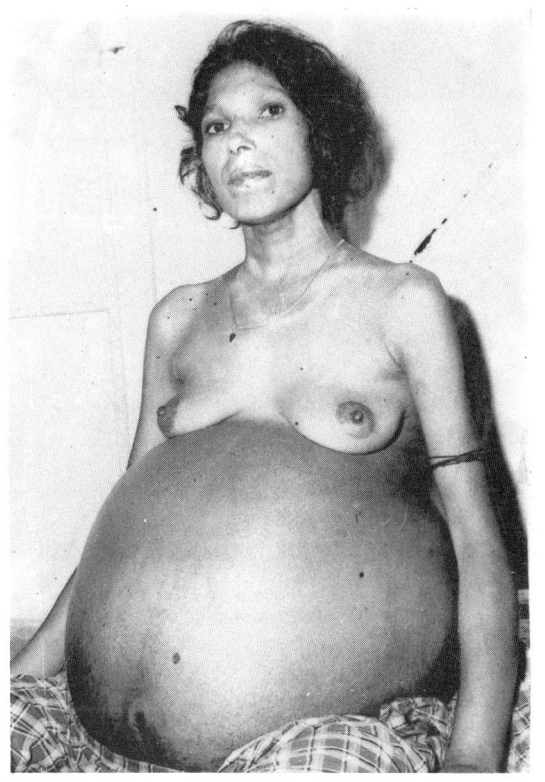

Massive Ascites with markedly engorged neck
veins

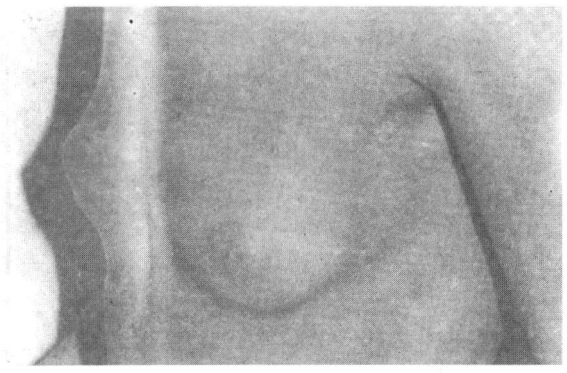

Bilateral Gynaecomastia

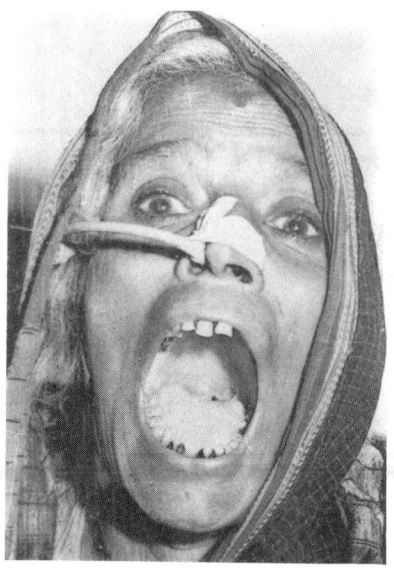

Palatal Palsy and Paralysed tongue

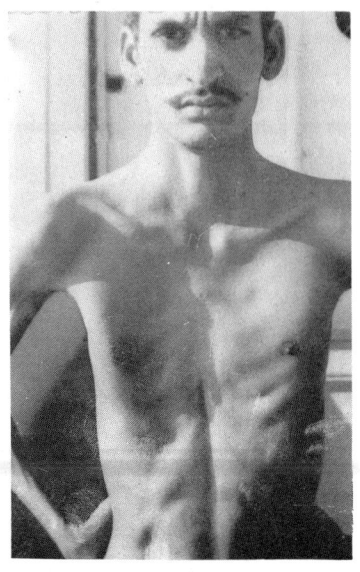

Pectus excavatum

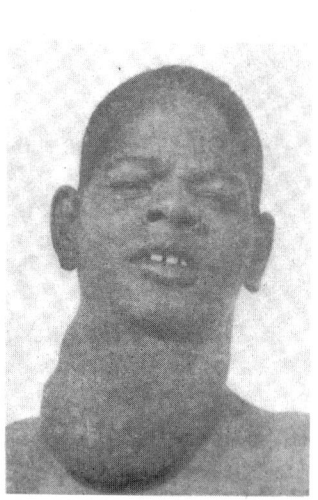

Goitre

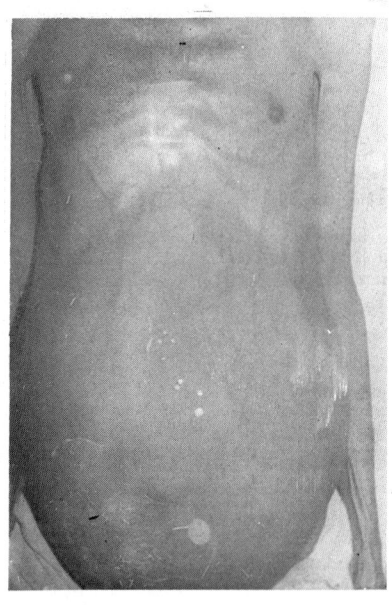

Ascites with prominent veins over abdomen

about the nature and duration of the symptoms. The mode of onset-sudden or gradual, and progression of symptoms has to be documented. Leading questions suggesting the answer are to be avoided. Direct questioning is necessary which prompts the patient to divulge relevant information. Often the patient considers certain information as personal, trivial or irrelevant, and may not tell. Direct questioning is necessary to draw out the family history, and past and personal history. In the process of a disorder certain symptoms may not be present in the patient, but still their absence should be recorded. They are referred to as negative symptoms. For example, the absence of sweating in a person having chest pain, and the absence of blood in the vomits are some examples that should be recorded as negative symptoms.

It becomes difficult to obtain coherent answers from the very young, the very old, the very sick, and the patients with memory deficit or mental changes, and the patients suffering from episodes of impairment of consciousness. In such instances the doctor has to turn to spouse, other family members or friends for obtaining relevant information.

Evaluation of the Information

While taking the history, one should be able to evaluate the information obtained. There are instances, where history may reveal the diagnosis even before the physical examination. In such instances, often the physical examination may not reveal any abnormality (for example, angina pectoris, trigeminal neuralgia, a convulsion or a fit) making the statement 'anamnesis everything, physical examination nothing' true.

Recording of the History

The history has to be written *in toto*, after uninterrupted and sympathetic hearing of the patient's narration. During this process, the doctor has the advantage of making observations on the patient such as stance and gait, build and shape on the patient (dwarf, excess height, obesity, wasting and skeletal deformities), mode of dress, hair, involuntary movement, face, voice and mental make up.

The history is recorded in the following manner:
1. preliminary data of the patient
2. presenting complaints: nature and duration (in chronological order)

3. history of present illness
4. history of past illness
5. family history
6. personal history

While writing the case sheet, irrelevant data has to be eliminated and the relevant data has to be written logically and succinctly. It comes with experience and knowledge of diseases. A brief summary of all essential features of the history must be made at the end of the case record.

THREE

INTERROGATION AND CASE SHEET WRITING

> "Computers may be fed with information and come up with diagnosis, answers, but a computer is only as good as the information that is fed into it. This information is what an experienced physician considers significant, which may not be what the relatively uninformed patient thinks must be important. The personal contact between physician and patient with all its infinite variety of approach, of personality, of articulateness and of sympathy, empathy, or apathy on both sides, must surely be the saving grace of medicine in the technological era, and from now on, for all time".
>
> *Edwin R. Bickerstaff and John A Spillane (1988)*

Preliminary (Biographic) Data

The name, age, sex, occupation and address of the patient are noted at the beginning of the case sheet. Different age groups are more susceptible to certain disease states than others.

The developmental abnormalities, if any, in infancy are noted. Infectious diseases are common in childhood. Peptic ulcer and chronic myeloid leukaemia are common in middle age. Degenerative diseases of vessels and neoplastic conditions are common in the elderly age group. Certain diseases such as haemophilia, gout, ankylosing spondylitis, and pseudo-hypertrophic muscular dystrophy are peculiar to the male sex. Thyroid disorders, systemic lupus erythematosus (SLE), and primary pulmonary hypertension are frequently seen in women. The occupations expose individuals to certain hazards like lead poisoning (in painters and plumbers) and pneumoconiosis due to exposure to dust (silica, coal).

The residence of the patient will enable the doctor to follow the case, and inform relatives about the seriousness of the patient's condition, at the same time, recording in which locality the disease is endemic or has assumed an epidemic proportion. The geographical history of the patient is essential. Also the places he has visited and stayed in India and abroad, should be recorded. Certain diseases are prevalent in certain parts of the country (filariasis in coastal regions of India, Kala-azar in Bihar, Lathyrism in Madhya Pradesh, Flurosis in Punjab, Andhra Pradesh and Karnataka, Kyasanur forest disease in Karnataka, and endemic goiter in mountainous regions).

On completion of the preliminary data, the details of the history are written as follows:

Presenting complaints: The nature and duration of each complaint has to be recorded in a chronological order. The 'presenting complaint' refers to the complaint, which has made the patient to seek help from the doctor. It should not include diagnostic terms.

The symptoms that have persisted for a long duration are to be written at the top, and the other complaints according to the duration in a descending order. The duration is calculated as the number of days, weeks or months, between the onset of the symptoms and the date of case taking. The complaints are written in the words of the patient. The recording will appear as follows: pain in the right side of the chest, six days; fever, six days; cough with expectoration, five days; and breathlessness, two days. The writing of the presenting complaints in a chronological order gives clues to the origin and progression of the disease.

History of Present Illness

The details of the present illness for which the patient has sought medical help are to be noted in detail. The duration, type of onset (sudden or gradual), frequency, treatment and its progression are recorded in a detailed manner. Each symptom is analysed in detail. There are no rigid rules and one has to vary the type of questioning, according to the case, so as to get the maximum information. If the patient has presented his complaint, with pain in the chest, the duration, type of onset, site, radiation, character, relation to exertion and breathing, aggravating factors (exercise, running, food intake), relieving factors (rest, drugs) and other associated symptoms (sweating, cough, breathlessness) are also to be enquired into and recorded.

The 'presenting complaints' give a clue to the system that is mainly involved. Depending on the system, the questions have to be framed and answers either in the affirmative, or in the negative, have to be recorded accordingly. A broad outline of the systemic symptoms is given as follows:

Cardiovascular System

Dyspnoea: duration, onset; sudden or gradual, relation to exertion, or noted on level or on climbing steps or hills, or at rest, Grading (New York Heart Association Functional Classification): I (on more than average work); II (on accustomed work); III (less than average work); IV (at rest), degree of activity necessary to produce dyspnoea, occurrence of dyspnoea at night (nocturnal) necessitating him to sit up in bed (orthpnoea).

Pain in the chest: Onset, duration (minutes or longer), frequency, site (deep seated, retrosternal) radiation (left shoulder, left arm, neck, throat, jaw, epigastrium, back), precipitation factors (4 E's-exertion, emotional stress, exposure to cold and/or hot, humid weather, or after eating a heavy meal), and smoking, relieving factors (rest or cessation of activity or withdrawal of stress or drugs), character (boring, constricting, vice-like, heaviness, tightness, squeezing, aching, burning), and presence of sweating.

Palpitations: mode of onset, sudden or gradual, duration of each attack, relation to posture, excitement, continuous or paroxysmal.

Associated symptoms: swelling of the feet, headache, dizziness, fainting attacks, fatigue, scanty, fever, cough, and haemoptysis.

Respiratory System

Cough: duration, relation to day and night, dry or productive.

Sputum: amount in 24 hours, character (mucoid, mucopurulent, purulent), relation to posture and time, smell.

Haemoptysis (coughing of blood), amount, colour, persistent or occasional, subsequent staining of sputum.

Dyspnoea: type of onset—sudden or gradual, duration, at rest or on exertion, relation to posture, association of wheeze, noisy breathing, persistent or paroxysmal, inspiratory or expiratory, relation to the season.

Pain in the chest: duration, site, type (dull, aching, pricking or stabbing), relation to cough and inspiration.

Fever: duration, onset—sudden or gradual, time of its occurrence (evening), low or high grade, associated rigors, sweating, night sweats.

Nasal discharge (rhinorrhoea), post-nasal drip (secretions dripping down the back of the pharynx and from upper respiratory passages), nasal obstruction, bleeding from the nose (epistaxis), nasal irritation, itching, sneezing, disturbances of smell.

Change in voice.

Loss of weight and appetite.

Alimentary System

Pain in the abdomen: duration, onset, location, radiation, character (dull, sharp, gripping, stabbing, cramping, burrowing, gnawing or colicky), severity, frequency and duration of each attack, relation to intake of food, factors of aggravation, and relief (food, alkali, milk, vomiting or defecation).

Appetite: loss, decrease, increase.

Weight: loss, increase, stationary.

Vomiting: frequency, amount and colour of the vomitus, relation to pain and food, presence of nausea, forcibility.

Intake of alcohol irritant food, drugs.

Haematemesis (vomiting of blood): amount, colour, appearance like 'coffee ground', presence of food particles, clots, malena (passage of black or tarry stools), intake of drugs (aspirin, corticosteroids, non-steroidal anti-inflammatory drugs).

Diarrhoea: recent or of long duration, intermittent or persistent, number, time of occurrence, relation to food, consistency of the stools (formed, unformed, frothy, watery), presence of mucus, blood, oil or fat, tenesmus (pain during defecation).

Constipation: normal habit, recent or long standing, use of purgatives, alternate with diarrhoea, passage of small hard dry stools.

Dysphagia (difficulty in swallowing): for solids, or liquids, stickiness in the retrosternal region, its site-high or low, painful swallowing (odynophagia), intake of corrosive poison or hot liquids, or in patients with AIDS with candida or herpes simplex infection.

Jaundice (icterus): duration, onset, progression, colour of urine (brown or reddish brown) and stools (light grey or clay colour), fever, intake of drugs (chlorpromazine, methyl testosterone, PAS, sulpha drugs), injections, blood transfusion, and itching, accompanying symptoms (pain, fever, and chills) incidence in other members of the family or neighbourhood.

Digestion: indigestion, belching (eructation), flatulence (or gaseous distension in the abdomen), sense of fullness, passage of flatus, water, brash, heartburn.

Bleeding per rectum: colour, fresh, or tarry, presence of piles (haemorrhoids), prolapse, pain, pruritus.

Ulcers in the mouth, bleeding gums.

Nervous System

Paralysis: sudden or gradual, complete (paralysis) or incomplete (paresis), paralysis of one half of the body (hemiplegia), one extremity (monoplegia), all the four limbs (quadriplegia) or lower extremities (paraplegia), sequence of involvement of limbs, premonitory symptoms of headache, giddiness, heaviness of the limbs, progressive or stationary motor paralysis—cortical or spinal.

Convulsions (fits): age of onset, frequency, aura (visual, auditory or uncinate), type of movements—localised or generalised, sustained (tonic) or intermittent (clonic) muscular contractions, site of commencement, loss of consciousness, history of fall, injury, biting of tongue, froth, incontinence of urine or faeces, headache or sleep after the seizure.

Headache: location, frequency, duration, time of occurrence, constant or paroxysmal, association of vomiting.

Involuntary movements: tremors, chorea, hoarseness of voice, disorders of speech, vomiting, disturbances of vision, blurring, photophobia (extreme sensitivity to light), diplopia (double vision), deafness, tinnitus (a ringing sensation in the ears), otalgia (pain in the ear), vertigo (dizziness, giddiness), frequency, its relation to posture, otorrhoea (ear discharge).

Myopathy: weakness and wasting of the muscles.

Sensory disturbances: numbness, parasthesia (tingling sensation), anaesthesia (loss of sensation), hypaesthesia (decease in tactile sensation), or hyperesthia (increased sensation of the skin).

Bladder: control over micturition, incontinence, precipitancy, hesitancy, dribbling of urine.

Bowel habits.

Alteration of consciousness (drowsiness, stupor, coma).

Fever: pain in the back and gait.

Renal System

Pain: location (costovertebral angle, lumbosacral region, suprapubic region), severity, type (dull, sharp or colicky), radiation (groin, testes or vulva).

Micturition: amount (large or small volumes) of urine, frequency (day and night), urgency, hesitancy, colour (clear, high coloured, cloudy, smoky), haematuria (blood in the urine at the onset, throughout or at the end of urination), pyuria (pus in the urine), passage of sand, dysuria (discomfort or pain during micturition), dribbling, incontinence (lack of control of bladder) and chyluria (milky urine).

Puffiness of the face, swelling of the feet.

History of upper respiratory catarrh, scabies, intake of analgesics.

Associated symptoms: fever, rigor, headache, vomiting, convulsions, visual disturbances, thirst, appetite, dyspnoea.

Genital System

Urethral discharge, swelling of testicles, sore (ulcer) on the penis, and scrotal swelling in men, and gynaecologic complaints in women.

Vaginal discharge (colour, amount or time of occurrence in relation to menstrual cycle), dysmenorrhoea (painful or difficult menstruation), metrorrhagia (bleeding or spotting of blood in the interval between menstruation) and post-coital bleeding.

Haemopoietic System

History of bleeding tendency, loss of blood, intake of drugs (aspirin, chloramphenicol), petechiae, bruise, piles, colour of stools, operations, injury, menstrual history, pregnancies, abortions, breathlessness, palpitation, headache and swelling of feet.

Locomotor System

Pain in the bone or joints: constant or noted on movements, shifting from one joint to another (migratory, flitting), type of joints involved (small or large).

Swelling, deformity, fractures, disability.

History of rheumatic fever, urethral discharge (male), leucorrhoea (female), tuberculosis, syphilis, trauma.

Muscle-weakness, difficulty in movements, wasting and hypertrophy of the muscles.

Cramps in calf muscles (precipitated by walking, relief by rest), numbness in the extremity, discomfort, ulceration, atrophy of digits, nails, necrosis.

Skin

Exposure to irritants, chemicals, intake of drugs, history of allergy, discolouration of skin, excessive dryness or sweating, texture of the skin, itching, loss of hair.

Exposure to sexually transmitted diseases with special emphasis on HIV/AIDS.

Eruptions—onset, duration, remissions and relapses, itchiness, appearance at one time or in crops, progression, bleeding, scaling.

In addition to the systemic symptoms, certain general constitutional symptoms (loss or gain in weight, amount and time interval, loss of appetite, loss of weight, fever, rigors, weakness) are to be enquired into. It is also necessary to enquire into some of the symptoms that are intermittent (relapses and remissions) with their relation to time, and seasons and events in the patient's life have to be ascertained.

After enquiring into the details, pertaining to the system of the presenting illness, other common symptoms of the different systems are to be determined and recorded.

History of Past Illness

The student has to enquire into, and record.

1) The history of the previous illness, occurrence of similar manifestations in the present illness, diseases of childhood, injuries, allergy, operations and any transient minor illness or procedure such as diplopia or tooth extraction.

2) The duration of the illness and treatment received (medication, surgery, radiotherapy, psychotherapy, and adverse reactions to the medication).

3) The previous diagnosis has to be verified by asking certain pertinent questions, regarding the symptomatology experienced by the patient.

4) The previous history of exposure to sexually transmitted diseases especially HIV infection, rheumatic fever, tuberculosis, jaundice, diabetes, pneumonia, hypertension, exposure to radiation, injections and blood transfusion.

5) The number of pregnancies (gravida), and deliveries (para), stillbirth and miscarriages and complications of pregnancy, in case of married women.

6) The previous admissions to the hospital or treatment from a doctor.

Family History

a) The patient's position in the family and marital status.
b) The health of parents, sisters, brothers, and in married persons the health of spouse and children.
c) The age and cause of death of all first degree relatives in the family.
d) The family of diabetes, tuberculosis, allergic and bleeding disorders, hypertension, coronary artery disease, cerebrovascular accidents, convulsions, mental illness and cancer are to be specifically enquired into to find out existence of any diseases in the family relevant to the patient's illness.
e) Enquiry about consanguinity is needed in certain rare hereditary diseases.

Social and Personal History

The nature of occupation, exposure to fumes and dust, education and social background, work environment and attitude to work, hobbies, sport, domestic relationship and surroundings, animals at house, recent visits to any endemic areas have to be enquired into. The history of taking alcoholic beverages (type and amount consumed) or use of tobacco (number of cigarettes or *bidis* smoked per day, and duration) and the habits of sleep and eating, micturition and defecation, have to be found out.

The history of the intake of drugs (tranquillisers, barbiturates, amphetamine, laxatives) has to be recorded.

The dietary history requires recording, consisting of the type and quantity of food consumed, with special emphasis on the intake of first class proteins, milk and milk products, fresh vegetables and fruits.

In women, the menstrual history, age of onset of menarche, menstrual interval, duration and amount of flow, last menstrual period, premenstrual tension, pain at the time of periods and use of contraceptives have to be specifically enquired into. In those who have attained menopause (cessation of menstruation), the duration should be asked.

At the end of the case sheet, the salient features of the history have to be summarized. It becomes a problem-oriented record enabling to attend those problems individually while organizing the treatment.

FOUR

GENERAL EXAMINATION

> *"Symptoms are the body's mother tongue; signs are in a foreign language"*
>
> *John Brown (1810-1882)*

Physical examination is carried out under two heads: general and systemic. To start with, a general survey of the patient is made by inspection, and later by palpation. The patient is examined in good light and in a comfortable position. The physical examination begins as soon as the patient enters the examination room, and while he is recounting the history, the general appearance, gait, posture, dress, speech, intelligence and emotional state are observed.

After the history, the patient is surveyed from scalp to the sole systematically, and the abnormalities are noted. The apparent age, general appearance, posture, stature, constitution, nutrition, general survey of the skin including the temperature, head, face, neck, ear, nose, throat, eyes, oral cavity, lymph nodes, extremities and genitalia in males are surveyed.

Then the various systems are examined by the use of the classical methods of examination: inspection, palpation, percussion and auscultation. The history points to the system affected. Generally that system is examined to begin with, and to be followed by the examination of other systems.

General Appearance

While looking at the general features, the age and the general appearance of the patient have to be recorded. The patient may look ill or anxious or breathless or may show evidence of distress or agony from pain. In neurotic individuals the general appearance does not conform to the symptoms described in superlatives.

Posture

The posture assumed by the patient in the bed (*decubitus*), on sitting and on standing has to be noted. The patient may adopt certain peculiar positions to get relief from his troubles. A healthy individual can alter the positions without any discomfort.

The body is flexed and immobile in Parkinsonism while standing. The knees are slightly flexed, the shoulders are drooped and the chin flexed. The upper limbs are slightly flexed at the elbows, and hands at the metacarpophalangeal joints; however, there is extension at the wrists and interphalangeal joints. An old hemiplegic on standing keeps the upper limb adducted at the shoulder, flexed at the elbow, pronated and flexed at the wrist, and the lower limb hyperextended. The hip is adducted, the foot is often inverted and plantar flexed. Marked lordosis is noted on standing in pseudohypertrophic muscular dystrophy and achondroplasia. Schizophrenic individuals maintain the same posture for a long time. In ankylosing spondylitis, the spine is held rigidly. Patients suffering from arthritis keep the limbs in a position of maximum comfort.

Normally, the various parts of the body and the limbs are held at rest. They may show involuntary movements (tics, chorea). In chorea, the patient is unable to sit still. In epilepsy, there may be tonic movements (persistent contraction of the muscles) followed by clonic movements (alternate contraction and relaxation of the muscles).

In tetanus, the spine is bent backwards and in extreme cases the body may be arched resting on the occiput and the heels (opisthotonus). Such a position may be observed in meningitis. In meningitis, the patient lies curled up on one side, turning away from the light. Hysterical persons exhibit a variety of bizarre postures, which cannot be explained on an anatomic or physiologic basis.

Patients having left heart failure and pulmonary venous hypertension exhibit orthopnoea. Orthopnoea is a postural dyspnoea that occurs when the patient is recumbent and is relieved by elevating the head and upper part of the body. Paroxysmal nocturnal dyspnoea (due to the reabsorption of dependent oedema that has developed during the day) occurs after the patient has been asleep for a few hours. The patient suddenly awakens with breathlessness and gets up and out of bed for relief.

A patient suffering from congenital cyanotic heart disease (Fallot's tetrology, named after Etienne-Louis Fallot, a French physician) may assume a squatting position (sitting on the heels with knees pressed against the chest). The patient suffering from heart failure, bronchial asthma and ascites sits up in the bed with arms resting on the pillow. The gravitational effects increase the congestion of the lungs when the patient lies flat in heart failure. Patients having mediastinal tumours and aortic aneurysm assume a knee-elbow position and lower their heads over the bed. In pericardial effusion the patient finds relief when leaning his body forward. The patient prefers to sit up with the legs hanging down and the head resting on the knees in thromboangiitis obliterans. Patients with pulmonary arterio-venous (AV) shunt or left atrial myxoma feel comfortable on lying down (platypnoea), and the position assumed is opposite of orthopnoea.

Patients may become breathless on lying in a lateral position (trepopnoea). The patient with pleurisy, pleural effusion and pneumothorax finds relief by lying on the affected side. This enables free expansion of the normal lung. It restricts the movement of the lung on the side of pleurisy and decreases the pain. The patient with cavitation in the lung may prefer to lie on the side that does not provoke coughing. The patient with a severe febrile illness with clouding of consciousness, often lies flat and log-like.

The patient with acute myocardial infarction may appear restless, anxious, and agitated, often thrashing about in bed in an effort to find a more comfortable position. On the other hand persons having angina pectoris that is related to exertion tend to remain quiet and sit or stand still in an effort to get relief, recognizing that any movement may increase chest pain.

The patient with an acute abdomen with peritonitis is compelled to lie on the back with one or both legs drawn up ('double-up'), and the patient is quiet. The patients with acute appendicitis or acute cholecystitis, clasp with the hand the right iliac fossa or right hypochondrium, respectively.

A seriously ill patient may not show any movement. The patients with colic, and coronary heart disease appear restless and toss in the bed from side-to-side. In hemiplegia, the affected side does not show any movement. There will be abnormal flaccidity of the arm and leg on the affected side. The limbs do not show any movement in paraplegia. The limbs are held in an extended position when the pyramidal tracts have been affected alone (paraplegia in extension). The limbs assume an attitude of flexion when there is involvement of the extrapyramidal tracts below the vestibular nucleus (paraplegia in flexion). It indicates greater severity of the lesion of the spinal cord than paraplegia in extension.

Injury to the deep cerebral hemisphere or upper brain stem may be associated with decorticate posture (arms flexed, legs extended) or decerebrate posture (arms and legs extended). Spinal cord injury is associated with flaccid paralysis.

In situations of paralysis of a group of muscles, an unopposed contraction of other muscles causes the limb to assume an abnormal position. Later fibrotic changes develop in the paralysed muscles and their tendons to result in true contractures.

Stature

The length of various parts of the body is measured, while giving an opinion on the stature (body proportion). Normally the span (length between the tips of the middle fingers of both outstretched and abducted upper limbs) is equal to the total height of the body (heel-to-vertex). Height represents a balance between growth velocity and bone age maturation. Bone age is a reflection of the integrated hormonal environment consisting of sex steroids, thyroid and growth hormones. The measurement of the upper segment (from the top of the head to the upper margin of symphysis pubis) is equal to the measurement of the lower segment (from upper margin of the symphysis pubis to the sole of the foot) in adults.

The individual with an increase in the stature above the normal standards of age, sex and race is referred to as a giant. The person is called a dwarf if the stature is decreased.

Gigantism: If the anterior lobe pituitary hyperactivity occurs before puberty (before attainment of full length of long bones), the individual presents features of gigantism. When the hyperactivity is noted in the adults it results in acromegaly. The pituitary giant has a well proportionated body and is tall.

Eunuchoid giants are individuals who are tall and lean due to delayed epiphyseal closure. There is sexual infantilism. The span is greater than the total height. The lower segment is greater than the upper segment. Marfan's syndrome (described by Antonio Marfan, a French paediatrician) and Klinefelter's syndrome (XXY) (described by Harry Klinefelter Jr, a US physician) show the span to be greater than the height.

Dwarfism: The dwarfs show stunted growth (short or small stature) when compared to persons of the same race and age. Infantalism is a term used for dwarfs showing retardation of muscular, mental and sexual development. Their upper segment is greater than the lower and the height longer than the span.

An infantile type of body proportion is seen in cretinism, juvenile myxoedema and achondroplasia. In Frohlich's syndrome (described by Alfred Frohlich, Austrian pharmacologist in US) the span is greater than the height and the lower segment greater than the upper segment similar to that of eunuchoid.

The common causes of dwarfism are:
1) Racial (pygmies, Gurkhas) or familial of psychosocial, or constitutional delay of growth and development
2) Chromosomal: Mongolism, Turner's (named after Henry Turner, US endocrinologist) syndrome.
3) Ateleiotic: A proportionate body but small in all its parts and appears as a pocket edition of adults.
4) Endocrine: Hypopituitarism (short stature with infantilism), cretinism, juvenile myxoedema, prolonged corticosteroid therapy.
5) Neurologic: craniopharyngioma.
6) Skeletal: Achondroplasia (short bowed legs with short arms), osteogenesis imperfecta, rickets, osteochondrodystrophy, Pott's (named after Sir Percivall Pott, a British surgeon) disease.
7) Systemic diseases: congenital heart disease, chronic renal failure, impaired nutrition, malabsorption syndrome, tuberculosis, bronchial asthma, cystic fibrosis, renal tubular acidosis, congenital syphilis.

Constitution (Somatototype)

There is a great variation of the body build from individual to individual. There appears to be a definite relation between the constitution and the disease. On the basis of general configuration of the individual, the constitution can be classified into the following four general types. However many individuals fall in between these types.
1) *Sthenic type:* The individual will have an athletic constitution with good musculature, broad shoulders, flat abdomen, average height, and subcostal angle will be a right angle.

2) *Hypersthenic (pyknic) type:* The individual is short and stocky and demonstrates a tendency towards obesity. The neck is short and thick, the chest broad and short and a thick abdominal wall. The subcostal angle is greater than the right angle (obtuse).

3) *Hyposthenic:* The individual is tall and thin. The shoulders are narrow. The chest is flat. The musculature is poorly developed. Underweight. The abdominal wall is thin and the lower abdomen is protuberant. The subcostal angle is less than a right angle (acute).

4) *Asthenic:* The individual gives an exaggerated feature of hyposthenic type.

Depending on the preponderance of the primary germ layer, the individuals can be grouped into three somatotypes (body configuration).

1) *Endomorph:* soft round contours and well developed cutaneous tissue. The extreme variety is considered obese and will have weight above the standard weight (hypersthenic).

2) *Mesomorph:* stocky and muscular (sthenic).

3) *Ectomorph:* Long, lean and lanky (hyposthenic and asthenic).

In any individual, usually there is no pure variety of morphism (body configuration). Individuals are either ecto-meso or meso-endo etc., thus have a mixed morphism (somatotypism, Sheldon). Certain diseases are common with a particular somatotype in a patient.

Endomorph: diabetes mellitus, hypertension, complicated obesity, osteoarthritis, gall stones.

Ectomorph: peptic ulcer, mental disorders, neurologic disorders, ulcerative colitis, irritable colon.

Mesomorph: musculo-skeletal disorders.

Nutrition

The person with normal nutrition has a normal weight and comparable with those of similar age, sex and height. The state of nutrition depends on the muscles and fat in the body and is estimated by assessing whether an individual is overweight or underweight. An underweight individual has a weight less by 20 per cent of the standard value. Such individuals appear emaciated and show loss of subcutaneous fat. The thickness of the subcutaneous fat is measured using the triceps fold of fat by skin fold calipers.

Those with overweight have an excess of fat and are referred to as obese when they have excess weight of over 20 per cent of the expected value. The distribution of the excess subcutaneous fat may be generalized (exogenous obesity from overeating) or limited to certain regions (endogenous obesity). The distribution in the latter instance, may be central, involving the trunk and neck (Cushing's syndrome named after Harvey Cushing, a US surgeon, adrenogenital syndrome), grible type involving the lower abdomen, hips and thigh (Frohlich's syndrome) or trochanteric involving the buttocks (hypogonadism).

The build (frame) refers to the skeletal growth based on the constitutional and hereditary characters. Nutrition indicates the general growth including skeleton, fat, muscle and is dependent on the intake of food including first class proteins and vitamins. Hence the patient may be well built and poorly nourished. The poorly nourished individuals appear thin, lean and are underweight. Those showing excessive loss of subcutaneous fat, loose skin and wasting of muscles are referred to as emaciated. Cachexia implies serious wasting. It is seen in conditions with chronic febrile states, HIV / AIDS, pulmonary tuberculosis, cancer, type 1 diabetes mellitus, thyrotoxicosis, chronic diarrhoea, anorexia nervosa, chronic renal disease, leukaemia and long standing muscular dystrophy.

Body Mass Index

In adults it is possible to determine the relationship between body weight and height by finding out whether the weight is appropriate for height. It refers to the body-mass index (BMI) and it is calculated by the formula mentioned below:

$$BMI = \frac{Weight\ (kg)}{Height\ (m)}$$

BMI varies from 20 to 25 in men and 18 to 24 in women. Those who are less than normal range are having weight loss and those greater than 30 are obese.

Skin

The skin is examined under adequate illumination during the general examination of the patient. All anatomic areas from the scalp to the soles of the feet are to be seen in a systematic way and later the skin is palpated. The skin may be affected *per se* or as a result of systemic diseases.

The following important features are looked into: texture, colour, eruptions, sweating, cleanliness, hair and temperature.

Texture: Normally the skin is stretched smoothly over the subcutaneous tissue. It is soft and elastic. The skin exhibits abnormal elasticity in Ehlers-Danlos syndrome—a connective tissue disorder, described by Edvard Ehlers, Danish dermatologist and Henri Danlos, French dermatoligist. The skin is thick and well keratinized in the male and it is softer in the female. If a fold of the skin is pinched up and then released, it assumes its original shape quickly. It loses its elasticity and becomes loose and wrinkled in a wasting disease, old age and dehydration. In ichthyosis the skin is furrowed and scaly. Acromegaly is associated with thickened, greasy and loose skin. The skin is dry, thick and cold in myxoedema. Thyrotoxicosis is associated with moist and warm skin. Anxiety states exhibit cold and moist skin. There is marked thickening of the skin in systemic sclerosis. It is inelastic and stretched tightly. In long-standing cases of rheumatoid arthritis the skin appears taut and thin. In oedematous conditions the skin is stretched and shiny.

Oedema: An abnormal accumulation of fluid in the subcutaneous tissue, resulting in swelling of the tissues is referred to as the oedema. The oedema is visible when 8 kg or more water has collected in excess and distributed in the subcutaneous tissue. Protein concentration of the oedema fluid determines its viscosity. Oedema fluid with low protein usually pits on pressure. It can be demonstrated by pressing lightly or firmly with the thumb over a bony prominence-like medial malleolus or over the shin of the tibia. It leaves a pit that persists for a while. The skin is glossy and gives a doughy feel. However, in very long standing cases of oedema it may not be possible to demonstrate pitting.

The common conditions giving rise to the oedema are heart failure, nephrotic syndrome, cirrhosis of the liver, hypo-proteinaemia, and beri beri. Oedema may be drug induced following therapy with nifedipine or non-steroidal anti-inflammatory drugs (NSAIDs). In patients with heart failure and in hypoproteinaemia, oedema is noted over the dorsum of the feet, around the ankles, and ascends to the legs and thighs (dependent oedema). In those who are confined to bed, the oedema is noted over the sacrum (sacral oedema) from gravitational effect. Oedema is a late sign of heart failure; it frequently involves the right leg prior to left leg. The oedema may be recognized over the abdominal wall. The renal oedema (acute nephritis) manifests first in the face by puffiness. It is marked in the morning. In cirrhosis, the fluid collection is noted in the peritoneal cavity initially and later over the feet. When the oedema is gross, there may be a rupture of the skin with oozing of the fluid.

The oedema is non-pitting in lymphatic obstruction (filariasis, carcinomatous metastasis, Milroy's disease, described by William Milroy, US physician), myxoedema and systemic sclerosis. When the oedema involves the whole body, it is referred to as anasarca (dropsy).

The oedema may be unilateral in venous or lymphatic obstructions of the limb. In venous obstruction (deep vein thrombosis, varicose veins, removal of veins at coronary artery bypass surgery) the oedema is pitting and the veins are prominent over the region. In long standing lymphatic obstruction the oedema is non-pitting. The hair follicles stand out giving an appearance of an orange. The oedema may be confined to the territory of the superior vena caval drainage (puffiness of the face, and oedema of the upper limbs) in conditions of superior vena caval obstruction.

Subcutaneous emphysema: A characteristic crackling sensation is felt on palpation in subcutaneous (surgical) emphysema (entry of air from the respiratory passages) or in gas gangrene.

Colour: The normal colour of the skin depends on the amount of pigments like melanin, carotene and the haemoglobin of the red cells, and the state of the skin capillaries. The colour varies in an individual according to his race and hereditary factors.

Abnormalities of melanin: Normally the skin contains varying amounts of melanin (brown pigment). There may be depigmentation from congenital deficiency of the pigments, and the skin appears white. It may be generalized (albinism) or localized (leucoderma). Vitiligo shows patches of white and darkly pigmented skin (leuco-melanodermia). In leprosy hypopigmented and hypoanaesthetic areas are seen. Post-Kala azar dermal leishmaniasis shows localized hypopigmentation in the face and upper chest. Hypopituitarism and hypogonadism are associated with diminished pigmentation to result in pale skin.

An increased pigmentation may be noted over a localized area due to the effect of physical irritants (exposure to ultraviolet light, X-ray irradiation, heat wave) or from chemicals (silver nitrate). In pellagra, the skin becomes rough, cracked with hyperpigmentation over the exposed parts of the body (hands, forearms, feet, legs and neck). It is noted on the extensor surfaces of the limbs symmetrically. In Addison's disease (described by Thomas Addison, English physician), brownish pigmentation is noted on exposed areas, axilla, palmar creases and buccal mucous membrane. A generalized pigmentation is noted in haemochromatosis (greying-bronze colour with a metallic sheen), malabsorption syndrome, in chronic arsenic poisoning (often covered areas more than exposed parts), argyria (diffuse slatey-grey hue from deposition of silver), and in malignant cachexia. A slate-like colour of the skin, hands, and nose may occur in patients receiving amiodarone therapy.

Areas of hyperpigmentation may be noted over the face and dorsum of the hands in conditions of nutritional types of anaemias. Moles (pigmented naevus) appear as dark brown spots. They may be flat or raised above the surface. Sometimes they are hairy. *Café au lait* spots may be noted in neurofibroma (Von Recklinghausen's disease, described by Friedrich von Recklinghausen, a German physician). Chronic venous congestion in lower parts of the legs in patients with varicose veins may result in pigmentation. Arterial obstruction results in blackness of the skin (gangrene). Pigmentation may be noted in the axilla in conditions of abdominal cancer, cancer of the lung and breast (acanthosis nigricans).

Abnormalities due to carotene: People who take food rich in carotenes (carrots, oranges and egg yolk) exhibit a yellow coloured skin. It is especially noted in the palms and soles. It does not stain the sclera unlike jaundice. Diabetics look yellow because of carotene disturbances.

Abnormalities of haemoglobin and of the skin capillaries: An extreme pallor is noted in anaemia. Pallor of the skin may be temporary due to shock, haemorrhage and intense emotional disturbance, or permanent due to anaemia or peripheral vasoconstriction. Even though pallor is considered synonymous with anaemia, not all pale persons are anaemic. Pallor is better appreciated in conjunctivae and mucous membrane than skin. A pale skin from diminished pigmentation is noted in hypopituitarism and hypogonadism.

Flushing: Transient capillary dilatation results in flushing of the skin and is commonly noted in the head and the neck. It may be due to emotional disturbances ('blushing') or hormonal imbalance at menopause ('hot flushes'). High fever, hyperthyroidism and conditions with retention of carbon dioxide, are associated with generalized flushing. Carcinoid syndrome, polycythaemia, prolonged corticosteroid therapy and alcohol intake may be associated with flushing. Flushing may be provoked by alcohol in Hodgkin's disease.

In fever, the face may appear flushed due to the capillary dilatation. It may be noted in overheating, and in the areas of inflammation. In polycythaemia vera the skin appears purple. Pallor may be seen locally in a limb to which blood supply is interrupted, and in the fingers or toes due to arterial spasm (cold, Raynaud's disease, described by Maurice Raynaud, a French physician). The presence of jaundice may tint the skin from lemon yellow (haemolytic jaundice) to dark yellow and greenish colour (obstructive jaundice). Its presence has to be noted in daylight. Generally, it is associated with yellowish discolouration of the sclera.

Cyanosis: When the level of deoxygenated haemoglobin exceeds 5 gm per 100 ml (30 per cent) of blood in the superficial vessels, it gives a dusky blue colouration to the skin and mucous membrane. It is recognized as cyanosis and is looked for in the regions with an increased capillary network (cheeks, ears, lips, oral mucosa and nail beds) and in the hands and feet where the skin is thin.

There are three types of cyanosis: peripheral, central and mixed. Peripheral cyanosis, is observed in the peripheral circulatory failure, and on exposure to cold, causing peripheral vasoconstriction. As the blood flow is slow there is extraction of a greater amount of oxygen from the capillaries thus reducing the haemoglobin to a marked extent. It is also noticeable in conditions with a low cardiac output. Cyanosis is recognized in cool areas of the nail beds, the outer-aspect of the lips, outer surface of the ear lobes and cheeks. The extremities are cold but the tongue is not cyanosed. Warming improves peripheral cyanosis but worsens central cyanosis.

In central cyanosis, the amount of desaturated haemoglobin in the arterial blood is elevated. It is due to improper oxygenation of the blood in the lungs (alveolar hypoventilation, ventilation-perfusion imbalance, shunt and diffusion abnormalities), or from the mixture of arterial and venous blood in the heart from right-to-left or, veno-arterial shunts, or acute left ventricular failure. Central cyanosis is obvious when the arterial oxygen saturation has fallen below 80 per cent that corresponds to a PaO_2 (arterial oxygen tension) of 50 mms Hg of less. The cyanosis may be evident in any part of the body, but in particular warm well perfused regions like the mucosa of the tongue, oral cavity, ear lobes, tips of the nose and fingertips. Central cyanosis is also a feature of polycythaemia due to an increased concentration of haemoglobin accompanied by increased level of reduced haemoglobin. Cyanosis depends on the absolute amount of deoxyhaemoglobin and not on relative amount. Hence patients with polycythaemia become cyanosed with mild hypoxaemia, whereas patients with anaemia do not develop cyanosis till hypoxaemia is severe. The extremities are warm. A combined form of central and peripheral cyanosis may be noted in chronic cor pulmonale (mixed cyanosis).

A differential cyanosis is a condition where the toes appear cyanosed. Usually they are not clubbed. The hands are normal and it is encountered in the reversal of shunt due to pulmonary hypertension developing in patent ductus arteriosus (PDA). The left hand may become cyanosed when the ductus is located at the branching part of the left subclavian artery. A regional cyanosis is encountered in Raynaud's disease, arterial occlusion and thrombophlebitis. The presence of abnormal haemoglobin such as sulphaemoglobinaemia (reduced haemoglobin combining with hydrogen sulphide, enterogenous cyanosis) and methaemo-globinaemia (following administration of sulphones, sulphona-mide, phenacetin, primaquin and aniline dyes) may give a blue tint to the skin. These conditions do not respond to administration of oxygen. Methaemoglobinaemia gives a chocolate hue, hence referred as chocolate cyanosis. A generalized cherry-red discolouration of the skin is noted in carbon monoxide poisoning. There is no cyanosis, as carboxyhaemoglobin prevents reduction of oxyghaemoglobin.

There can be permanent bluish discolouration of the skin due to deposition of blue pigment (pseudocyanosis). It is seen in exposure to metals used in therapy (silver and gold salts), or drugs such as minocycline, amiodarone, chloroquin and phenothiazine.

Other conditions: Spider naevi—Spider angioma appear as small red spots consisting of a central arteriole with radiating branches.

When pressure is applied over the central arteriole with the head of a pin, it becomes blanched. The presence of spider naevi is located in the face, upper limbs, and upper part of the trunk in the territory of superior vena caval drainage. They appear in conditions associated with liver cell failure, pregnancy, starvation and intake of oral contraceptives.

Telangiectasia: Telangiectasia refers to multiple localized dilatation of the vessels and capillaries in the skin and mucous membranes (hereditary haemorrhagic telangiectasis) and systemic sclerosis).

Bleeding: The bleeding in and under the skin may occur spontaneously, or after slight trauma, or as a manifestation of systemic diseases such as acute leukaemia, purpura, Ehlers-Danlos syndrome, scurvy etc. These reddish purple spots do not blanch on application of pressure and are called purpura. Often mosquito bites are confused for purpura. On application of pressure they can be made to disappear. The bleeding spots may be very small, less than 3 mm in diameter (pin head) or from capillary haemorrhage (petechiae) or large exceeding 3 mm in diameter from bleeding from a large vessel (ecchymosis). When the collected blood results in a fluctuant swelling with elevated skin it is referred to as haematoma. Petechiae can be made to appear on application of pressure around the arm by the sphygmomanometer cuff and raising the pressure above the systolic level. It indicates an increased capillary fragility.

Eruptions: The skin may exhibit various types of rashes or eruptions. It is an important sign in exanthematous fevers and drug reactions. When the eruptions are present, their description must indicate their location, type, colour and itchiness. Their distribution may be symmetrical (internal cause) or asymmetrical (external cause); localized or widespread; and centrifugal (smallpox, erythema multiforme) or centripetal (chickenpox, pityriasis). They may be noted on flexor (atopic eczema of children) or extensor (psoriasis in adults) surfaces. There are two types of skin lesions: primary and secondary.

The primary lesions may be in the form of macules, papules, nodules, vesicles, or pustules. Macules are present as circumscribed areas of variable size up to 1 cm in diameter with an alteration of colour and without any elevation (leucoderma, mole, measles, glandular fever, syphilis, typhoid fever, purpura, erythema, leprosy). They can be seen but not felt. Papules are circumscribed eruptions less than 0.5 cm in diameter raised above the skin (acne, lichen planus, warts, follicular keratitis, smallpox, chickenpox, psoriasis, measles, eczema). Their surface may be round, flat or pointed. The term maculopapule refers to a raised and discoloured circumscribed lesion. When the diameter of the papule is greater than 1 cm, it is called a nodule. It appears like a circumscribed large palpable mass (leprosy, syphilis, neurofibroma, erythema nodosum, Kaposi's sarcoma, described by Moritz Kaposi, Austrian dermatologist, subcutaneous nodules of rheumatoid arthritis and adenoma sabaceum). It is firm to touch. It may arise from the skin or subcutaneous tissue.

A wheal is a transiently raised skin with central pallor. It is caused by acute oedema of dermis. Urticaria are red wheals anywhere in the body and are accompanied by itching. Neurofibroma consists of sessile or pedunculated nodules of various sizes over the skin in different parts of the body. If the size is greater than 1 cm it is called a tumour. These papular eruptions may be clustered together as disc-shaped lesions referred to as plaques (psoriasis, morphea). Linear yellow plaques may be seen on the eyelids as a manifestation of disturbed lipid metabolism (xanthoma palpebrarum).

Small blisters are called vesicles and are not larger than 0.5 cm in diameter (herpes zoster, herpes simplex, small pox, chicken pox, and sudamina). They contain serous fluid. In herpes zoster a crop of vesicles appear on an erythematous base and are distributed in the course of sensory nerves unilaterally in a girdle-like manner. The vesicles are called pustules if they contain pus (acne vulgaris, small pox, folliculitis). The malignant pustule of anthrax exhibits a black center with surrounding redness. It must be noted the lesion is neither malignant nor purulent. The vesicles larger than 0.5 cm are referred to as bullae (pemphigus, bullous impetigo, superficial burns, scalds). They may be unilocular or multilocular. They may contain serous, seropurulent or haemorrhagic fluid.

The secondary lesions appear as a result of the changes taking place in the primary lesion. The macular and papular lesions may exhibit scaling of the epidermis (desquamation). The dried flakes (scales) are silver white and dry in psoriasis. The scales are adherent in lichen planus. The epidermal cells may adhere together with the dried fluid of vesicles, pustules and bullous lesions resulting in the formation of scabs or crusts (impetigo). They may

Primary Skin Lesions.

Lesion	description	example
Macule	circumscribed area of alterd colour without any elevation	café au-lait spot
Papule	circumscribed eruptions of < 0.5 cm	acne
Vesicle	fluid-filled small blister < 0.5 cm	herpes simplex
Bulla	vesicle > 0.5 cm	pemphigus
Pustule	vesicle containing pus	folliculitis
Plaque	confluence of papules with flat top	psoriasis
Nodule	large, solid deep-seated round mass > 1 cm	erythemanodosum
Wheal	elevated lesion with central pallor and red margin	urticaria
Scale	desicated thin plate of cornified epidermal cell	icthyosis

be red from haemorrhage, or yellow-green from pus. The infiltration into the skin around the primary lesions gives a leathery feeling. There may be excessive pigmentation. The lesions may undergo ulceration (destruction of the whole thickness of an area of the skin by infection, ischaemia, injury or neoplasm) or heal resulting in a scar (following primary syphilis on the penis, lupus vulgaris, post-operative scar). There may be a hypertrophy of the scar tissue (keloid).

Sweating: Increased sweating (hyperhidrosis) is observed in conditions following the subsidence of pyrexia, anxiety states and hyperthyroidism. Sweating characteristically occurs during sleep in pulmonary tuberculosis. Localised loss of sweating (anhidrosis) may be found in hypopigmented areas of leprosy and in conditions associated with interruption of the sympathetic nerve. The skin is dry in dehydration, ichthyosis, xeroderma, high fever and hypothyroidism. Cold clammy skin is encountered in shock and hypoglycaemia.

Cleanliness: There may be evidence of hyperpigmentation of the skin due to prolonged lack of bathing. The infestation of the body with parasites of scabies and pediculosis should be looked for. Scabies presents with excoriated papules (due to intense itching) in the webs of the fingers, wrists, axillae, groin, genitalia, legs and feet. It is associated with burrows (short linear straight or sinuous elevations of the outer epidermis and are coloured black) in the skin. Pediculosis affects the hair on the scalp, body, axillae and pubic region. Pigmentation may be seen with chronic infestation by body lice Excoriation due to scratching may occur from irritation of the skin. It can occur in certain rashes, obstructive jaundice, polycythaemia vera, and Hodgkin's disease, described by Thomas Hodgkin, British physician. Pruritus is common around external genitalia in diabetes.

Hair

There is a great variability of the colour, texture and density of hair over the scalp. It is genetically determined and is of a racial character. There may be balding and recession of hair at the temples and a graying of the hair prematurely.

At puberty the axillary and pubic hair grows in both sexes. In addition, in the male, hair appears over the face, chest, abdomen and limbs. The pubic and abdominal hair, merge in the males. In the female the pubic hair has a horizontal upper level. In hypothyroidism, hair is thick, coarse and scanty, especially over the frontal region, and there is loss of hair in the lateral-third of the eyebrows. In leprosy there is a loss of hair in the lateral third of the eyebrows, eyelashes and hair over the depigmented areas. There may be an absence of hair over the face, axillae and pubic regions in hypogonadism and hypopituitarism.

The loss of hair may be complete (*alopecia totalis*) or localized (*alopecia aerata*) over the scalp. A scarring alopecia is noted following destruction of hair follicles as in burns, X-ray irradiation, or herpes zoster ophthalmicus. A traction alopecia occurs in the presence of normal scalp skin. The hair is silky in Down's syndrome, described by John Down, English physician. Patchy localized loss of hair is noted in nervous children, in taenia capitis (ring worm) and rarely in secondary syphilis. An abnormal growth of hair is referred to as hirsuitism and it has special importance in women and children. An excess hair may be noted over the moustache area and beard in post-menopausal women. It is noted in Cushing's syndrome, prolonged use of corticosteroids, and precocious puberty. There is loss of hair in hypothyroidism, chronic liver diseases, severe iron deficiency anaemia, Addison's disease and administration of antimitotic drugs. There can be loss of hair from the legs in men as a feature of arterial insufficiency.

Temperature

The skin has to be felt to find out the skin temperature. The skin is warm in pyrexial states, hyperthyroidism and it is cold in peripheral circulatory failure and myxoedema. The foot is cold in obstruction to the arterial supply.

The normal temperature is 37°C (98.6°F) with a range from 35.6 to 37.2°C (98-99°F) when taken from the mouth. Though by keeping the palm of the hand, a rough idea of the temperature is made, it is advisable to record the temperature with a centrigrade clinical thermometer. Before its use, the thermometer should be washed with water, and the mercury column brought down by shaking it. The thermometer should be kept beneath the tongue and the mouth closed. It must be allowed to stay for more than a minute. The temperature can also be recorded by keeping the thermometer in the axilla. In children it can be recorded by placing it in the fold of the groin with the thigh flexed on the abdomen or by inserting it into the rectum. Rectal temperature should be taken in comatose and elderly patients. The temperature of the mouth and of the rectum are half a degree higher than that of the axilla or groin. The temperature is also measured by infrared technique at the tympanic membrane. It gives the core temperature at hypothalamus as both have a common blood supply.

The temperature may be normal, increased or decreased. When there is an elevation of the body temperature (above 37.7°C or 99°F) in a resting individual from the normal range, it is referred to as fever or pyrexia.

The daily four-hourly record of the temperature, on a graphic chart gives information on the course of the fever (Wunderlich curves, named after the person who first introduced temperature records in the hospitals). On the basis of it, the fever has been classified into the following types (Figs. 1a and 1b).

1) *Remittent:* A persistently elevated temperature which shows wide fluctuation and exceeds 2°C in a day without touching the normal. Generally the evening temperature is higher than that recorded in the morning (for example, malaria, tuberculosis, acute rheumatic fever, sepsis). Occasionally it may be inverted (tuberculosis, typhoid).

2) *Intermittent:* The temperature rises to a variable height and it touches the normal level for several hours daily (malaria, sepsis, abscess). The paroxysm of raised temperature may come down to baseline every day (quotidian) or every alternate

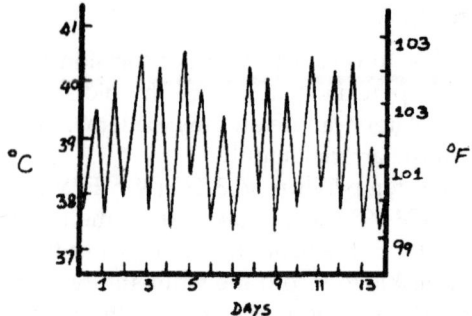

Fig. 1a Remittent fever.

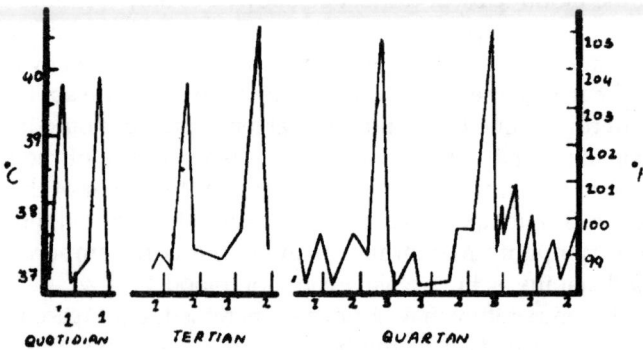

Fig. 1b Intermittent fever.

day (tertian) or after every 72 hours (quartan). Tertian fever is noted in infections from *P. falciparum*, *P. vivax* and *P. ovale*. Quotidian fever is noted in *P. malariae* infection. A daily remission may be noted in mixed infection.

3) *Continuous:* The temperature remains elevated for many days without showing much fluctuation (less than 1°C) for example, untreated typhoid fever, subacute infective endocarditis, bacterial pneumonia, miliary tuberculosis, HIV infection, urinary tract infection and brucellosis.

4) *Relapsing (periodic):* Febrile state for several days alternating with variable periods of apyrexia (Hodgkin's disease, rat bite fever, small pox, relapsing fever, brucellosis, undulating fever, dengue fever).

5) *Irregular:* The temperature that does not fall into any of the above categories, and shows marked variability.

The condition is referred to as hypothermia when the temperature is below 35°C (95°F), and it is called hyperpyrexia when it rises above 41°C (106°F) for example, malaria, heat stroke, pontine haemorrhage.

The temperature may rise suddenly (pneumonia, acute pyelonephritis, certain types of malaria) or gradually (typhoid, brucellosis, falciparum malaria). In many instances chills or rigors herald the onset of fever (lobar pneumonia, malaria, puerperal sepsis, after blood transfusion, urinary tract infection and cholecystitis). Heat is conserved while the temperature rises to a new level and the skin vessels get constricted making the body feel cold and the patient to shiver (rigor). In children and infants the onset may be associated with convulsions.

The fever may subside either by crisis or by lysis. In crisis the temperature falls to a normal level suddenly (lobar pneumonia, malaria, administration of antipyretics or antibiotics). In malaria initially there is rigor lasting for an hour or two. The patient shivers with cold and covers himself with many blankets. There may be sweating. Soon the temperature rises to 40°C or more, and the skin becomes dry and flushed. After about four hours there is profuse sweating and the temperature comes down quickly to normal or subnormal level. Such a sudden defervescence is not seen in urinary tract infections or septicemia.

In lysis the temperature gradually falls to a normal level in the course of some days (enteric fever). The subsidence of fever may be associated with sweating (tuberculosis, rheumatic fever, pneumonia, malaria). Two peaks of fever in a day occur characteristically in miliary tuberculosis and kala azar. Fever may persist for several weeks in HIV infection.

Pyrexia of unknown origin (PUO) is a constantly elevated body temperature of more than 37.5°C persisting for more than 2 weeks with no diagnosis after initial investigations.

Normally for each half degree centigrade rise of temperature the pulse rate quickens by 10 beats. The pulse rate quickens out of proportion to the temperature in cases of rheumatic fever, tuberculosis, and thyrotoxicosis (relative tachycardia). The pulse and temperature relationship is not maintained in cases of typhoid fever, meningitis, cerebral abscess, dengue fever and in viral infections where the pulse rate is relatively slow when compared to the temperature (relative bradycardia). With every half a degree rise of temperature the respiratory rate increases by four cycles.

In *Streptococcus pneumoniae* pneumonia, the respiratory rate shows a disproportionate rise when compared to the temperature. Fever occurs in a wide variety of conditions and the cause must be ascertained carefully.

The body temperature is referred to as subnormal when the temperature is below 36.6°C (98°F). This can be a sudden or gradual development. It develops acutely in peripheral circulatory failure, following myocardial infarction, metabolic acidosis, overwhelming infections, and after prolonged exposure to cold. It can develop gradually in patients with hypothyroidism and chronic wasting diseases.

Gynaecomastia

Gynaecomastia is a unilateral or bilateral enlargement of the breast in males simulating that in the female in size and shape due to hyperplasia of the duct, epithelium and periductal stroma. Firm hyperplastic mammary tissue can be felt under the nipples that is not adherent to the nipples and deep structures. The condition may be physiologic (adolescence) or pathologic. Some of the pathologic conditions are; Klinefelter's syndrome, testicular feminisation, secondary testicular failure, true hermaphroditism, testicular tumours, cirrhosis of the liver, adrenal tumours, and leprosy. It may be noted sometimes after the intake of diethylstilboestrol, digoxin, gonadotrophins, spironolactone, cimetidine, alkylating agents, isoniazid, methyldopa and tricyclic antidepressants.

Head

There is a great variability in the size and shape of the skull from person to person. The circumference of the skull is measured along a horizontal line connecting the supraorbital ridges in the front and the occipital protuberance at the back. It measures 56 cm in an adult and is 46 cm at the age of one year.

The skull may be long (dolichocephaly) or round (brachy-cephaly). The general contour may be small and round as in microcephaly, craniostenosis and Mongolism. The skull may be abnormally large and globular (macrocephaly). The condition may be congenital or acquired from hydrocephalus, acromegaly, osteitis deformans or gargoylism. In achondroplasia the skull appears large compared to the short limbs of the individual, and the bridge of the nose is depressed. In hydrocephalus the head is large and the forehead appears bulged. The eyes are pushed downwards exposing the upper part of the sclera. In children the sutures remain separated and the fontanelle bulge. In osteitis deformans, there is a disproportionately large head compared to a small face and the skull is greatly distorted with an increased transverse diameter. The forehead is prominent. In acromegaly, the head and the face are large and the supraorbital ridges are prominent and the lower jaw is elongated.

The shape of the skull is altered in various disorders. In oxycephaly, the skull is elongated vertically (tower skull). The forehead is wide and the orbits are shallow resulting in protruded eyeballs. In rickets, the skull appears square or flat, with prominent frontal and parietal eminences. In congenital syphilis, there are prominent frontal eminences (bossing) and a sunken bridge of the nose. A large skull with a depressed bridge of the nose and prominent supraorbital ridges, is seen in gargoylism. In Mongolism, the skull is small and round. The eyes are tilted inwards and downwards. The nose is broad and flat.

On palpation a localized tenderness may be elicited at the site of inflammation (sinusitis, mastoiditis) or tumour deposits. There may be depression, from depressed fractures or swellings (sebaceous cysts, osteoma, secondaries). In hyperparathyroidism, the bones appear soft and fragile. Generally, the cranial sutures unite by the sixth month after birth, and the anterior fontanelle close by the sixteenth month. A premature closure is noted in oxycephaly. A delayed closure is seen in rickets, congenital syphilis, cretinism and hydrocephalus. The fontanelle, bulge from raised intracranial tension as in hydrocephalus, and meningitis, or, get sunken, as in dehydration. Temporal artery may be palpably enlarged and tender in cranial arteritis.

A tympanitic note is elicited in internal hydrocephalus and it gives a cracked-pot sound in children with separation of the sutures from raised intracranial tension, congenital syphilis, rickets and fracture of the skull. Auscultation should be made by placing the stethoscope over the temple, closed eyes, preauricular area, mastoid, occiput and the crown regions. A generalized systolic bruit may be heard in arteriovenous malformations, carotid-cavernous fistula and Paget's disease, named after James Paget, English surgeon. Aneurysm of the internal carotid artery in the cavernous sinus may produce a bruit over the eyeball. Bruit of glomus jugulare is heard over mastoid.

Movements: The head may be fixed exhibiting rigidity of head and neck (meningitis, tetanus, diseases of cervical spine, and spasm of neck muscles). It may be retracted backwards in meningitis. There may be sudden jerky repetitive movements (habit spasms, tics and chorea). In senility and Parkinsonism there may be movements of the head sidewards, backwards or forwards (titubation). There can be head-nodding movement secondary to ballistic form of severe aortic regurgitation, often refered as de Musset sign, after a French poet, Alfred de Musset.

Face

The inspection of the face gives clues to many systemic diseases. The following abnormalities of the facial appearance are noted: colour, contour, oedema, symmetry and expression. Some of the important facies are described.

Acromegaly: Massive face with coarse features, prominent nose and forehead, protruded lower jaw and prognathism.

Cushing's syndrome: Round face (moon facies) with plethoric (flushed) skin, prominent cheeks, acne, hirsutism.

Myxoedema: Pale, dull somnolent appearance exhibiting lack of intelligence, swollen eyelids, thick dry skin, loss of hair of the lateral third of the eyebrows, slow mental reaction.

Cretinism: Pale, dull appearance, broad flat nose, thick lips, protruded tongue, scanty hair.

Anxious facies: Pale, anxious look, sweating, noted in nervous individuals.

Thyrotoxicosis: Staring look with wide palpebral fissures, prominent shiny eyes, infrequent blinking, lid retraction, quick movements of the eyes, restlessness.

Parkinsonism: Expressionless and immobile face (mask-like facies), and infrequent blinking.

Myasthenia gravis: Drooped eyelids and jaw, blank expression of the face.

Facial palsy: Unilateral loss of wrinkling of forehead, wide palpebral fissure, flattened nasolabial fold, drooping of the angle of the mouth.

Hippocratic facies: Sunken eyes, hollow cheeks, parched dry skin, pinched nose. It is observed in severe dehydration and wasting diseases.

Leonine face: Flat nose, thick skin with nodules and thinning of the eyebrows (Leprosy).

Tetanus: Tonic spasm of the muscles, raised eyebrows, drawn out angle of the mouth, difficulty to open the mouth (trismus).

Systemic sclerosis: Markedly thinned and tight skin with difficulty in opening the mouth.

Mongoloid face: Stupid look, medial epicanthic folds along the upper lid, slanting eyes, open mouth, broad fissured tongue, disproportionately small oval head, slopping forehead, a flattened occiput, low set ears with small lobules.

Hyperteleorism: Widely set eyes, depressed nasal bridge, and frontal bossing. Cardiac abnormalities associated with hyperteleorism are pulmonary stenosis especially in association with atrial septal defect (ASD), Down's syndrome, Noonan syndrome, Hurler's syndrome, and supravalvular aortic stenosis.

Cardiovascular disorders: The conditions may be associated with pinkish purple patches over the cheeks (mitral stenosis), pallor (aortic regurgitation), cyanosis (cyanotic heart diseases), puffiness of the face, oedema of the upper limbs (superior vena caval obstruction), moon face (pulmonary stenosis).

'Elfin' facies: a broad high forehead, puffy cheeks, low ears, hyperteleorism, an upturned nose with long vertical groove between nose and mouth (filtrum), a wide pouting mouth and hypoplastic mandible (supravalvular aortic stenosis).

Nephritic facies: Pale puffy face, swollen eyelids noticeable more in the morning.

Tabetic facies: Bilateral partial ptosis with wrinkled forehead, elevated eye brows.

Systemic lupus erythematosis (SLE): Well circumscribed, scaly patch in butterfly distribution on either side of the nose.

Eyes

The eyes may often give an indication of an underlying general endocrine or neurologic diseases. The expression of the face is reflected in the eyes. The eyes are bright and staring in hyperthyroidism; dull in hypothyroidism. In psychoneurotic disorders they are bright and alert, and present a vacant look in optic atrophy, mental deficiency and coma. The eyes may be fixed in ophthalmoplegia. The following parts of the eyes are examined: eyebrows, lids, palpebral fissure, conjunctiva, sclera, cornea, pupils, iris and lens.

Eyebrows: There may be a loss of eyebrows especially in its outer third in conditions of myxoedema, leprosy and secondary syphilis. There may be oedema in and around the eyelids especially in the infraorbital region. The loose areolar tissue facilitates the accumulation of the fluid. The eyelids are swollen in acute nephritis, nephrotic syndrome, angioneurotic oedema, myxoedema (deposition of muco-proteins) and trichinosis. Unilateral swelling of the eyelids may arise from the inflammatory conditions, in and around the eyelids and in cavernous sinus thrombosis.

Lids: During inflammatory conditions of the lids (blepharitis) the borders of the lids appear red and swollen around the base of the eye lashes and may be covered with dry crusts. Painful swelling from infection of the hair follicles may appear at the margin of the inflamed lid as in a stye or hordeolum. Non-tender hard nodules from obstruction of the sebaceous duct, may be noted in the region, away from the margin of the lid (chalazion). Vesicles over an erythematous base may occur on the eyelid in herpes zoster ophthalmicus. The lid margins may be everted (ectropion) or inverted (entropion). There may be contraction of the sphincters of the eyelid (blepherospasm) causing narrowing of the orbital fissure and the eyes may be turned away from the light (photophobia) in meningitis, in inflammatory conditions affecting the eyes and in riboflavin deficiency.

Yellow plaques consisting of deposits of lipoid material referred to as xanthelasma, may be seen especially in the skin of the upper eyelids, at the inner canthus, in some middle aged and elderly individuals. Sometimes the condition is associated with hyperlipidaemia.

Normally the upper eyelid covers the upper part of the cornea and the lower eyelid covers the portion up to the junction of the cornea and sclera (limbus). There may be an inability of the lids to close the eye due to the paralysis of orbicularis oculi (facial palsy) resulting in a wide palpebral fissure. The upper eyelid may descend like a curtain in front of the eye and narrow the palpebral fissure (ptosis). It may be unilateral or bilateral. Ptosis is noted in paralysis of the oculomotor nerve or of cervical sympathetic chain and in ocular myopathy. In Mongolism (Down's Syndrome) the palpebral fissure is narrow, slanting and obliquely placed. There is a fold of skin (epicanthic fold) along the upper lid.

Eyeballs: The eyeballs may be displaced forward to an abnormal degree (proptosis) and is referred to as exophthalmos, when it is associated with a wide palpebral fissure. Bilateral proptosis may occur in congestive heart failure. Exophthalmos may be bilateral (hyperthyroidism, oxycephaly) or unilateral (AV fistula, cavernous sinus thrombosis, retro-orbital tumours and aneurysms).

In hyperthyroidism, there is retraction of the upper lid and lower eyelid exposing the sclera above or below the cornea while gazing straight ahead (lid retraction, Dalrymple sign, named after John Dalrymple, English oculist), infrequent blinking of the eyelids (Stellwag's sign, named after Carl von Carion Stellwag, Austrian ophthalmoligist), failure of the upper lid to follow the movement of the eyeball when the individual looks down (lid lag, von Graeff's sign, named after German ophthalmologist), absence of frontal wrinkles when the patient looks upwards (Joffroy's sign, named after Alexis Jaffroy, French physician) and failure of convergence of the eyes when the patient is asked to look at the finger brought in front (Moebius sign, named after Paul Moebius, German neurologist).

The eyeballs may appear retracted into the orbit (enophthalmos) in dehydration, wasting diseases and sympathetic paralysis. The decrease or increase of the intraocular tension can be ascertained by noting the degree of fluctuation while palpating the sclera with the index fingers through the upper lid when the patient is looking down. The eyeballs feel soft and inelastic in diabetic ketoacidosis, and dehydration, and hard in glaucoma.

Lacrimal gland: The lacrimal gland, has to be examined by pulling up the lateral part of the upper lid while the patient is looking downwards and inwards. The gland is swollen and tender in acute inflammation (dacryoadenitis). Chronic dacryoadenitis is associated with painless enlargement of lacrimal glands bilaterally as in reticulosis, tuberculosis and sarcoidosis. Proptosis may be noted in tumours of lacrimal gland.

Conjunctiva: The conjunctiva is looked at for its colouration. It consists of two parts: bulbar (visible) and palpebral (hidden) lining the eyeball and inner surface of the eyelids respectively. Normally it is pink; becomes pale in anaemia and yellow in jaundice. Conjunctiva loses its lustre and becomes dry (xerophthalmia) in vitamin A deficiency. There is abnormal dryness (conjunctivitis sicca) due to lacrimal gland diseases (Sjogren's syndrome, named after Henrik Sjogren, Swedish ophthalmologist, measles, or Stevens Johnson' syndrome, described by American paediatricians, Albert Stevens and Frank Johnson). In respiratory failure and polycythaemia, conjunctivae show a glistening appearance due to an increased vascularity.

To visualize the palpebral conjunctiva of the lower lids the index fingers of both hands are to be placed over the lower eyelids of both eyes, and depressed while the patient is asked to look upwards. To examine the palpebral conjunctiva of the upper eyelid, the patient is asked to look downwards, then with the right thumb placed at the upper part of the upper lid, it is pulled upwards so as to evert the eyelashes. The lashes are held between the forefingers and thumb of the left hand, and the lid is everted, by rotating it round the right thumb.

The conjunctiva may exhibit swelling (oedema, 'chemosis'), redness, excessive lacrimation and engorgement of the blood vessels (infection) from local inflammation. There is mucopurulent discharge in severe bacterial infection and the sticky purulent exudates may cause adhesion of the lids on waking. Viral infections are associated with slight serous discharge. In allergic conditions conjunctiva shows slight oedema with a milky hue. Hypo-proteinaemia or impaired venous drainage is associated with conjunctival oedema. Trachoma is associated with small pale follicles on upper palpebral conjunctiva. The presence of similar follicles in lower Palpebral conjunctive indicates allergic conditions or viral infection of the conjunctiva. A vascularised conjunctiva may grow on to the cornea from its medial side in a triangular fashion which may show progressive fibrosis (pterygium). There may be subconjunctival haemorrhages and petechiae (subacute infective endocarditis, septicemia, leukaemia, a bout of severe cough, fracture of skull, and bleeding tendency).

Sclera: Normally the sclera is uniformly white. It may become muddy (dirty brownish yellow) in some people. It is stained yellow in jaundice. Jaundice is looked for by observing the eyes of the patient in sunlight. The upper eyelids are raised when the patient is looking down. The tint may vary from lemon yellow to greenish yellow in colour. In osteitis deformans, the sclerae are thin and blue. Blue colour is imparted by the choroidal pigment beneath. Triangular white foamy plaques may be seen over the sclera in vitamin A deficiency (Bitot's spots, named after Pierre Bitot, French physician).

Cornea: Cornea is transparent. Inflammation of the cornea (keratitis) is associated with circumcorneal infection. There can be ulcerations. Cornea becomes hazy in deep keratitis. Cornea becomes opaque and glossy in keratomalacia. The cornea may exhibit small (nebulae) or big (leucomata) opacities consisting of fibrous tissue due to the old injuries or previous infection. An opaque white ring of lipoid material develops near the periphery of the cornea with advancing age (arcus senilis). If arcus is seen in young and middle aged patients, it is referred to as arcus juvenilis, and is sometimes results from hyperlipidaemia. A golden-brown Kayser-Fleisher ring, described by Bernhard Kayser and Bruno Fleisher, German physician, may develop at the periphery of the cornea in hepatolenticular degeneration (Wilson's disease, named after Samuel Kinnier Wilson, English neurologist) due to deposition of copper, and it is appreciated by slit-lamp.

Iris: The colour of the iris is variable and the colouration of the eye is dependent on its colour. The inflammation of the iris (iritis) may be associated with circumcorneal injection. It may exhibit white specks on the posterior surface of the cornea and exudates in the anterior chamber which may be purulent in bacterial infection (hypopyon). Iritis occurs in rheumatoid arthritis, ulcerative colitis and sarcoidosis. In albinism there is loss of pigment of the iris. Eye gives a pink appearance. There is impaired vision and nystagmus. The pupils may be dilated or constricted, equal or unequal, regular or irregular. The irregularity may be a sequelae to iritis or tabes dorsalis.

Lens: The lens becomes opaque (cataract) in old age and in conditions of diabetes. There can be a curious movement of the iris due to ectopia lentis in Marfan's syndrome, described by Antonin Marfan, French paediatrician.

Intraocular tension: Intraocular tension is raised in glaucoma and is reduced in dehydration, diabetic coma and myopia. It is recognised by palpating the eyeballs as follows: the middle, ring, and little fingers of both hands are placed on the patient's eyebrows while both index fingers elicit fluctuation by placing them gently on the patient's closed eye (Fig. 2).

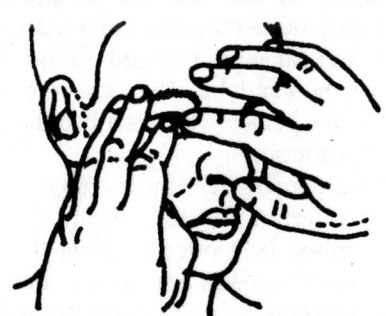

Fig. 2 Determination of intraocular tension.

Red eye: Ocular inflammation presents in the form of a red eye. There is either conjunctival or ciliary injection by the dilated posteror conjunctival or anterior ciliary vessels respectively. Subconjunctival haemorrhage is another cause of red eye. Conjunctivitis, keratitis, iritis, and acute glaucoma produce a red eye. These conditions are distinguished by the following features:

	Conjunctivitis	Keratitis	Iritis	Acute glaucoma
Pain	variable severity	moderate to severe	dull	sudden, severe
Vision	unaffected	loss	reduced	marked loss
Discharge	sticky	minimal	–	–
Pupils	normal	normal	small irregular	dilated and fixed

Examination of Ear, Nose and Throat

Ears

The inspection of the lateral and medial surfaces of the cartilaginous auricle (pinna), mastoid process, external auditory meatus and the tympanic membrane has to be made while examining the ears. The auditory and labyrinthine functions are tested while examining the auditory nerve.

The congenital malformations like the absence of a part of an ear, absence of well-defined lobes, presence of an accessory auricle, prominent ear or displaced ear, fusion of the ear to the face and the position of the ear, in relation to a line drawn through the canthi of the eyes have to be noted (malformed and low set ears). In Down's syndrome the ears are low set and the auricles are usually large and the lobules may be rudimentary of absent. There may be creases in the ear lobes extending more than half of the diagonal length of the ear lobe. They are referred to as Frank creases, named after the person who described them as a risk factor for coronary artery disease.

There may be tenderness over the tragus in the inflammatory conditions of the external auditory meatus. The presence of mastoiditis is recognised by tenderness over the mastoid region on application of pressure. Pre-auricular and post-auricular lymphadenitis and parotitis result in tenderness in front and behind the ear. The lobules of the ear appear erythematous, shiny and thickened with plaques of infiltration over the ear (lepromatous leprosy). The presence of gout is shown by the presence of hard nodules (tophi consisting of sodium biurate) over the helix. There can be cyanosis on the periphery of the ear. There can be herpetic eruptions on the ear (Ramsay-Hunt syndrome, described by James Ramsay-Hunt, American physician).

The external auditory canal and tympanic membrane are to be examined with the use of the auroscope. Routinely they are examined with the help of a lighted torch. The pinna is gently pulled upwards, backwards and slightly laterally so as to straighten the external auditory canal. External meatus may be narrowed due to bony overgrowth (exostosis). The wax and desquamated epithelium may form hard plugs, and occlude the canal completely causing deafness. The presence of any discharge has to be looked into. Pus may be oozing from a ruptured furunculosis in the external auditory canal or through the perforated tympanic membrane from a middle ear infection. In a middle ear infection, the movement of the external ear is not associated with any pain, but the hearing is affected. Blood may be found discharging from trauma or from a fracture of the base of the skull. Normally the tympanic membrane gives a translucent greyish appearance. It loses its glistening appearance in otitis. This membrane may be bulged forwards and inflamed in suppurative otitis media. It may be retracted due to adhesions, as a result of previous infection of the middle ear. The membrane may show marginal or central perforation.

Nose

The nose is examined for its abnormality, discharge, tenderness over the paranasal sinuses, and patency of nares. The external appearance of the nose varies from individual to individual. In acromegaly, the nose may be enlarged due to thickening of subcutaneous tissue and bony overgrowth. Nose is broad in hypothyroidism. The nose is red, large and bulbous in rhinophyma.

Nose may be narrowed when there is chronic obstruction of the airways since childood. Due to erosion of nasal bones in congenital syphilis and leprosy, there will be a saddle-nose (depressed bridge of the nose). There can also be damage and destruction of the skin and underlying tissue of the nose in tuberculosis (*lupus vulgaris*) and sarcoidosis (*lupus pernio*). Lupus erythematosus causes a butterfly erythematous lesion on the nose with its wings spreading out over the cheeks. In rosacea there is reddening of the nose and cheeks with a 'butterfly-wings' appearance. In pellagra, the skin appears dry, cracked and hyperpigmented in the same region. The nose is flattened in cleft palate deformity.

The *ala nasi* may be active during respiration in conditions of pneumonia, cardiac failure and bronchial asthma. It enables one to open the nostrils wide during inspiration. Infection of the sinuses is revealed by the presence of the tenderness on application of pressure with the thumb over the maxillary and frontal sinuses (roof of the orbit). The patency of the nares is tested by closing each nostril in turn, by compression of the *ala* with the thumb while the patient is breathing through the other, with the mouth closed. A unilateral obstruction may be evident in deviated septum, foreign body, and polyp. In acute rhinitis, the obstruction is bilateral.

There may be discharge from the nose. It may be watery (coryza, allergic rhinitis, mucopurulent sinusitis, CSF rhinorrhoea), or blood (trauma, ulcers, foreign body, hypertension, typhoid, rheumatic fever, and haemorrhagic conditions). The nose bleeding is referred to as epistaxis.

The nasal vestibule is examined using a bi-valved speculum. For routine examination, the tip of the nose is pushed up with the thumb, and then examined with a light. The nasal septum may be deflected. It may be perforated (syphilis, non-specific ulcer) or may show the presence of a cleft palate. In Wegener's granulomatosis, named after Friedrich Wegener, a German pathologist, the nasal septum and the cartilage may get perforated leading to saddle nose deformity. There may be evidence of polyp (moist greyish swelling), a foreign body, ulcers and bleeding points on the nasal septum. Normally the nasal mucosa is pale pink and moist. The mucosa may be red and inflamed (acute rhinitis), pale and swollen (allergic rhinitis) or greyish and swollen (chronic rhinitis). The olfactory function is examined while testing the olfactory nerve (see page 220).

Throat

The throat is examined in good light-preferably, daylight. The patient is asked to open the mouth wide and say a prolonged 'ah-h-h', enabling the elevation of the soft palate and uvula. To have a better view, the tongue may be depressed by placing firmly a tongue depressor in its middle. The examiner has to concentrate his look, on the soft palate, uvula, palatine arch, tonsils, and posterior wall of the pharynx.

The oropharynx is situated behind the soft palate and the tonsillar fossa. The posterior wall of the pharynx is covered by mucosa with multiple tiny adenoid swellings. In acute pharyngitis, the mucosa is red, shiny and swollen. The wall appears bulged inwards in retropharyngeal abscess. In herpangina (Coxsackie virus infection) vesicles may be evident on the wall. The infection of the nasopharynx may be revealed by the presence of tricking of mucopus on the posterior pharyngeal wall (postnasal drip).

The tonsils are located in the tonsillar fossa between the pillars of fauces as oval masses of lymphoid tissue. They vary in size. The size of tonsils is greater during childhood. The tonsils enlarge and become red in acute tonsillitis. There may be whitish (glandular fever) or yellowish (streptococcal tonsillitis) exudates coming from the crypts. There will be a collection of pus surrounding the tonsil in peritonsillar abscess. In diphtheria, a dense greyish white membrane appears on the tonsils, pharynx, soft palate and uvula. It is lightly raised above the surface and is firmly adherent. On removal of the membrane there will be bleeding. In acute septic inflammatory conditions the mucosa is bright red and swollen with a greyish white exudates (Vincent's angina, named after Henri Vincent, a French physician, streptococcal infections, agranulocytosis, infectious mononucleosis).

The palate is inspected for its colour, continuity, ulcers, vesicles and patches. The hard palate covering the anterior three-fourths of the roof of the mouth may show a median defect (cleft palate), perforation (tertiary syphilis, necrosis of bone following radiotherapy), ulcers, petechiae (thrombocytopaenia, glandular fever, rubella and streptococcal tonsillitis), patches or pigmentation. The palate may be highly arched and this is appreciated by looking at the roof of the palate. Often it coexists with an arachnodactyly. The uvula may be elongated or bifid. The mobility of the soft palate and uvula is tested while testing the IXth and Xth cranial nerves.

The voice may reveal hoarseness in acute and chronic laryngitis, tuberculosis, tumours, incomplete paralysis of the vocal cords and myxoedema. There may be stridor (noisy respiration) due to obstruction in the larynx or trachea.

Cheeks

The cheeks may show wasting, change in colour (pallor or flushing) and swelling. They are pale in anaemia and hypopituitarism, pale and puffy in nephrotic syndrome and may exhibit malar flush in mitral stenosis. Systemic lupus erythematosus may exhibit red raised eruptions on the bridge of the nose extending on to the cheeks. Facial paralysis leads to obliteration of the nasolabial fold on the affected side. The cheeks are sunken in dehydration and wasting diseases. There may be unilateral or bilateral enlargement of parotid glands (infective parotitis, suppurative parotitis, Mickulicz's syndrome, anaemia, diabetes mellitus, sarcoidosis, chronic alcoholism, cirrhosis of the liver, salivary duct calculus, Sjogren's syndrome, intake of iodides, and mixed parotid tumour). There may be dilated small veins as punctuate red or purple spots (telangiectasis) on the face in cirrhosis of the liver, chronic alcoholism or as a hereditary condition.

Chvostek's sign: When the region in front of the external auditory meatus is tapped with the finger the facial muscles on that side may go into momentary contraction pulling the mouth to that side. It is due to the stimulation of the hyperexcitable facial nerve and is seen in tetany. The sign is named after Franz Chvostek, Austrian surgeon.

Lips

A deep cleft may be seen in the upper lip on one, or both sides, as a congenital defect (cleft lip). The normal pink colour of the lips becomes dark brown in chronic smokers. Alterations in colour may be congenital. The redness is increased during inflammation (cheilitis). The lips are pale in anaemia and blue in cyanosis. These alterations are obvious early over the lips than in other sites. These signs are masked by lipstick, and *pan* chewing.

The lips are dry in fever, toxaemia, exposure to cold, dehydration and diabetes mellitus. In angioneurotic oedema, insect bites and inflammatory conditions, they show a marked swelling. The lips are thick in acromegaly and hypothyroidism. Small vesicles on an erythematous base appear over the lips in herpes febrilis (simplex). They soon burst to form scabs (cold sore). Such lesions may also occur on other parts of the face. Herpes simplex is noted in respiratory infection. There may be collection of epithelial debris, food and bacteria on the lip (sordes) as a manifestation of prolonged fevers and renal failure.

The lips show brown or bluish-black pigmentation in Addison's disease. There may be circumoral brown or black pigmentation from underlying small bowel polyposis. The lips may be kept separated (open mouthed) in conditions with nasal obstruction, facio-scapulo-humeral muscular dystrophy, cretinism and Mongolism. The angles of the mouth may appear deviated to one side suggesting facial palsy on the opposite side. In severe airways obstruction, the patient exhibits pursing of the lips. The lips are tightly held at the height of inspiration and are narrowly held apart during expiration.

The lips exhibit soreness with redness, crusting and fissures. They are more common at the corners of the mouth (angular stomatitis). Protein energy malnutrition and deficiency of B complex especially riboflavin are frequently associated with angular stomatitis and the fissures on the line of closure of the lips. Angular stomatitis may also occur from ill-fitting dentures and from candida infections (thrush). There may be ulcers on the lips. Epithelioma can develop as an indolent, flat and shallow ulcer on the lower lip away from the midline. Extra-genital chancre may appear as a small, firm, indurated lesion on the upper lip. The saliva may be drooping from the mouth (Parkinsonism, cerebro-vascular accident, organophosphorus insecticide poisoning).

There is paralysis of the lips in the nuclear lesions of hypoglossal nerve (progressive bulbar palsy). There is difficulty in opening the mouth due to the spasm of the muscles of mastication (classically in tetanus it is called trismus). It is noted in mumps, ankylosis of the mandible and systemic sclerosis. The lips are puckered in the latter condition. The lower lip is pendulous showing part of the mucus membrane and it is noted in myopathic facies.

Oral Cavity

The oral cavity is examined in bright light. It may reveal manifestations of local diseases or signs of systemic diseases. The teeth, gums, tongue, inner surface of the lips, cheek, and palate (see examination of the throat) are to be examined carefully. The patient is asked to open the mouth wide. To visualize the palate, the head has to be tilted backwards.

Buccal Mucosa

The buccal mucosa is normally pink in colour. It becomes bright red in inflammatory conditions and pale in anaemia. Aphthous ulcers appear as small superficial, painful ulcers with surrounding hyperaemia. They can be demonstrated on the inner side of lips by holding and everting the lower lip with the index finger and thumb of both hands. The oral mucosa may show a brown pigmentation in Addison's disease. There may be white patches raised above the surface like small milk curds from monilial infection. The patches are difficult to remove. Their presence may be a manifestation of HIV infection. Leukoplakia exhibits presence of white opalescent plaques in the inner aspect of the cheeks.

The mouth may be dry (xerostomia) or may show excessive secretion of saliva (ptyalism). There may be small bluish-white spots, over an erythematous base on the buccal mucosa opposite the molar teeth, in the early stages of measles before the appearance of rash (Koplik's spots, named after Henry Koplik, a US paediatrician). The orifice of parotid duct, opposite the maxillary second molar tooth appears inflamed in mumps.

The Breath

The character of the breath has to be assessed and it gives diagnostic clues. In individuals with bad oral hygiene, stomatitis, carious teeth, pyorrhoea, chronic gingivitis, septic tonsils, atrophic rhinitis, suppurative disorders of the lung, gastric carcinoma and intestinal obstruction, and breath is associated with a foul smell (halitosis).

The odour of alcohol is easily recognised on breath. There is a fishy or ammoniacal odour in uraemia, fruity or acetone smell in diabetic ketoacidosis, and 'mousy' odour (fetor hepaticus) in liver cell failure. The intake of alcohol, or administration of paraldehyde gives the breath a characteristic odour. The intake of organophosphorous insecticides gives a garlic odour to the breath. A putrid smell is imparted to breath in lung abscess. Infected bronchiectasis gives a stale fecal smell to the breath.

Teeth

On opening the mouth, the teeth are inspected. The primary teeth are 20 in number and the permanent 32. Sometimes the third molar of the lower jaw remains unerupted. When natural teeth are present, the inspection should be made for their number, presence of any irregularity, cavities due to their decay (caries) and the relation of the teeth to each other. The cleanliness, staining (poor dental hygiene, brown in smokers, horizontal grey band in children receiving tetracyclines), presence of tartar (precipitate of calcium salts of saliva), exposure of the roots and presence of false teeth or dentures have to be noted.

The upper central permanent incisors are peg-shaped and notched in congenital syphilis (Hutchinson's teeth, named after Sir Jonathan Hutchinson, an English surgeon). The first permanent molars may even be dome-shaped (Moon teeth, named after Henry Moon, an English surgeon). In acromegaly the teeth are widely spaced and the enlarged lower jaw projects forwards (prognathism). In endemic flurosis chalky white patches are noted on the teeth and the enamel is mottled. Sometimes the teeth are pitted and exhibit brown staining.

Gums (Gingivae)

The gums are normally pink in colour and they adhere closely to the necks of the teeth. The gums become pale in anaemia, blue in cyanosis, and bright red in inflammation (gingivitis). There may be a bluish black pigmentation in a linear fashion along the edge of the gums in lead poisoning, or after prolonged use of bismuth preparations. It is pigmented in Addison's disease. The gums are swollen and spongy as in scurvy, and bleed on pressure. The gums show hypertrophy in pregnancy, acute leukaemia, and in phenytoin toxicity. There is recession of the gums from the teeth in advanced age and in chronic periodontitis. Bleeding gums are encountered in leukaemia and purpura. In Vincent's gingivitis the gums show ulceration and are covered with greyish white slough and give a foul odour. In pyorrhoea, there is oozing of pus on pressure from the region between the gums and teeth. Alveolar or dental abscess shows localized swelling of the gums and sometimes swelling of the face.

Tongue

The tongue is inspected, by asking the patient to protrude it forwards. It appears to be deviated towards the side of a paralysed hypoglossal nerve. Such deviation to the affected side is also encountered in hemiplegia and in carcinoma, when it affects the side of the tongue and the floor of the mouth. A darting movement may be observed in chorea. Tremors may be noted in Parkinsonism, chronic alcoholism (delirium tremens), thyrotoxicosis or nervousness. Fasciculations on the affected side of the tongue are seen in the lesions of the hypoglossal nerve or in its nucleus.

The following features are looked for during inspection of the tongue:

1) *Colour:* The tongue is pink normally. It is pale in severe anaemia, blue in cyanosis (always central in origin), megenta coloured in riboflavin deficiency, bright red in superficial glossitis and pellagra. It may show patchy pigmentation from birth. There may be a black or brown pigmentation in people taking iron preparations or in Addison's disease respectively.

2) *Dryness or moisture:* Normally the tongue is moist and papillae are visible on its dorsum. It becomes dry in dehydration. Dryness is evident in mouth breathers also.

3) *Cleanliness:* The tongue may be clean or may show the presence of fur (coating). The fur consists of epithelial cells, food particles and bacteria. The tongue appears coated in pyrexial states, lack of hygiene, heavy smokers, mouth breathers, edentulous individuals and in people on a prolonged milk diet. In typhoid the coating is central. The tip and margins of the tongue are free of fur. In advanced renal failure and acute intestinal obstruction a brownish coating is noted over the dry tongue. Fungal infection is associated with a brown fur ('black hairy tongue') and is due to elongated growth of the filiform papillae without desquamation.

4) *Size:* The tongue may get enlarged (macroglossia) due to endocrine (acromegaly, cretinism, myxoedema), metabolic (primary amyloidosis) or developmental (Mongolism) abnormalities or due to tumours (haemangioma, lymphangioma). The tongue may get swollen suddenly and become painful from angioneurotic oedema. It shows evidence of atrophy in lesions of the hypoglossal nerve and in progressive bulbar palsy. It appears small in states of dehydration.

5) *Mobility:* The tongue is immobile in bilateral hypoglossal nerve paralysis. There may be an inability to protrude the tongue completely in tongue-tie (short *frenum lingue*) or in advanced malignancy of the tongue affecting the floor of the mouth.

The tongue appears protruded in cretinism and Mongolism.
6) *Surface:* Normally the papillae are evident over the dorsum of the tongue. In conditions of anaemia, pellagra and sprue, the filiform papillae are atrophic and give the surface smooth or bald appearance. There is hypertrophy of the fungiform papillae in scarlet fever and the tongue is red (strawberry tongue). The tongue may show many hollows and deep fissures (congenital, chronic superficial glossitis). In chronic superficial glossitis, the fissures run longitudinally and the papillae are not normal. The surface shows white opaque areas of the thickened epithelium (leukoplakia). In congenital fissuring, the surface shows many irregular, often symmetrical horizontal folds, and the papillae are normal.

Geographic tongue refers to the appearance of a map on the tongue, due to localized irregular red areas of desquamation of filiform papillae surrounded by a whitish-yellow border. The condition is a symptomless inflammatory disorder. Children with pyrexia may exhibit a similar appearance of the tongue. In conditions of B-complex deficiency, Vincent's stomatitis, aphthous stomatitis, multiple small ulcers are seen over the tongue. The tongue may be covered with white patches in thrush. In leukoplakia, firmly adherent whitish opaque crusts are seen.

When the patient is asked to touch the palate with the tip of the tongue, its undersurface can be viewed. It demonstrates the *frenum lingue* and the opening of the submandibular duct on either side of its base. The sublingual veins are prominent in the elderly. The mucosa gives a yellowish tinge in patients with jaundice. Ulcers may be seen over the *frenum lingue* in patients with persistent coughing (whooping cough). There can be cystic swellings in the floor of the mouth: ranula or sublingual dermoid. Ranula develops due to an obstruction to the duct of a mucous gland and it is a bluish white translucent swelling of variable size. Sublingual dermoid gives a round opaque swelling beneath the mucosa.

The patient is asked to protrude the tongue fully to one side when the mouth is widely open, to look at its side and at its lateral undersurface for the presence of an ulcer. Benign ulcers (inflammatory or traumatic) are superficial. They are painful and do not show any induration. Carcinomatous ulcers are hard and indurated and the edges are everted and raised.

Neck

Inspection of the neck is done to note the general appearance, presence of any asymmetry, swellings, enlargement of the thyroid gland, lymph nodes, submandibular salivary glands, blood vessels, trachea, movements of the neck, muscles and superficial nerves. During inspection the patient must sit relaxed with hands resting on his thighs. The patient may be asked to keep the neck in a slight extension and this puts the sternomastoid muscles under tension. The inspection is carried out under adequate light by standing in front of the patient, then on turning the neck to the sides. The neck is palpated gently in the submandibular region, anterior and posterior triangles, suprasternal and supraclavicular regions. Swelling in the neck is generally felt from behind.

The neck is thin and long in asthenic individuals; short and thick in hypersthenic individuals. There may be webbing of the neck (Turner's syndrome, named after Henry Turner, a US endocrinologist). There may be an abnormal deviation of the neck with rotation of the head to one side (wry neck or torticollis). There may be oedema (anasarca, superior vena caval obstruction), deposition of fat in the supraclavicular region (Cushing's syndrome) or fullness (emphysema, myxoedema). The sterno-mastoid muscles may be seen active by elevating the upper part of the chest in conditions of respiratory distress. The larynx can be moved from side to side and it produces crepitus. A pharyngeal mass can displace it and reduce the sensation.

There may be rigidity with an inability to flex and turn the neck (meningitis, tetanus and disorders of cervical vertebrae). In conditions of arthritis affecting the cervical spine, the neck is fixed and there is an inability to move the head in any direction. The muscular spasm affecting the sternomastoid and trapezius is likely to pull the head to one side resulting in asymmetry of the neck. In meningitis, the neck is held in extension and appears arched in extreme cases.

Thyroid Gland

The thyroid gland consists of two lobes connected by an isthmus. It is attached to the thyroid cartilage and to the upper end of the trachea. The thyroid gland is not visualized normally. When it is enlarged (goitre), it presents in the form of a swelling or fullness in the midline of the neck, and it moves on deglutition.

The patient is asked to swallow sips of water or saliva keeping the neck in a slightly extended position. The base of the neck in the midline is watched for the movement. The lobes of the thyroid, are situated by the side of the thyroid cartilage, and upper tracheal cartilages. The isthmus connecting the lobes lies across the trachea just below the cricoid cartilage. Slight enlargement of the thyroid is often better seen than felt.

The gland may be felt standing either in front of or behind the patient. While standing behind the patient (Fig. 3) the tips of the index, middle and ring fingers of both hands are placed on either side of the trachea below the thyroid cartilage and the patient is asked to swallow. By gentle rotary movements of the fingers the consistency, surface and nodularity can be made out. A thrill may be felt in gross vascularity.

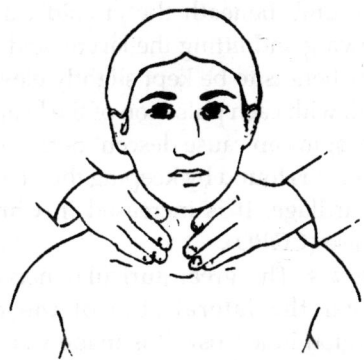

Fig. 3 Palpation of thyroid gland from behind.

The following manoeuvre is employed to feel the lobes: The neck is flexed towards the side of palpation. When the right lobe is palpated, the lobe is pushed forward by placing the fingers of the right hand behind the sternomastoid muscle, and the lobe is felt with the left hand. The palpation is facilitated, by asking the patient to swallow. A similar procedure is adopted while palpating the left lobe with the right hand. The lobe is pushed forward with the left hand. The thyroid gland may be felt as a firm mass with a smooth surface. The gland may show uniform enlargement (goitre, thyrotoxicosis) or the presence of nodules.

The lower pole of the lobe is not felt when the enlargement has extended into the thorax and its presence is made out, by percussion over the manubrium sterni which gives a retrosternal dullness. The gland should be auscultated for the presence of systolic bruit. It has to be distinguished from the transmitted cardiac murmur along the carotid artery.

Pulsations: The pulsations are visible at the base of the neck and may arise from the jugular veins and/or carotid artery. The carotid arterial pulsations may be so prominent as to be called throbbing or dancing carotids in aortic regurgitation (Corrigan's sign, described by Sir Dominic Corrigon, an Irish physician). Similar pulsations may be evident in hyperdynamic circulatory states. Cardiac arrhythmias, if present, are evident during the inspection of the carotid artery.

Tracheal tug: In aortic aneurysm, the pulsations may be transmitted to the trachea. It is appreciated by placing the forefinger and thumb beneath the cricoid cartilage, while the patient is swallowing and lifting the larynx and trachea upwards. The chin of the patient is to be kept slightly elevated. A tug is felt distinctly as a pull with each pulsation of the heart. The downward pull of the diaphragm can cause descent of the trachea and larynx during inspiration. It is found by keeping the tip of the index finger in the thyroid cartilage. It is increased in Chronic Obstructive Pulmonary Disease (COPD).

Superficial nerves: The great auricular nerve may stand out prominently over the lateral side of the neck across the sternomastoid region in leprosy. It is made visible by turning the head to the opposite side. The thickened nerve can be rolled under the fingers.

Lymph Nodes

The enlarged lymph nodes may be visible when the neck is inspected. Sometimes, the enlargement may be so gross, as to give rise to a distortion of the normal contour of the neck. While making the general examination, the lymph nodes in the three common sites are looked for routinely. Those sites are cervical, axillary and inguinal regions. When certain specific diseases are suspected, other sites are looked for i.e., supratrochlear glands in secondary syphilis, mesenteric lymph nodes in tuberculous lymphadenitis, or Virchow's (German pathologist) glands in the neck in carcinoma of the stomach or testis (Fig. 4).

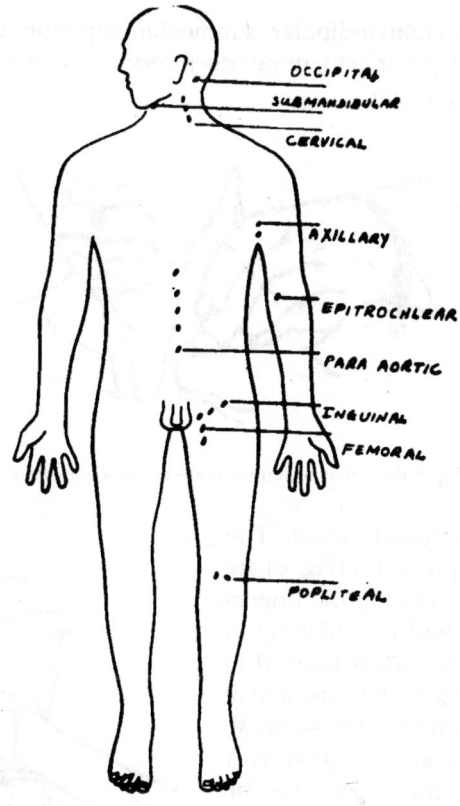

Fig. 4 The lymph nodes: common sites of palpation.

Inspection and palpation are the two methods applied in the examination of the lymph nodes.

Cervical lymph nodes: The cervical glands are palpated from behind while the patient is seated (Fig. 5). Both hands are placed on either side of the neck, and the nodes are felt by making slow rotary movement of the fingers. They are felt systematically and compared on either side. The nodes can be felt by standing in front of the patient also. One hand fixes the head and the nodes are felt with the other hand. To palpate the upper deep cervical nodes, the head is turned to the same side to relax cervical fascia and then the glands are felt underneath the sternomastoid, along the internal jugular vein. The cervical glands are felt in the following order from behind: occipital, posterior auricular, preauricular, submandibular, submental, superior cervical along the external jugular vein, upper deep cervical, lower deep cervical and supraclavicular.

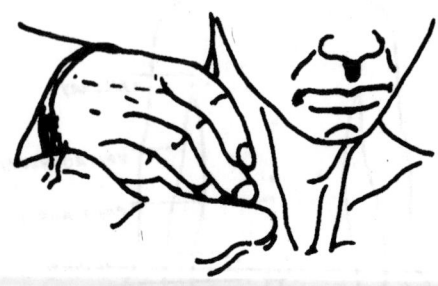

Fig. 5 Palpation of lymph node on scalenus anterior.

Axillary lymph nodes: The axillary lymph nodes (Fig. 6) are examined by placing the fingers against the chest wall high up in the axilla. The arm is allowed to hang by the side. The patient may be seated or supine. The pectoral, central, apical and posterior axillary glands are to be palpated.

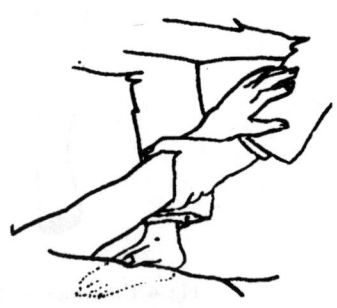

Fig 6. Palpation of axillary lymph nodes.

Inguinal lymph nodes: The inguinal lymph nodes in the groin are felt while the patient is recumbent. The glands are arranged in horizontal and vertical sets. They are felt on both the sides. The femoral glands are felt in the femoral triangle.

Normally the lymph nodes are not palpable in the adults. When they are enlarged the following points are to be noted: site, number, size, consistency (hard, firm or soft), tenderness, discrete or confluent, mobile or fixed over the underlying structures, the attachment to the overlying skin and fluctuation.

The enlargement of the lymph nodes may be localized or generalized. The lymphadenopathy may be due to infection (acute or chronic), hypersensitivity, reticuloses, lymphatic leukaemia or metastases from malignant diseases.

The inflammatory changes in the nodes result in their enlargement. They are soft and tender. There may be evidence of red streaks in the overlying skin indicating the presence of lymphangitis. The skin is red and hot. The primary site of infection has to be looked for in the territory of the lymphatic drainage. Sepsis may result in the formation of abscesses giving a fluctuation.

In tuberculosis, though a systemic disease, the glands are noted commonly in the cervical region, behind the sternomastoid. They are discrete in the early stages and soon become matted together due to periadenitis. They become fixed to the deeper tissue and overlying skin. Later they become fluctuant, following caseation burst, and form an ulcer which ultimately heals to result in a sinus, in some cases. Previous infection especially untreated may be diagnosed by the presence of pigmented fixed scars over the skin.

The primary stage of syphilis gives rise to a painless enlargement of the glands commonly in the inguinal region. They are discrete, firm and shotty, non-adherant to the skin and adjacent tissues. In secondary syphilis, the enlargement becomes generalized. The supratrochlear nodes are enlarged and are palpable in the region above the medial epicondyle when the elbow is semiflexed (Fig. 7). In filariasis the inguinal lymph nodes are frequently enlarged. In Lymphogranuloma venereum (LGV), the inguinal lymph nodes are enlarged and tender. They are adherent to the skin. They may show fluctuation and may break open leaving a draining sinus. Past infection may leave behind mild or symptomless enlargement of lymph nodes in the groin. HIV infection presents with generalized lymphadenopathy. HIV infection in the beginning presents as an unexplained lymphadenopathy.

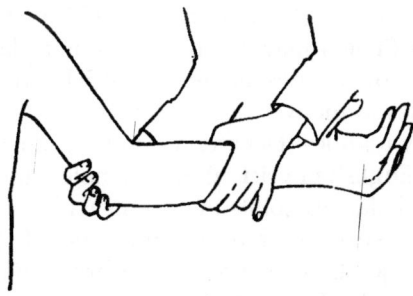

Fig. 7 Palpation of supratrochlear lymph nodes.

There will be a localized enlargement of the lymph nodes in metastatic carcinoma. The glands are stony hard with irregular margin, non-tender, and fixed to the deeper tissues and attached to the overlying skin. The primary is to be sought in the draining area. In lymphoma (commonly Hodgkin's disease), the glands are discrete, non-tender, firm with a rubbery feel, and fixed to the deeper structures in late stages. Rubbery enlargement of lymph nodes without tenderness may be noted in granulomatous conditions (tuberculosis, sarcoidosis), glandular fever and leukaemia. Para-aortic lymph nodes become palpable only in the presence of their marked enlargement, as in lymphoma.

Lymphatic leukaemia manifests with a generalized enlargement of the lymph nodes of various sizes (1-3 cm), non-tender, firm, discrete and freely mobile. In acute lymphatic leukaemia, the cervical lymph nodes are frequently involved. They show slight to moderate enlargement, and are tender.

Examination of the Hands

There may be developmental anomalies of the fingers and hand. The hand may be absent with only rudimentary fingers. There may be absence of fingers, or the fingers may appear as short stumps. There may be supernumerary fingers or thumb (polydactyly) or fusion of the fingers (syndactyly). The fingers appear long, thin and tapering (arachnodactyly) in hypogonadism, Marfan's syndrome and hyperthyroidism. In the broad hands of acromegaly or hypothyroidism the fingers may appear thick, spade-like with a square tip.

There may be evidence of trophic changes in the form of ulcers, and/or loss of the tips (leprosy, syringomyelia or following injury). In Raynaud's disease, thromboangiitis obliterans and arterial embolism, the fingers may be shrivelled and black (gangrene). The existence of scabies is recognised by the presence of vesiculopustules in the webs of the fingers.

Small bony nodules (Heberden's nodes, named after William Heberden, an English physician) may be noted at the bases of the terminal interphalangeal joints in patients with osteoarthritis. The fingers show spindle-shaped swelling of the proximal interphalangeal joints in rheumatoid arthritis and there may be ulnar deviation of the fingers from the metacarpophalangeal joints in long standing cases. Small tender transitory nodular swellings

(Osler's nodes, described by Sir William Osler, Canadian-born physician who worked in Canada, US and UK) and hypothenar eminences in subacute infective endocarditis.

The hands may assume various shapes. Radial, ulnar and median nerve paralysis produce wrist drop, claw hand and ape hand deformities respectively.

Wrist drop: There is flexion of the wrist with an inability to extend.

Claw hand: There is hyperextension of the metacarpophalangeal joints with excessive flexion of the interphalangeal joins especially of the ring and little fingers.

Ape hand: The thumbs remain in the same plane as other fingers.

The other shapes, the hand can assume are;

Carpopedal spasm: The fingers are adducted together covering the flexed and adducted thumb. The fingers appear rigid and terminal phalanges are hyperextended and wrist flexed. Such an obstetric position of the hand is seen in tetany. A sphygmomanometer cuff may be applied around the arm and inflated above diastolic blood pressure for three minutes to induce such a spasm (Trousseau's sign, described by Armand Trousseau, a French physician)

Trident hand: In achondroplasia, all the fingers are of similar size and diverge from one another.

Cretinism: Cretins exhibit a square palm with short fingers.

Duputren's contracture: The fibrous thickening of palmar fascia results in the flexion contracture of the fingers on the palm especially of the ring and little fingers. The condition is inherited and may be noted in alcoholic cirrhosis of the liver. It was described by Baron Gillotime Duputren, a French surgeon. Injuries in the region of the elbow or a very tight dressing at that region, may result in the flexion of the writs and fingers (Volkmann's contracture, named after Richard von Volkmann, a German surgeon). The small muscles of the hand may show wasting to a variable degree and give a flattened appearance to the hand.

The palms appear pale in anaemia, white in Raynaud's disease, red and warm in cirrhosis of the liver. In thyrotoxicosis the hands are warm and moist. The hands become cold in peripheral circulatory failure, Raynaud's disease, neurocirculatory asthenia, myxoedema and chronic wasting diseases. In fever, the hands are warm and dry.

The skin over the dorsum of the hands becomes rough with pigmentation and cracks (pellegra). The skin appears taut and shiny in systemic sclerosis, and the finger tips are tapered. The fingers may have a nicotine stain in heavy smokers.

Nail

A nail consists of the nail plate, nail folds (proximal and lateral), matrix (lunula) and nail bed. There can be detachment of the nail bed from the nail plate (onycholysis) and it is seen in dermatophytic infections, psoriasis, trauma, contact dermatitis and tetracycline intake followed by exposure to sun. Inflammation of the nail folds is referred to as paronychia, and it occurs from bacterial and candidial infections. A nail is examined for thickening, thinning, pitting, clubbing and discolouration. The nails may exhibit transverse, or longitudinal ridges, or furrows in infective diseases. Nail growth may be temporarily arrested in severe illness and a transverse ridge appears when they start their growth (Beau's lines, named after Joseph Beau, a French physician). They may become lusterless and friable with heaped scales in taenia unguiium. The nails may be deformed, pitted and yellow in colour in psoriasis, mechanical trauma and eczema. A nail may be destroyed in severe lichen planus or epidermolysis bullosa. Some nails may be absent in genetic nail-patella syndrome. The nails may become white or demonstrate clubbing or assume a spoon shape. There will be bluish discolouration of the finger-tips in cyanosis. Small linear haemorrhages are noted beneath the nails in trauma, psoriasis, trichinosis and rheumatoid arthritis and subacute infective endocarditis (splinter haemorrhages).

There is abnormal whiteness of the nails in chronic liver cell failure. In hypoalbuminaemia, the nails may show double white horizontal bands, parallel to the lunule. Transverse white lines may be noticed in the nails after ingestion of arsenic, thallium, fluoride and in severe systemic disorders such as myocardial infarction, acute and chronic renal failure and in patients receiving chemotherapy for malignancy with multiple drugs such as methotrexate, doxarubicin, cyclophosphamide, vincristine, bleomycin and prednisolone.

Yellow nails may develop from diffuse yellowish discolouration of the nail plates (yellow-nail syndrome) and it is seen in lymphatic obstruction associated with pleural effusion. The nails appear yellow in heavy smokers and individuals working with photographer's colour developing solutions.

Clubbed digits: Hippocratic (named after Hippocrates, Father of Medicine, who lived in Island of Cos during 460–375 B.C.) nails. They refer to a bulbous enlargement of the terminal phalanges of the digits especially on the dorsal surface by an overgrowth of fibroelastic tissue in the nail bed. It is noted in the fingers as well as toes. Generally it is bilateral. Occasionally it can be unilateral, and even unidigital.

A variety of subacute or chronic diseases affecting the respiratory, cardiovascular, hepatic and alimentary systems may be associated with clubbing. About 80 per cent of acquired clubbing is related to intrathoracic disorders. The condition can exist in an idiopathic or hereditary form. The latter condition develops during childhood in the absence of any associated disease state. Rarely clubbing may be limited to the toes only in association with patent ductus arteriosus (PDA) with reversal of blood flow and in infected abdominal aortic prosthesis.

In the early stages of clubbing, there is an increase in the thickness of the connective tissue in the nail bed (normal 2 to 4 mm) due to an interstitial oedema and cellular infiltration. Later it is replaced by collagen fibres. Minimal clubbing is recognised by applying gentle pressure to the proximal nail just beyond the cuticle (Fig. 8). It gives an impression as if the nail is floating on a spongy pad

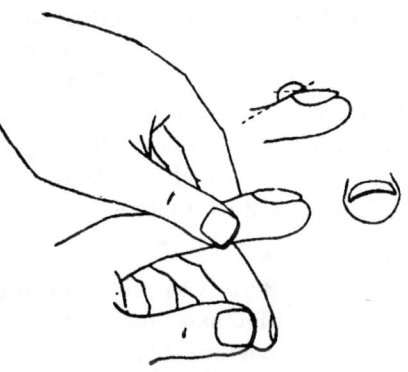

Fig. 8 Clubbed digit-method of examination.

(soft clubbing). Mild clubbing is associated with obliteration of the normal angle between the base of the nail and the proximal skin. It can even be recognised by bringing the dorsal surfaces of the terminal phalanges of the middle fingers against each other. There is disappearance of a diamond-shaped window that is normally seen in the presence of mild enlargement of the soft tissue at the base of finger nails (Schamroth's sign, after a South African Physician).

In marked clubbing, the connective tissue changes extend throughout the digits bringing about alteration in the shape of the finger-tips. The underlying bone is normal. The enlargement is uniform with an increase in the curvature of the nail in its longitudinal and transverse axes (hard clubbing, watch glass type). It may be restricted to the proximal portion (parrot's beak) or to the mid-portion (drum-stick type) of the distal phalanx. These differences in the types of clubbing have no clinical significance. The nails become shiny. Clubbing is recognised by looking at the digits from the side (profile sign).

The clubbing is assessed objectively either by measurement of the hyponychial angle between the nail and the proximal skin or the interphalangeal depth ratio by viewing the index finger from the side against a dark background.

The hyponychial angle is formed by joining a point of the distal finger crease and a point on the thickened skin underlying the free edge of the nail (hyponychia) to a point at the cuticle and normally it is 180° or less. The angle is increased in clubbing as the enlargement of the soft tissue at the base of the nail tends to lift the cuticle away from the underlying bone. It increases the angle and the depth of the finger tip (phalangeal depth ratio). It is assessed by measuring the depth of the distal phalanx (DPD) at the cuticle in relation to the depth at the distal interphalangeal joint (IPD). Normally the ratio of DPD to IPD is less than 1.0 and it is increased in clubbing.

Bilateral
1) *Respiratory:* Chronic suppurative diseases—lung abscess, bronchiectasis, cystic fibrosis, and empyema thoracis, bronchogenic carcinoma, chronic mesothelioma of the pleura, chronic fibrocaseous tuberculosis, idiopathic interstitial pulmonary fibrosis.
2) *Cardiovascular:* Congenital cyanotic heart disease, subacute infective endocarditis, aortic aneurysm, PDA, AV malformations.
3) *Liver and gastrointestinal:* Cirrhosis of the liver, chronic diarrhoea, ulcerative colitis, Crohn's (named after Burill Crohn, a US physician) disease, iliitis (malabsorption syndrome), polyposis of the colon, gastrointestinal neoplasms.
4) *Miscellaneous:* Polycythaemia, chronic pyelonephritis, thyrotoxicosis with pretibial myxoedema, hypervitaminosis A,

syringomyelia, old hemiplegia, toxic exposure to vinyl chloride, arsenic, mercury and phosphorous.

5) *Hereditary:* Variable clubbing in different digits, which appears during puberty and does not disappear.

6) *Idiopathic:* Associated with thickening of the skin and excessive sweating over the face.

Unilateral

Aneurysm of the arch of the aorta and its branches, casualgia, arteriovenous fistula, apical lung lesions (tumours and fibrosis), old hemiplegia.

Unidigital

Following injury to the finger or its nerve supply.

The clubbed digits may be associated with periosteal new bone formation particularly of the long bones of the distal extremities (radius, ulna, tibia and fibula). There is symmetric arthritis commonly of the ankles, knees, wrists, and elbows, increased thickness of the soft tissues in the distal third of the forearms and legs and signs of autonomic disturbances in the hands and feet such as flushing, blanching, parasthesias, and profuse sweating. The condition is referred to as hypertrophic osteoarthropathy (Marie-Bamberger's disease, named after Pierre Marie, a French physician and Eugene Bamberger, an Austrian physician). It is encountered in the malignancy of the lung and mesothelioma of the pleura.

Koilonychia (spooning of the nails): Iron deficiency anaemia leads to a malnutrition of matrices of the nail plates. The nails become thin, flat and brittle. There is loss of normal luster and the nails become pale. They become concave, hollow in the center with the nails edges being raised in the periphery. Rarely the condition may be congenital or may occur after trauma to the fingers. Occasionally, koilonychia may be associated with Plummer-Vinson syndrome (named after Henry Plummer, a US physician, and Porter Vinson, a US surgeon), haemoglobinopathies, polycythaemia, post-gastrectomy state, haemochromatosis, acromegaly, hypothyroidism, hyperthyroidism, coronary artery disease and lichen planus.

Male Genitalia

The methods of inspection and palpation are employed while examining the male genitalia. It is a good practice to examine the genitalia, inguinal regions, perineum and rectum together as they can be examined in one exposure of the region.

The following structures of the male genitalia are examined: penis, scrotum, and prostate. The prostate is examined while making an examination per rectum (*see* page 98).

Penis: The size of the penis and presence of ulcers over the penis are looked for. The external genitalia is infantile until puberty. The genitalia may remain extremely small in hypopituitarism, hypothyroidism, and enuchoidism. In precocious puberty, the penis is large for the age of the individual. After puberty there is growth of pubic hair and it extends up in a triangular fashion towards the umbilicus. The hairs become sparse in old age, and in cirrhosis of the liver. The penis and scrotum may appear oedematous in ascites. Their size may be increased in elephantiasis affecting the region. The collection of fluid in the tunica vaginalis of the testis results in hydrocoele. The swelling shows a fluctuation. It is non-tender and its upper limit can be made out. Unlike inguinal hernia it does not exhibit any expansile impulse.

Normally the prepuce (foreskin) of the penis can be retracted over the glans penis. It facilitates examination of inner lining of the prepuce, the glans penis, the coronal sulcus and the external urethral orifice (meatus). The prepuce should be brought forward after examination. It prevents occurrence of paraphimosis (painful oedema of glans). The glans is exposed in an uncircumcised individual. It is not possible to retract the prepuce in phimosis and there is narrowing of the preputial orifice. Normally the external urethral orifice opens at the tip of the glans. There may be deficiency of the ventral (hypospadias) or dorsal (epispadias) wall over the urethra resulting in the opening of the external urethral orifice in the midline of the ventral or dorsal surface of the penis respectively. In gonococcal urethritis, there may be a purulent discharge from the meatus.

The presence of ulcers in the region of coronal sulcus, inner surface of prepuce, or glans are to be looked for (primary syphilis, cancer penis, LGV, chancroid). A single painless small ulcer with densely indurated margins and base, occurs in syphilis. In cancer, the growth may be cauliflower-like or it may appear as an indurated ulcer. In LGV, the ulcers are multiple and are also found in the region of the groin, perineum and the anus. There will be multiple punched out ulcers in chancroid.

Scrotum: Scrotal skin should be inspected for any redness, swelling or ulcer. There may be burrows and excoriated papules of scabies. The contents of the scrotum are palpated gently between the thumb and fingers of both hands. The testis is freely mobile in the scrotum. It is a firm, ovoid structure and gives an unpleasant sensation to the individual when felt. The epididymis is a soft nodular structure and lies above and behind the testis.

The testis should be looked for in the inguinal region or in the groin, if it is not felt in the scrotum (undescended or retractile testis). There may be evidence of hermaphroditism with the presence of testis and female external genitalia. The testis is swollen and tender in epididymo-orchitis. In cancer, testis becomes heavy and painless. The testicular sensation is lost early. The testicular sensation is lost in tabes. The testis becomes atrophied in old age, following trauma, leprosy, cirrhosis of the liver, following radiation and sometimes following herniorraphy, mumps, orchitis, anterior pituitary deficiency and Klinefelter's syndrome. Multiple round firm, nodular swellings may be noted over the scrotum (Sabaceous cysts).

In tuberculosis and filarial funiculitis, the epididymis is moderately enlarged and craggy and spermatic cord becomes thickened. The scrotum should be examined while the patient is standing for presence of varicocele.

Examination of Legs and Feet

The shape, deformities and swelling of the legs and feet are to be examined carefully. The lateral popliteal nerve is felt in the lateral side of the popliteal fossa for thickening (leprosy). The disorders affecting the bones like rickets, osteomalacia, osteitis deformans, achondroplasia and osteogenesis imperfecta can result in genu valgum or genu varum deformities. In genu varum, there is outward bowing of the legs with separation of the knees widely (bow legs). In genu valgum (knock knee), the knees are close as the femur is directed medial-wards more than normal and the feet are placed separately.

There may be absence of toes (congenital or as a result of injury, leprosy, amputation), fusion of toes or supernumerary toes. There may be evidence of localized hypertrophy of the toes. In acromegaly the bones of the feet show marked enlargement with hypertrophy of the skin and subcutaneous tissue. The longitudinal arch of the foot may be lost resulting in flat foot (*pes planus*), or exaggerated as in claw foot (*pes cavus*). The big toe is turned outwards at metatarsophalangeal joints in *hallux valgus*. Talipes equinovarus (club foot) is a common congenital deformity with the soles of the feet turned inwards. The patient walks on the lateral side of the feet. A variant of this deformity may result in the patient walking on his toes or heels.

The presence of oedema, clubbing of the toes, pulsations of arteries (dorsalis pedis and posterior tibial), thickened nerves (lateral popliteal), gangrene of the toes or of the foot, ulcers and swellings have to be looked at carefully. The trophic ulcers are noted on the foot. Small tender subcutaneous swellings are noted on the front of the legs bilaterally in erythema nodosum. Bulbous swelling and ulcer may appear around the ankle and foot as a result of guinea worm infestation.

Venous Disorders

The veins may undergo dilatation and tortuosity (varicose veins), they may become inflamed (phlebitis) and show evidence of thrombosis. These conditions may coexist or develop one upon the other. Due to gravity, the legs are affected more often than the arms.

Varicose Veins

The superficial veins of the lower extremity may become prominent, tortuous and dilated. They are referred to as varicose veins. They are made prominent by asking the patient to stand. It affects the saphanous venous system. The greater saphanous vein lies on the anteromedial aspect of the thigh and leg. The lesser saphanous vein lies on the posterolateral aspect of the calf. There may be pigmentation, oedema, or ulceration in the region of medial malleolus in long standing venous stasis.

Trendelenburg's (described by Friedrich Trendelenburg, a German surgeon) test helps in assessing the efficiency of the valves in the long saphanous vein. The vein must be emptied, by raising the leg when the patient is supine. Pressure should be applied on the saphanous opening so as to occlude the upper end of the vein. Then the patient has to stand while the pressure is maintained on the vein. In the presence of incompetent valves the vein fills from above, the moment pressure is released.

Thrombophlebitis

The leg veins may exhibit thrombosis and the veins involved may be superficial or deep. The condition may develop suddenly with inflammatory signs (thrombophlebitis), or gradually and may remain silent (phlebothrombosis). The condition has to be noted with care in patients who are bedridden for a long time, in patients after pelvic or abdominal operations, after childbirth, and in patients with congestive heart failure, carcinoma of the pancreas and bronchogenic carcinoma. Venous thrombosis is also noted in women taking oral contraceptives.

In superficial thrombophlebitis, there will be redness, warmth, swelling and tenderness near the affected veins. The vein feels cord-like on palpation. The superficial veins appear distended and do not collapse when the leg is extended. Deep vein thrombosis may show the presence of tenderness in the region of calf on pressure. On sharp dorsiflexion of the foot with slightly flexed knees, there will be marked tenderness in the calf muscles (Homan's sign, described by John Homan, a US surgeon). The procedure is not recommended as there is a chance for the clot to get dislodged.

Documentation

The physical signs are to be documented under general examination and systemic examination in a systematic manner. The record should reflect what one has observed and not the inference drawn from it. Diagrams should be used to illustrate abnormal physical signs.

FIVE

ABDOMEN

> *"If the physician is to understand the correct meaning of health,*
> *he must know that there are more than a hundred, indeed more*
> *than a thousand, kinds of stomach; consequently, if you gather*
> *a thousand persons, each of them will have a different kind of*
> *digestion, each unlike the other"*
>
> Paracelsus (1493-1541)

The front and the back of the abdomen are examined by using the methods of inspection, palpation, percussion and auscultation.

Divisions of abdomen: The abdomen is divided into nine quadrants by two horizontal and two vertical imaginary lines (Fig. 9). The upper horizontal line is drawn across the abdomen at the lowest point of the tenth costal arch (subcostal line), and the lower horizontal line at the level of anterior spine of the iliac bones (interspinous line). The two vertical lines drawn on either side as extension of the midclavicular line to the middle of the inguinal ligament, roughly lie at the level of the lateral border of the *rectus abdominis* muscle.

The nine quadrants are the right and left hypochondriac, lumbar and iliac regions on either side and the epigastric, umbilical and hypogastric regions in the centre from above downwards (Fig. 9). The important viscera underlying these regions are as follows:

Right hypochondrium: Right lobe of the liver, gall bladder, hepatic flexure of the colon, part of the duodenum, part of the right kidney and the suprarenal gland.

Epigastrium: Pyloric end of the stomach, duodenum, part of the liver, pancreas and aorta.

Left hypochondrium: Stomach, spleen, splenic flexure of the colon, tail of the pancreas, upper pole of the left kidney, and the suprarenal gland.

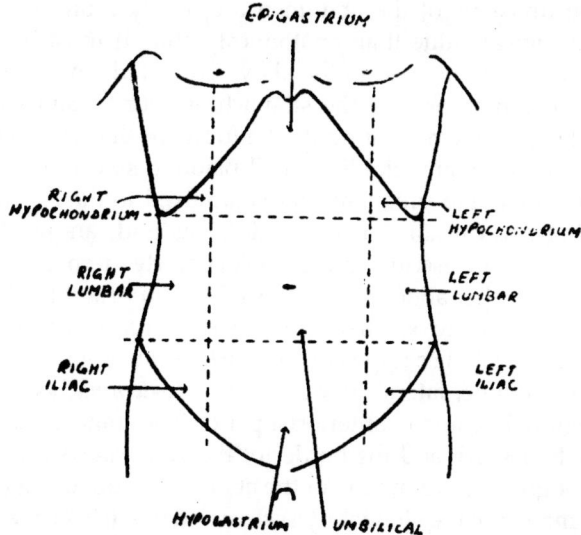

Fig. 9 Abdominal quadrants.

Right lumbar: Ascending colon, lower half of the kidney, part of the duodenum and jejunum.

Umbilical: Transverse colon, lower part of the duodenum, jejunum and ileum, mesentery, omentum and aorta.

Left lumbar: Descending colon, lower half of the left kidney, part of the jejunum and the ileum.

Right iliac (inguinal): Caecum, appendix, lower end of the ileum, right ureter, right ovary in the female, and right spermatic cord in male.

Hypogastric (suprapubic): Urinary bladder, ileum, and pregnant uterus.

Left iliac: Sigmoid colon, left ureter, left ovary in female, and left spermatic cord in male.

The anterior surface of the abdomen can also be subdivided into four quadrants by drawing a perpendicular line from the tip of the xiphisternum to the symphysis pubis through the umbilicus and a horizontal line crossing at the umbilicus. The quadrants are referred to as right upper, right lower, left upper and left lower quadrants. Epigastrium is composed of the medial halves of the right and left upper quadrants.

These divisions of the abdomen are purely arbitrary and it has more clinical value than anatomical value. It must be noted that the viscera mentioned in the above are not always correct as some of the structures like the stomach, intestines, and kidneys are mobile and may not constantly be found in the same regions. However some organs like liver, gall bladder, spleen, distended urinary bladder, and pregnant uterus are fixed to the regions.

Land marks: Certain anatomic divisions and landmarks are frequently used to describe the location of pain, tenderness, rigidity, swellings and other abnormal findings. The important landmarks in the abdomen are xiphisternum, costal margin, umbilicus (variable, generally lies opposite the fourth lumbar vertebra), *linea alba* in the midline, lateral border of *rectus abdominis*, symphysis pubis, inguinal ligament, anterior superior iliac spine, renal angle between the last rib and the border of the *sacrospinalis* muscle.

Although the examination of the abdomen is done as a part of the examination of the alimentary system and of the liver, it enables the examination of other important structures of the haemopoietic system (spleen), genitourinary system (kidney, urinary bladder, uterus, ovary and testes) concurrently. The examination of the abdomen includes the examination of the various systems.

Inspection

The abdomen is inspected in good light while the patient is lying flat on his back with the arms loosely by the sides, and the head resting on a pillow. The abdomen is uncovered from the costal margin to the pubic symphysis. The patient should be encouraged to relax and breath quietly through the mouth. Often a small talk or restatement of history aids in relaxing the patient. The examiner should sit at the right side of the patient with his head only slightly above the abdomen and look for the presence of visible peristalsis, pulsations, or any swellings. The presence of hernia and engorged veins are recognized better when the patient stands erect.

Attitude

A patient writhing in bed and unable to find a comfortable position may he having intestinal obstruction. A patient lying with lower extremities flexed and avoiding any motion may be having peritonitis.

Contour of the Abdomen

Normally the abdomen is bilaterally symmetrical and the contour may be flat, round, or scaphoid. In a flat abdomen, the anterior abdominal wall extends in a horizontal plane from the level of the costal margins and the pubic symphysis. It is normally seen in well-nourished individuals and in athletes. A round abdomen refers to the generalized distension showing a convexity to the horizontal plane. It is seen in younger children and in adults from excess deposition of fat in the subcutaneous tissue, or from lack of activity and muscle tone. The convexity is marked at the level of umbilicus in recumbent position and it moves downwards by gravity to the infraumbilical region in erect position. In scaphoid (sunken) abdomen the anterior abdominal wall is hollowed in, and presents a concavity to the horizontal plane when looked at from the sides. It is seen in thin individuals of all ages, and in individuals suffering from dehydration, malnutrition, advanced stages of starvation and malignant diseases, particularly carcinoma of the stomach or oesophagus.

Distension: The abdomen may show generalized distension in conditions such as obesity (fat), ascites (free fluid in the peritoneal cavity), tympanitis (gas in gastrointestinal tract), pregnancy (foetus), fecal impaction, and massive cysts (e.g. ovarian cyst, pancreatic cyst). These conditions are often described as six f's, "fat, fluid, flatus, foetus, faeces and fatal growth". In ascites, there is uniform distension of abdomen with bulging flanks. In tympanitis, the flanks are not bulged. The distension in the lower half of the abdomen may be due to pregnancy, distended bladder, uterine, or ovarian tumours. The upper half of the abdomen may show distension from tympanitis, pancreatic cyst or carcinomatosis. In obesity, the abdomen is protruded forwards uniformly. The skin folds are exaggerated and the fat deposit can be lifted with the skin.

A localized asymmetrical bulge may occur from enlargement of the organs, such as the liver and the spleen, in their respective quadrants. The liver and the spleen move with respiration, due to their connection with the diaphragm. The distended stomach, obstruction of the small and large bowels, and distended urinary bladder result in localized, often symmetrical prominence of the abdomen in the epigastrium, umbilical region, flanks and hypogastrium respectively. Kidney swellings may appear either in the lumbar region or in the back. Sometimes, the abnormality of the spinal curvature may be responsible for asymmetry of the abdominal contour. Extreme lordosis may give a false impression of distended abdomen.

The recti muscles may get separated in the midline (divarication of the recti) due to the weakness of the muscles. When such a patient in a recumbent posture tries to raise his head from the pillow, a part of the abdominal contents protrudes forward between the recti. This is evident in ascites and in women who have borne children. A bulge containing pieces of extra-peritoneal fat or omentum may appear in the epigastric region as ventral (epigastric) hernia.

Skin

The skin is observed for the presence of scars, striae, rashes, veins, oedema and pigmentation.

Scars: There may be scars over the abdominal wall due to the previous operations, trauma, burns, or branding. The operative scars may be noted in the upper and lower midline, the right paramedian region, the right subcostal region, in the inguinal regions and the suprapubic region. Traditional surgical scars indicate the likely type of surgery. The site may be weak and result in hernia (incisional). When there are scars due to minimal access laparoscopic surgery, enquiry should be made on the type of surgery undertaken.

The branding marks of different sizes and shapes may give a clue to the probable site of the lesion. Sometimes, there is a dense deposition of fibrous tissue at the site of the scars to result in keloids.

Striae: The inspection of the lower abdomen may demonstrate striae (vertical, often wrinkled streaks) due to prolonged stretching of the skin, with rupture of the elastic fibres in the reticular layer of the skin. They indicate a recent change in the size of the abdomen and are frequently the result of repeated pregnancies, or loss of weight in a previous ascites, or obesity, wasting diseases and severe dieting. The striae are pink when recent, and white when old (*striae atrophicae* or *gravidarum*). White purple striae are noted in Cushing's syndrome and on prolonged corticosteroid therapy.

Pigmentation: The skin appears smooth, stretched and shiny in a distended abdomen from any cause. It becomes lax and wrinkled in cachexia, after childbirth, and after removal of fluid from the peritoneal cavity. Dark pigmentation is seen in the midline below the umbilicus as a sign of pregnancy (*linea nigra*). There may be pigmentation in the region of the belt area as a result of tying a *dhoti* or *saree* tightly around the abdomen. Repeated application of heat with a hot water bottle, heat pad or earthen pot (*kangri*) may result in brown mottled pigmentation (Erythema *ab igne*). Rarely multiple small hard nodules may be seen in the skin from haematogenous metastasis. Haemorrhagic pancreatitis may be associated with discolouration of flanks (Turner's sign, named after a British surgeon Gilbert Gray Turner) due to ecchymosis. Similarly there can be periumbilical discolouration which was initially described in ectopic pregnancy (Cullen's sign, named after Thomas Cullen, an American surgeon). Ecchymosis may be noted in splenic rupture, rectus sheath haematoma, perforated duodenal ulcer, ruptured abdominal aortic aneurysm, ischaemic bowel disease and following liver biopsy.

Hair: The distribution of hair should be noted. Normally in women the pubic hair is roughly triangular with the base above the symphysis whereas in men it is diamond shaped, often extending up to the umbilicus. Chronic liver diseases and endocrine abnormalities alter the distribution and quantity of hair.

Movements of the Abdominal Wall

The abdominal wall moves freely with respiration. During inspiration, the abdominal wall becomes prominent due to downward movement of the diaphragm and is indrawn during expiration. It is equal on both sides. The movement is more obvious in men (abdominothoracic respiration) than in women (thoracoabdominal or costal respiration). An underlying inflammation of the viscera, or of the peritoneum, or swelling causes restriction of the movement with respiration. The movements are less prominent in ascites and in pregnancy. In generalized peritonitis the movement is markedly diminished or absent ('still abdomen'). Spasmodic movements of the abdominal wall are evident during hiccoughs.

The normal excursion of the abdominal wall becomes reversed in diaphragmatic paralysis. This is evident in unilateral phrenic nerve paralysis as a *see-saw* movement. The free movement of the right cupola of the diaphragm, appears like a wave in the lower part of the right thorax when viewed tangentially in daylight (Litten's sign).

Umbilicus

The umbilicus is situated in the centre of the abdomen and appears slightly indrawn. The umbilicus is displaced downwards in ascites, and pushed upwards in gravid uterus and in tumours of the ovary and the uterus. In ascites, umbilicus is stretched transversly and gets everted, due to increased intra-abdominal tension. It may be the seat of a hernia. Umbilical hernia is confirmed by the presence of an expansile impulse on coughing. In obesity or in gaseous distension, the umbilicus is depressed. There is longitudinal stretching of the umbilicus in ovarian cyst. A major intraperitoneal haemorrhage may cause a bluish discolouration of the umbilicus. There can be periumbilical discolouration from ecchymosis. Hard cutaneous or subcutaneous nodules may be found in umbilical region from metastatic carcinoma arising from stomach, colon, pancreas or ovary (sister Mary Joseph's nodule, named after an Americun nun and medical worker). There can be an accumulation of inspissated desquamated epithelium and other debris in elderly obese individuals (*omphalolith*).

Veins

Normally the veins in the abdominal wall are not visible. Small thin veins may be noted over the subcostal margins. The veins stand out clearly when engorged. The presence of distended veins over the abdominal wall indicates obstruction to the flow of the blood through the portal vein or inferior vena cava. The obstruction is likely to be great if there is greater distension and more numerous veins. In obstruction to the portal vein (portal hypertension), veins are visible in the epigastrium and very rarely they appear as tortuous, dilated veins radiating from the umbilicus (*caput medusae*). Collateral veins appear in the flanks in the obstruction in the inferior vena cava or common iliac veins.

The direction of the flow of the blood in the superficial veins is determined in the following manner: A vein without any tributaries in its vicinity, is selected. The examiner applies both index fingers firmly on the vein. Then the lower finger (right) is drawn away a few centimeters, thus emptying the blood by 'milking' it from the intervening segment of the vein. While maintaining the same pressure with the upper finger (left), the lower finger is lifted. The vein remains empty if the blood flow is

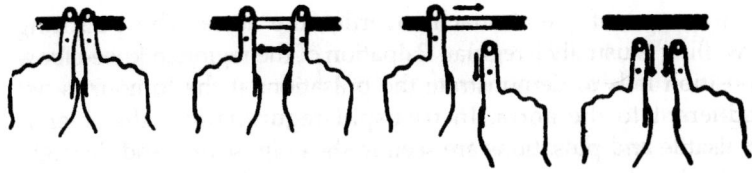

Fig. 10 Direction of blood flow in the superficial veins.

not in that direction. Then the lower finger is kept at the lower site and the upper finger is removed. The blood appears to flow down from above if the blood flow is in that direction (Fig. 10).

Normally the blood flow in the veins is away from the umbilicus, i.e., the upper abdominal veins carry blood upwards to the superior vena cava and the lower abdominal veins drain downwards to the inferior vena cava. The blood flow continues to be normal in all directions, away from the umbilicus in portal obstruction. The obstruction of the vena cava alters the flow direction in these veins. The veins fill from below upwards in the inferior vena cava, and above downwards in the superior vena cava. The blood flow is reversed in the veins below the umbilicus in the inferior vena caval obstruction, and in the superior vena caval obstruction the blood flow is reversed above the umbilicus. Inferior vena caval obstruction leads to oedema of the limbs.

Distended Veins in the Abdominal Wall.

Abnormality	Portal vein obstruction	IVC obstruction
Prominent veins	epigastrium	flanks
Direction of flow of blood	away from umbilicus	above downwards below umbilicus
oedema of lower limb	may be present	present

Pulsations in the Epigastrium

The aortic pulsations may be visible in the epigastric region in thin-built, nervous individuals. It is due to transmission of aortic pulsations through the abdominal wall. Vigorous pulsations may be noted in aortic regurgitation, thyrotoxicosis, anaemia, neurocirculatory asthenia, and right ventricular hypertrophy. Expansile pulsations are evident in aneurysm of the abdominal aorta, and the widened aorta can be felt. The pulsations may be transmitted to the anterior abdominal wall when a tumour (carcinoma of the stomach) overlies the aorta. The pulsating swelling is usually irregular. Palpation of the region in knee-elbow position fails to demonstrate the pulsations if the tumour is not adherent to the aorta. In tricuspid regurgitation, the liver is pulsatile and pulsations are seen in the epigastrium and the right hypochondrium.

Peristalsis

Normally the peristaltic waves are not seen, except in those with a thin abdominal wall, or in those with cachexia. Generally visible peristalsis is considered an important evidence of obstruction to the stomach or bowel. The examiner must sit bringing the eyes to the level of the abdominal profile and spend a few minutes watching the abdomen.

In pyloric obstruction, there may be fullness in the left side of the upper abdomen from a distended stomach and peristalsis may be visible. Peristalsis can be augmented by giving the patient water to drink or by gentle kneeding of the abdomen. The peristaltic waves begin as raised areas in the wall in the left hypochondrium, and gradually move across the upper abdomen to the right hypochondrium. Sometimes, in gross dilatation of the stomach the wave passes down the hypogastrium and then ascends towards the right side of the epigastrium. Long standing obstruction with severe distension of the stomach may produce a splashing sound on shaking the abdomen (succussion splash). In obstruction at the ileocaecal valve, or tuberculous stricture of terminal ileum, the peristaltic waves appear prominently around the umbilicus, and the distended coils of the small intestine are seen lying parallel, one above the other giving a 'ladder' pattern down the centre of the abdomen. Peristaltic waves are noted in the peripheral part of the abdomen in obstruction in the large intestine and the peristaltic waves move from right to left in the upper abdomen. Intestinal peristalsis may be noted in elderly women with a lax abdominal wall. However there is no organic disease.

Back

The back of the abdomen, is formed by the posterior wall of the abdomen and the spine. It is inspected while the patient is in a sitting position. Normally the contours of both sides are symmetrical in the absence of any disease, or developmental defects. The usual concave curvature may be full due to a swelling of the kidney (hydronephrosis, polycystic kidney, infection of the perirenal tissue, tumours of the kidney or cold abscess). Aneurysm of the abdominal aorta may cause fullness and pulsations in the left side.

Spider naevi: Cutaneous angiomas that blanch on pressure over the central arteriole that feeds the clump of dilated blood vessels are to be looked for in the upper extremities, face, neck, chest and upper abdomen. They are noted in cirrhosis of the liver, infective hepatitis, rheumatoid arthritis and pregnancy.

Other Sites

The groins and scrotum in a male are to be inspected for the presence of herniae and swellings. The position of both testes has to be determined.

Palpation

Palpation of the abdomen is carried out to confirm the findings of the inspection, to detect and evaluate tenderness, muscle guarding and resistance, to feel the individual organs, and to note the presence of abnormal swellings or fluid.

Procedure: While palpating the abdomen, the examiner should stand or sit on the right side of the patient who is lying flat on his back with the head slightly raised and arms to the sides. However the palpation is carried out better by sitting beside the patient. The patient is asked to turn his face to one side and breath slowly and deeply, keeping the mouth open to facilitate the abdominal type of respiration. The knees must be drawn upwards to obtain adequate relaxation of the abdominal muscles. Sometimes it is desirable to divert the attention of the patient by engaging him in a conversation.

Palpation is carried out in 4 steps:
1. superficial palpation
2. deep palpation
3. dipping
4. ballotment

Superficial Palpation: The hand should be warmed by rubbing it with the other, and is placed flat on the surface of the abdomen and not at right angles. The wrist and forearm remain in the same horizontal plane. The fingers should be slightly flexed at the metacarpophalangeal joints and approximated. It enables the palmar aspect of the fingers to mould itself to the abdominal wall and participate in the palpation. The palpation is not done with the tips of the fingers but with the movements at the metacarpophalangeal joints. The hand is moved over various quadrants of the abdomen in a systematic manner, by gently pressing into the abdominal wall to a depth of about a centimeter. The flat of the hand is lifted up each time when a new area is palpated. The normal anatomical structures beneath the palpating fingers are visualized.

Tenderness: Tenderness appears as pain on pressure. Deep tenderness is encountered in inflammatory lesions of the viscera and their covering peritoneum. A light palpation is begun from an area remote from that of pain complained by the patient. It enables to locate the areas of tenderness, muscle spasm and rigidity, and solid masses. Further it helps in getting the confidence of the patient. While palpating the abdomen, the facial expression of the patient has to be watched, to determine the presence of tenderness, which will be revealed when he winces on palpation of the tender area. Tenderness should not be mistaken for cutaneous hyperaesthesia and tenderness in the superficial tissue of the abdominal wall.

Pain and rigidity: Normally the abdomen feels soft and gives an elastic feeling. The palpation does not cause any pain. An increased resistance or tenseness may be felt, and it may persist even after getting adequate relaxation of the abdominal muscles. The tenderness from a reflex contraction of the muscles of the abdominal wall may vary from guarding to a board-like rigidity. It may be localized or generalized. Visceral pain is generally midline in location and vague in character. The patients may exhibit generalized discomfort. Parietal pain is localized and precisely defined. The pain is directed, often with involuntary guarding, rigidity or rebound. Pain is always associated with tenderness, however, intestinal ischaemia elicits severe pain but little tenderness. Patients with musculoskeletal abdominal pain may exhibit tenderness that is exacerbated by Valsalva manoeuvre, after Antonio Valsalva, an Italian anatomist, consists of forcible exhalation effort against a closed glottis or straight leg raising manoeuvres.

The areas of tenderness (Ligat's sign) and the point of its maximum intensity should be clearly demarcated. The rigidity and tenderness in a localized area like the right iliac fossa, right hypochondrium or epigastrium is due to acute appendicitis, acute cholecystitis or perforated peptic ulcer respectively. In generalized peritonitis, there will be a board-like rigidity of the abdominal wall. It may be encountered in tetanus also. Tuberculosis enteritis gives a doughy feel of the abdominal wall.

Sometimes pressure on one side of the abdomen with the finger tips will result in pain in a different region due to the transmission through a gas filled intestine to the site of tenderness. This is referred to as **rebound tenderness.** In another variety, pain occurs following release of pressure due to rebound of tissue in the affected region. In acute appendicitis, there is tenderness in the right iliac fossa while palpating the left iliac fossa (Rovsing's sign, named after Niels Rovsing, a Danish surgeon).

Abdominal wall: While palpating the abdominal wall, pitting oedema may be noted due to collection of fluid in the subcutaneous tissue. It is best demonstrated by pinching a fold of the abdominal wall. A crackling sound and tactile sensation (crepitus) may be felt in **subcutaneous (surgical) emphysema** or gas gangrene. It is due to displacement of bubbles of gas or air in the subcutaneous tissue or in the underlying muscles. The presence of epigastric and umbilical hernia is confirmed by placing the hand over the regions, while the individual is asked to cough. An impulse is felt on the swelling. Omentum, intestine or fluid may form the contents of the hernial sac.

Deep palpation: After winning the confidence of the patient and after delineating the areas of tenderness, deep palpation is to be carried out with firm pressure. If the patient is still holding the abdomen rigid, the examiner has to press hard on the lower sternal region with his left hand while proceeding with palpation of the abdomen with his right hand. The attempts to inspire against pressure will relax the abdominal muscles. During deep palpation the approximated fingers are pressed more deeply. The examining fingers slant inwards and move back and forth. The radial border of the index finger is moved upwards while the patient is asked to take a deep inspiration. It enables the examiner to feel the organs and muscles in the upper abdomen that are coming down with inspiration. Sometimes when there is a marked resistance or necessity to feel a deep-seated organ, abdominal pressure has to be used, and both hands are to be superimposed. In this **double handed (reinforced) palpation,** the tips of the left fingers exert pressure on the terminal interphalangeal joints of the examining right fingers, which enable them to feel the outline of the underlying structures.

Abdominal mass: In thin built individuals, the abdominal aortic pulsations may be felt in the epigastric region, and also the lower lumbar vertebral bodies. Sometimes in normal individuals, the sigmoid colon and the caecum may be felt as ill-defined masses in the left and in the right iliac fossae respectively. The impacted faecal mass in the sigmoid colon and in the descending colon may give an erroneous impression of a mass, especially in chronically constipated individuals. In such instances, it is desirable to feel the abdomen after giving an enema. The liver is felt below the right costal margin in infants, and sometimes its left lobe may be felt across the epigastric region below the xiphisternum. The distended bladder may be felt in the hypogastric region. Hence there is need to palpate the abdomen after emptying the bladder.

Points to be noted in Abdominal Mass.

Location
Size and shape
Surface, margin and consistency
Mobility and fixity
Tenderness
Pulsation

While a mass or a lump is felt during deep palpation, it has to be ascertained whether it is in the abdominal wall (intramural) or in the abdominal cavity (intra-abdominal). The left hand is placed over the forehead and the patient is asked to raise his head while the right hand is placed over the mass. The manoeuvre is to make the abdominal muscles tense (**rising test**). If the mass is in the abdominal wall it becomes more prominent on raising the head against resistance. The intra-abdominal mass becomes less prominent and the abdominal wall can be moved over the swelling.

Dipping and ballotment: In situations of ascites, dipping method or ballotment is used to delineate the floating mass. The fingers extended in a straight line with the forearm and perpendicular to the abdomen are suddenly flexed at the metacarpophalangeal joints, thus dipping into the abdominal wall towards the anticipated site of the organ or mass, and held there. If the organ or mass is freely moveable, it will move upwards due to the displacement of the fluid and is felt at the finger tips. Instead of single-handed ballotment, the manoeuvre may be done using both hands (**bimanual ballotment**). In that case, one hand pushes the anterior abdominal wall and the hand placed in the flank estimates the size of the mass.

Bimanual palpation is used while palpating a large mass, such as kidney, in the lateral sides of the abdomen. To feel the left kidney, the examiner inserts his left hand behind the left costal margin and palm of his right hand downwards over the abdominal wall with the tips of fingers curling posteriorly. With each deep inspiration, the two hands are brought close together, the lower one lifting the organ and the upper one pushing in, so as to appreciate the structure.

Description of the swelling: The swelling in the abdomen may arise from enlargement of an organ (liver, spleen, kidney, lymph nodes) or distension of a hollow viscera (intestine, bladder, uterus) or from growths. When a mass is felt the following features are noted: it's position, size, shape, consistency (soft, firm, hard or cystic), surface (smooth, nodular, irregular), margins (sharp, round), tenderness, mobility and its direction, influence of respiration, pulsations, extension under the costal margin or pelvic cavity and continuity with other organs and attachment to the anterior abdominal wall.

Generally the swellings are interpreted on the basis of their anatomical location in the abdominal cavity. The structures related to the diaphragm (liver, spleen and stomach) show downward movement during inspiration. They can't be moved by the palpating hand. The swellings of mesenteric origin, is not influenced by respiratory movements, but can be moved freely by palpation (tumours of small intestine or transverse colon, cysts in mesentery, secondary deposits in omentum).

An attempt has to be made to 'get above' the swelling when it is in the upper abdomen, and 'get below' when the swelling is in the lower abdomen. This enables one to find the upper, or the lower border of the swelling, as it disappears under the costal margin or into the pelvic cavity respectively. It is not possible to 'get above' in upper abdominal swelling of hepatic, splenic, renal or gastric origin. Similarly it is not possible to 'get below' a lower abdominal swelling of the bladder, uterus and ovary.

The swelling may be completely fixed if it has a retroperitoneal origin (pancreas) or when it is the result of the chronic inflammation affecting other organs (diverticulitis of the sigmoid colon). The tumour that has spread to the abdominal walls or abdominal organs does not exhibit any mobility.

Pulsation: The swelling in the upper abdomen may exhibit pulsations. It becomes necessary to determine whether it is transmitted pulsation from the underlying aorta or itself exhibiting expansile pulsation. Two fingers are to be placed on the swelling. They remain parallel if they are transmitted pulsation and they get separated if the pulsation is expansile, as in aneurysm. The abdominal aorta is felt just above the umbilicus. The pulsations of the aorta are to be felt by slowly inching the thumb of the left hand toward the aorta and the finger-tips of the right hand toward the aorta and then the width has to be measured.

Liver

The palpation is started from the right iliac fossa and moved gradually upwards towards the right costal margin, while looking for the liver. Often the enlargement, is missed by palpating the liver too close to the costal margin. The lower border is felt by placing the palm flat outside the rectus muscle with its edges parallel to the costal margin. The patient is asked to take a deep breath, and the fingers are pressed firmly inwards and upwards into the abdomen. The edge moves down, and if palpable it rides over the radial border of the index finger (Fig. 11). Sometimes, it may be necessary to place the left hand beneath the right flank, and press upwards, while the liver is felt by the right hand. The edge of the liver has to be felt by moving the hand from the lateral (hypochondrium) to the medial (epigastrium) region. Normally liver has a sharp edge and is firm and regular.

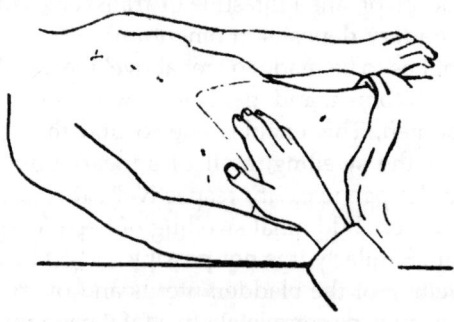

Fig. 11 Palpation of the liver.

The degree of enlargement is expressed in terms of finger breadths, or, centimetres below the costal margin on the mid-clavicular line. It is referred to as mild, moderate or massive, depending on the extent of the enlargement. The liver may be palpable even without any enlargement, as in its downward displacement from massive pleural effusion, emphysema, kyphoscoliosis or from visceroptosis. The displacement of the upper border is noted by percussing down along midclavicular line.

The features of an enlarged liver enables one to arrive at the probable cause of the enlargement. The liver is massively enlarged in secondary deposits, reticulosis, amyloidosis, heart failure, amoebic abscess, and fatty or glycogen infiltration of the liver. The size of the liver is often proportionate to the degree of cardiac failure. Moderate enlargement of the liver is noted in obstruction of the common bile duct, and in presence of gall stones. The enlargement of the liver is mild-to-moderate in infective hepatitis.

The liver becomes tender in congestive heart failure, constrictive pericarditis, viral hepatitis, amoebic hepatitis and abscess. Enlarged liver is painless in malignant disease, cirrhosis, biliary obstruction, amyloidosis, leukaemia, Hodgkin's disease, and infiltrative diseases. The surface is smooth in hepatitis, heart failure, and amyloidosis, granular in cirrhosis giving an impression of 'rivers on a plain', and nodular in malignancy giving an impression of 'mountains on a plateau'. The consistency is soft in fatty infiltration, amyloidosis, infective hepatitis, acute kala azar and heart failure; firm in cirrhosis and hard in malignancy. The margin is rounded in congestive hepatomegaly. It is sharp in hepatomegaly with fibrosis.

The liver is markedly enlarged and pulsatile during systole in tricuspid incompetence, and it is recognized by placing a hand behind the lower ribs posteriorly, and the other anteriorly on the right hypochondrium. The hands separate with each expansile pulsation synchronous with the heart beat. Localised expansile pulsations may be encountered in hepatic infiltrates.

Common causes of enlargement of the liver are as follows:

1. Infections: viral hepatitis, amoebic hepatitis, malaria, kala azar, hydatid disease, tuberculosis, infectious mononucleosis, and amoebic liver abscess.
2. Congestion: portal hypertension, congestive heart failure, constrictive pericarditis.
3. Cirrhosis of the liver in early stages.

4. Toxic: hepatitis due to drugs.
5. Haematologic: iron deficiency anaemia, reticulosis, Hodgkin's disease, leukaemias, multiple myeloma, thalassaemia, myelofibrosis.
6. Metabolic: diabetes mellitus.
7. Infiltrative: fatty liver, sarcoidosis, lipoidosis.
8. Amyloidosis.
9. Biliary obstruction: stone, carcinoma, cholestatic hepatitis.
10. Tumours: primary (hepatoma), secondary deposits.

Gall Bladder

The gall bladder is felt as a smooth pear-shaped, soft, superficial swelling when distended, in the right hypochondrium at the outer edge of the right rectus muscle, near the tip of the ninth costal cartilage in the direction of the umbilicus. It moves with respiration. The swelling can be held between the thumb and the forefinger and can be moved from side-to-side. The upper border merges with the inferior border of the right lobe of the liver, or vanishes beneath the right costal margin. Very rarely the tongue-shaped projection of the right lobe of the liver, called Reidel's lobe may be mistaken for a gall bladder or a movable kidney.

An inflamed gall bladder (acute cholecystitis) presents tenderness when palpated. To elicit the tenderness, the patient is asked to take a deep breath while the right hand is placed beneath the costal margin at the level of the tip of the ninth costal cartilage. The descent of the inflamed gall bladder can be stopped by the fingers and the patient will have a sudden catch with an arrest of breathing (Murphy's sign, named after John Murphy, an American surgeon). A gall bladder may be felt in the absence of jaundice when there is mucocoele of the gall bladder. It develops from impaction of a gall stone in the neck of the gall bladder. Presence of a palpable gall bladder in the presence of deep jaundice, implies an obstruction to the common bile duct particularly by carcinoma of the head of the pancreas. This is possible only, if the gall bladder has not been fibrosed from cholecystitis due to stones within it (Courvoisier's law, after Ludwig Courvoiser, a Swiss surgeon). The obstruction of cystic duct by stone may be associated with enlargement of the gall bladder.

Stomach

There may be tenderness on deep palpation in case of peptic ulcer. It is felt on the left side of the epigastrium in gastric ulcer, and on the right side in duodenal ulcer. A mass may be felt in carcinoma of the stomach and there may be tenderness. A splashing sound may be felt and heard when the hand placed over the epigastric area on the left side is suddenly made to dip. It can also be elicited by gently rolling the patient from side to side. It is encountered in persons with a thin abdominal wall after food, and in conditions of pyloric obstruction.

Spleen

The spleen is normally not palpable and becomes palpable only when it is enlarged to twice its original size. It is felt with the right hand beneath the left subcostal margin while standing on the right side of the recumbent patient. The left hand is placed behind the lower ribs and is pressed medially and forwards while the patient is taking deep breaths. It is necessary to palpate the spleen with the right hand, moving it from the right iliac fossa. The hand is pressed while the patient is taking deep inspiration, and the hand is gradually moved upwards during expiration towards the left hypochondrium, keeping the fingers parallel to the costal margin (Fig. 12).

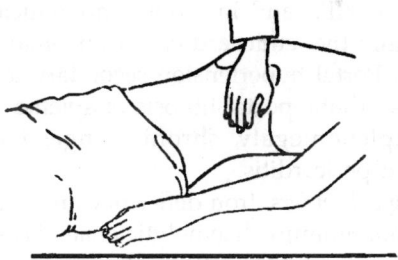

Fig. 12 Palpation of the spleen.

The sharp margin of the enlarged spleen is felt. A very large spleen can be missed completely if the hand is pressed down on top of it. Often a moderately enlarged spleen is made easily felt with the patient lying half turned to his right side.

When the spleen is grossly enlarged, it may occupy the left hypochondrium, left lumbar, umbilical regions and the regions beyond the midline of the abdomen as it grows downwards, forwards and medially. The mass is felt more superficially and has a sharp edge. It is easy to detect the notch in its lower medial border when the enlargement is great. However it is not always evident. It is not possible to insinuate the fingers between the subcostal margin and the enlarged spleen, thus, its upper border cannot be felt. Generally the spleen has a smooth surface, and the consistency is soft in cases secondary to infections, and firm in cases due to haematologic, myeloproliferative and infiltrative disorders. It moves well with respiration due to its close contact with the diaphragm and it is not possible to delineate the upper border of the swelling. It is not bimanually palpable. It is dull to percussion. Dullness is also found between the ninth and the eleventh ribs in the midaxillary line as the enlargement occurs in a superior and posterior direction, before it becomes palpable beneath subcostal margin. Percussion is less satisfactory than palpation in determining enlargement of the spleen. The mass may become tender if there is evidence of perisplenitis secondary to infection and a friction rub (splenic rub) is audible when auscultated over it.

The spleen is enlarged in the following conditions:

1) *Infections:* Acute-enteric fever, septicaemias, infectious hepatitis, brucellosis, acute malaria, acute kala azar, miliary tuberculosis, HIV, and infectious mononucleosis. Subacute-subacute infective endocarditis, chronic-malaria, kala azar.

2) *Congestive:* Portal hypertension secondary to cirrhosis of the liver, non-cirrhotic portal fibrosis or splenic vein thrombosis, tropical splenomegaly, chronic-congestive heart failure, constrictive pericarditis.

3) *Haematologic disorders:* Iron deficiency anaemia, megaloblastic anaemia, autoimmune haemolytic anaemias except sickle cell anaemia, haemoglobinopathies, thalassemia.

4) *Myeloproliferative disorders:* Leukaemia, lymphoma, reticulosis, myelofibrosis, polycythaemia rubra vera, essential thrombocythaemia

5) *Infiltrative conditions:* Amyloidosis, sarcoidosis, lipoid storage diseases.

6) *Connective tissue disorders:* Rheumatoid arthritis (Felty' syndrome, Still's disease), Systemic lupus erythematosus.

Although in the majority of the conditions, the enlargement of the spleen is slight or to a moderate extent, massive splenomegaly may be encountered in the following conditions: chronic malaria, kala azar, chronic myeloid leukaemia, portal hypertension, amyloidosis, some forms of lymphomas, myelosclerosis, and tropical splenomegaly.

In acute infections, acute leukaemias, and in iron deficiency and megaloblastic anaemia, only the tip of the spleen may be felt.

Kidney

To feel the kidney the left hand is placed posteriorly in the region between the last rib and the iliac crest just lateral to the paraspinous muscles while the patient is in a recumbent position and the head slightly raised on a pillow. The right hand is kept over the abdominal wall flat with the fingers pointing towards the costal margin without any movement. While in this position the patient is asked to take a deep breath, and the posterior abdominal wall is suddenly pushed up against the hand placed firmly on the abdominal wall in front. This manoeuvre enables one to feel the mass sandwiched between the two hands. This technique employed to feel the kidney is referred to as bimanual palpation. The right kidney is palpated from the right side and the left by standing on the left side of the patient. Sometimes the left kidney may be felt by standing on the right side. In such an instance, the left hand has to be brought across the abdominal wall and placed posteriorly (Fig. 13).

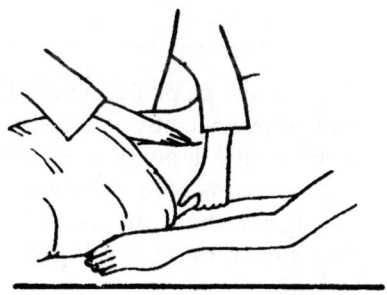

Fig. 13 Palpation of the kidney.

Normally the kidneys are not felt. When the kidney is enlarged it extends downwards and laterally in the loins. It is felt as a rounded ovoid firm mass. In hydronephrosis, it is firm with a smooth surface. It is nodular and felt bilaterally in polycystic kidneys. Hypernephroma appears hard, larger than normal, and slightly irregular. The floating kidney can be moved into different parts of the abdomen. It may be felt when the patient is erect and disappears on lying down (dropped kidney).

The distinction between the spleen and the left sided kidney is necessary. An enlarged spleen is a relatively superficial mass in the left hypochondrium. It enlarges downwards, forwards and medially. The fingers cannot be insinuated between the costal margin and the spleen. The spleen has sharp edges and a notch on the medial border. It moves well with respiration and is dull to percuss. It is not ballotable.

Differentiation of a Spleen from Left Kidney.

Clinical features	spleen	kidney
Anatomical location	superficial	deep
Shape	triangular	round
Insinuation of fingers beneath costal margin	not possible	possible
Direction of growth	downwards, forwards medialwards	downwards, laterally
Movement with respiration	well	slight
Edge	sharp	round
Notch on medial border	present	absent
Bimanual palpation	no	possible
Percussion	dull	band of colonic resonance
Fullness in loin	no	yes

The kidney is bimanually palpable and a ballotable mass. It is situated in the loin and moves slightly with respiration. The fingers can be insinuated between the upper pole of the kidney and costal margin. It enlarges downwards with a tendency to bulge into the loin. It has rounded edges without any notch. It is resonant in the front due to the presence of the colon. It presents with fullness and dullness in the loins.

The presence of any tenderness in the kidney region is noted by application of deep pressure at the costo-vertebral angle. A perinephric abscess may be mistaken for an enlarged kidney. The abscess is tender and it tends to point backwards.

Measurements

The following measurements are taken for the purpose of diagnosis of the abdominal conditions. The distance between the tips of the xiphisternum and the umbilicus; the umbilicus and the upper margin of symphysis pubis; and the umbilicus and the anterior superior iliac spine on either side. In ascites, the distance between the xiphisternum and the umbilicus, is greater compared to the distance between the umbilicus and the symphysis pubis. In tumours arising from the pelvic cavity or gravid uterus, the distance between the symphysis pubis and the umbilicus is greater, compared to the distance between the umbilicus and the xiphisternum. In ascites, the distance between the umbilicus and the anterior superior iliac spine on either side is equal. This distance on the side of ovarian tumour or cyst is greater than that of the opposite side.

The circumference of the abdomen at the supraumbilical (midway between the umbilicus and the xiphisternum), the umbilical and the infraumbilical (midway between the umbilicus and the pubic symphysis) regions is also taken. The supraumbilical girth of the abdomen is greater in ascites; growths arising from the pelvic cavity present a greater girth of the abdomen at the infraumbilical level. The upper part of the abdominal cavity is larger and more compliant than the pelvic part and increases in capacity accommodating free intraperitoneal fluid.

Tip of the ninth costal cartilage: The tip of the ninth costal cartilage is recognized, by drawing a line from the anterior superior iliac spine to the umbilicus, and extending it to the costal margin. Such a line touches the tip of the ninth costal cartilage at the costal margin. Generally the measurements of the liver or the spleen are taken from that point, and expressed in centimetres below the costal margin.

Urinary Bladder

The urinary bladder becomes palpable as a symmetric swelling in the suprapubic region, when it is full and in situations of retention of urine. It is felt as a smooth, firm, regular, oval shaped swelling arising out of the pelvis. It is not possible to get below the swelling though its upper and lateral borders can be easily made out. It is dull to percussion, and the individual gets a desire to micturate when pressed on the swelling. A bladder swelling usually disappears on passing urine.

The Aorta and Common Femoral Artery

The abdominal aorta can be felt a little above and to the left of the umbilicus in thin built persons. The fingertips are used for the purpose. The extended fingers of both hands held side by side are pressed deeply into the abdominal wall to feel the pulsations and its width (See page 82).

A large aortic aneurysm is felt as a mass pulsating in all its directions (expansile pulsation). The common femoral artery is felt by placing the pulps of the right index, middle, and ring fingers in the groin, just below the mid-inguinal point.

Percussion

Normally the abdomen is resonant to percussion. A light percussion is carried while the patient is lying on his back. Light percussion provides more information than heavy percussion. A tympanitic note is elicited due to the presence of gas in the stomach and intestines. The note is high-pitched over the loops of the small intestine and relatively low-pitched over the stomach. The pitch is intermediate over the colon. Gastric tympany is increased over a markedly dilated stomach from pyloric obstruction. Tympanitic notes over the abdomen become more pronounced in intestinal obstruction. The liver, spleen, kidneys, distended urinary bladder, tumour and enlarged glands give a dull note. Percussion acts as an accessory method to palpation in defining the outline of the enlarged organs.

Liver: The upper margin of the liver dullness is determined by percussing the right fifth intercostal space in the mid-clavicular line while the patient is breathing quietly, lying in the bed. Dullness normally lies at the level of the sixth rib. Percussion is continued downwards, and the dull note changes to tympany at the level of the costal arch, indicating the lower border of the liver. It gives information about the liver span (distance in centimetres between the upper and lower margins of the liver in the mid-clavicular line). Dullness below the level of the costal arch indicates hepatic enlargement. However, there is an exception. The upper and lower margins of hepatic dullness is abnormal in a normal sized liver that has been displaced downwards. There can be an upward displacement of the liver dullness in situations of hydatid cyst of the liver, or massive collapse of the lung, or pleural adhesions, or increased intra-abdominal pressure from pregnancy, ascites, gas or tumours. Obliteration of the normal liver dullness suggests free air in the sub-diaphragmatic region that has escaped following perforation of peptic ulcer or intestine, or recent laparatomy or laparoscopy. Absence of normal liver dullness is also encountered in atrophic liver, or over-inflated lungs, or right-sided pneumo-thorax or rarely from interposition of the hepatic flexure of the colon between the diaphragm and the liver (Chilaiditi's sign, named after Demetios Chilaiditi, an Austrial physician). A hyper-resonant note from pneumoperitoneum can be made more prominent by propping the patient towards a sitting position.

Subphrenic abscess: In conditions of subphrenic abscess, alternating areas of dullness and resonance may be noted due to the presence of liver, gas, and pus in the abscess cavity, and intestine.

Spleen: On the left side of the chest, the resonant note of the lung becomes tympanitic at the ninth intercostal space due to gas in the splenic flexure. Percussion of the spleen is done with the patient lying midway between the supine and the right lateral position. Normally the splenic dullness extends from the ninth to the eleventh rib in the left axillary line. As spleen moves freely with respiration, percussion has to be made during expiration and inspiration to establish the movement of the spleen with inspiration. An enlarged area of dullness points to enlargement of the spleen, or, of the left kidney. It is easily distinguished by percussing the abdomen with the patient in a supine position. The enlarged spleen lies anterior to the colon and it gives a dull note obscuring the tympany. The tympanitic note is unaffected in case of kidney, as the colon lies in its front.

Urinary bladder: The distended bladder from retention of urine (400-600 ml) gives a dull note. Its superior and lateral borders can be delineated from the adjacent bowel which is resonant.

Localised swellings: Other masses (lymph nodes, tumours) causing localized swellings in the abdomen give a dull note.

Ascites: Percussion gives a dull note over the flanks in cases of ascites. With an increase in the quantity of the fluid, the hypogastric region and flanks become dull giving a horse-shoe shaped dullness (Fig. 14). The dullness extends over a wide area when ascites becomes massive.

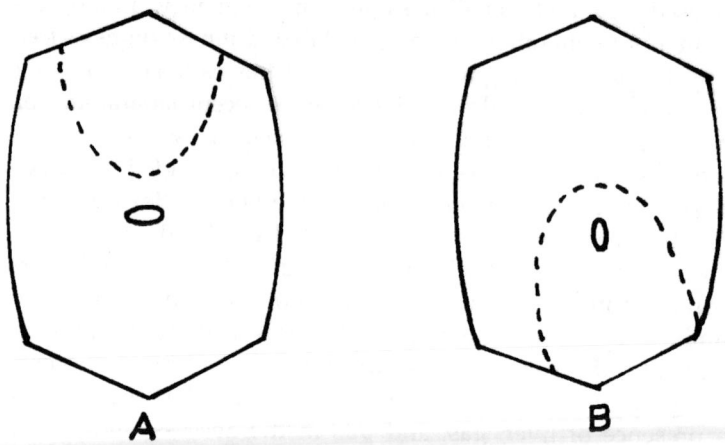

Fig. 14 Distension of abdomen (a) ascites (b) ovarian cyst.

Percussion helps to distinguish ascites from fluid in the abdominal wall, or inside a cyst. Due to the effect of gravity, fluid in the abdominal wall can descend to the flanks and produce dullness simulating that of ascites. Generally such a situation occurs as a part of anasarca and it pits on application of pressure. It is possible to demonstrate the presence of fluid in the peritoneal cavity in three different ways:

    1. 'fluid thrill'
    2. 'shifting dullness' and
    3. periumbilical dullness

1. Fluid Thrill (Wave)

When the patient is lying flat on his back the examiner places the palm over the flank on one side and flicks the opposite flank with the fingers of the other hand (Fig. 15). During this procedure, the patient is asked to press the abdomen by placing the ulnar border of his hand perpendicularly in the midline. This is especially necessary in the presence of excess fat, or oedema of the abdominal wall to dampen the transmission of the impulse through the fat of the anterior abdominal wall. The fluid wave transmitted through the fluid to the other side of the flank, is appreciated as a distinct impact by the palpating fingers. The method is useful in the presence of massive ascites, and it may not be elicited in moderate collection of fluid. 'Shifting dullness' helps in recognizing such a situation.

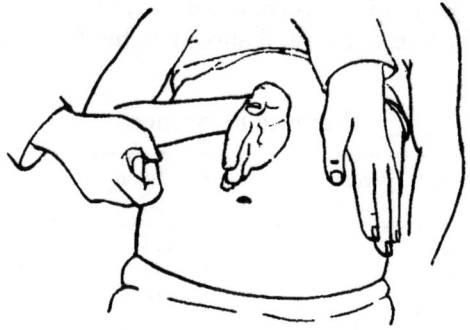

Fig. 15   Fluid thrill.

2. *Shifting Dullness*

The fluid moves to the flanks when the patient lies on his back, and it produces dullness laterally. At the same time a tympanitic note is elicited in the middle of the abdomen because of the underlying bowel. Free fluid in the peritoneal cavity shifts its position because of the gravity, when the patient turns on his sides. This principle is used in demonstrating the 'shifting dullness'.

The abdomen is percussed from the epigastric region towards the umbilicus. Then the percussion is continued with the finger running parallel to the long axis of the abdomen, towards either flank, where they become dull from the presence of the fluid and the line of dullness is noted. Without moving the pleximeter finger at one of the flanks, the patient is asked to turn to opposite side, and to wait for a minute enabling the descent of the fluid towards the dependent flank, and floatation of the coils of the intestine. The flank becomes resonant on percussion. The percussion is continued towards the opposite flank across the umbilicus keeping the patient in the same position. The dullness would appear to have risen from the original level in that side of the flank, and it will be nearer to the midline. The procedure is repeated on the other flank. The test for 'shifting dullness' is not performed on the side of the enlarged liver or spleen.

The 'shifting dullness' may be absent when there is too little fluid. It is absent in massive ascites, localized collection of the fluid as seen in cysts, and inflammatory adhesions of the peritoneum, and in individuals with a short mesentery. Rarely the fluid filled loops of the bowel may shift so as to bring alteration in the percussion note similar to that seen in the shifting of free fluid (pseudoascites).

Presence of Ascites.

Shifting dullness	fluid thrill	periumbilical dullness	inference on ascites	amount of fluid
present	present	–	present	moderate-to-massive
present	absent	–	present	moderate
absent	present	–	present	massive
absent	absent	present	present	very minimal
–	–	–	absent	no

3. Periumbilical Dullness

When the fluid is small in amount (less than 1 litre), it collects in the pelvic cavity and it cannot be demonstrated by 'shifting dullness'. It is demonstrable only by placing the individual in the knee-elbow position. This position will facilitate the drainage of the free fluid from the pelvis and from the gutters of the abdomen into the periumbilical region. Percussion has to be done from the flanks towards the most dependent part of the abdomen. There will be dullness in the periumbilical area in the presence of ascitic fluid.

Diffuse Enlargement of the Abdomen.

	ascites	large ovarian cyst	intestinal obstruction
prominence of abdomen	uniform	lower abdomen	upper abdomen
flanks	bulged	no bulge	no bulge
Umbilicus	transverse displaced down, everted	vertical and drawn up	normal or depressed
Palpation	–	large swelling arising from pelvic cavity	–
greaterabdominal girth distance between anterior superior iliac spine and umbilicus	supraumbilical equal on either side	infraumbilical unequal, greater on the side of swelling	–
Percussion note	dull in flanks	resonant in flanks	resonant throughout
Shifting dullness	present	absent	–
Fluid thrill	present	absent	–
Bowel sounds	normal	normal	increased

Ovarian Cyst

It is possible to distinguish an ovarian cyst from ascites by percussion. Though a fluid thrill can be elicited in an ovarian cyst, it is not associated with any dullness in the flanks. There will be a prominence anteroposteriorly. Unlike ascites, an ovarian cyst gives rise to dullness upwards. The dullness does not shift on altering the position. Fluid thrill will be present.

Auscultation

It is preferable to auscultate the abdomen before palpation and percussion as those procedures may alter the auscultatory findings.

The abdomen is auscultated for the presence of normal peristaltic sounds. They appear gurgling and bubbling (*borborygmi*) due to the peristaltic action of the intestinal wall on the contents (fluid and air) within. These sounds vary in their frequency, intensity and pitch. As they are produced by spontaneous physiologic activity, they appear at different places of the abdomen intermittently. The sounds are heard with greater intensity when the food is overdue. They are heard continuously over the ileocaecal region when the intestinal contents are passing through the ileocaecal valve nearly four to six hours after a meal. The peristaltic sounds are high-pitched, and are appreciated by placing the diaphragm of the stethoscope in one place lightly against the abdominal wall preferably to the right of the umbilicus ('abdominal post'), and listening for two minutes. There is no need to move the stethoscope from one site to another, as the sounds generated at one point of the intestine radiate widely over the entire abdominal wall.

The bowel sounds may be increased in hyperperistalsis with or without any obstruction in the bowel. There is an increased peristaltic activity in early pyloric or intestinal obstruction and loud gurgling sounds are heard as the exaggerated peristaltic waves attempt to push fluid and air against an obstruction. The sounds are high-pitched and splashing when the intestinal contents are passing through an obstruction in the small intestine. In such situations often the sounds are intensified during the waves of paroxysms and are accompanied by colicky abdominal pain. The abdomen is distended and is associated with vomiting.

Bowel Sounds.

Normal	intermittent gurgles
Small bowel obstruction	frequent loud gurgles
	coliky abdominal pain
Generalized peritonitis	silent

Peristaltic sounds are increased in frequency and intensity by diarrhoea, or after intake of laxatives, or from gastroenteritis with diarrhoea. Poor peristalsis is accompanied by weak sounds and it is noted in peritoneal irritation, and post-laparotomy. In such conditions, the peristaltic waves may be stimulated by flicking the abdominal wall with the finger and auscultated. The total absence of sounds speaks of a grave situation ('silent abdomen') and it is noted when the motility of the intestine is inhibited by inflammation (paralytic ileus as in generalized peritonitis), gangrene, or reflex ileus (after abdominal surgery), or an advanced stage of intestinal obstruction. The peristaltic sounds may also be absent in situations with marked electrolyte disturbances, in mesenteric artery thrombosis, during the course of severe pneumonia, uraemia, myxoedema or spinal cord injury. In pyloric stenosis, and in advanced intestinal obstruction, with markedly distended loops of intestine splashing sound is heard when the abdominal wall is depressed by the hand while listening through the stethoscope placed on the abdomen.

In addition to the visceral sounds (bowel peristalsis) other sounds audible over the abdomen have diagnostic significance. They are arterial sounds, venous hum, foetal heart sounds during pregnancy and parietal friction.

Other Sounds over the Abdomen.

Systolic bruit
Venous hum
Continuous murmur
Foetal heart sound
Uterine soufflé
Peritoneal friction rub
Puddle sign

Normally abdominal arterial sounds are audible. However, attempts are to be made to note the presence of a murmur or bruit especially in the hypertensive or arteriosclerotic patients. A bruit (pronounced as 'brooee') is a systolic sound created by turbulance in the flow of blood through a partially occluded or diseased artery. In French the word bruit means sound, and it is applied to first and second heart sounds, but the word is misused to mean an arterial murmur.

A loud systolic murmur is often heard over an aneurysm of the abdominal aorta or over an aorta compressed by an external mass and over the site of coarctation of abdominal aorta. It is heard when the bell of the stethoscope is pressed into the abdominal wall above and to the left of the umbilicus. In renal artery stenosis, a soft medium or low-pitched systolic murmur may be audible with a bell-type stethoscope near the umbilicus in the midline or laterally towards the flank or posteriorly in the renal angle. Unlike a transmitted cardiac murmur, the murmur of renal artery stenosis does not coincide with the apical impulse or the carotid pulse and is heard later. Vascular tumours of the liver may produce a continuous murmur with systolic accentuation. Presence of multiple bruits over the abdomen may indicate vascular disease suggesting ischaemia. Presence of AV fistula is associated with continuous murmur over the abdomen.

A venous hum increasing on inspiration in the region between the umbilicus and the xiphisternum over a small area may be heard from dilated periumbilical collateral veins connecting the portal and caval venous systems in the abdominal wall. It may be noted in Cruveilhier-Baumgarten syndrome, named after Jean Cruveilhier, a French pathologist and Paul Baumgarten, a German pathologist, or in obstructed portal circulation from cirrhosis of the liver, or over a hepatic haemangioma. Unlike arterial bruit, the venous hum is a continuous humming sound.

After 16 weeks of pregnancy, the foetal heart sounds and uterine soufflé are heard over the abdomen. The foetal heart sounds are heard like the ticking of a watch kept beneath a pillow. The site varies with the position of the foetus in the uterus. This is a definite sign of pregnancy. Uterine soufflé is a soft blowing murmur due to an increased blood flow through the dilated uterine vessels.

A peritoneal friction rub may be heard over hypochondriac regions in cases of abscess or tumour (hepatoma or metastatic carcinoma) of the liver and infarction of the spleen. Their location provides protracted excursion against peritoneal surface. These rubs may be made prominent by deep inspiration.

The abdominal sounds are high-pitched and are auscultated with a diaphragm type stethoscope. The bell type stethoscope is used to listen to arterial murmurs and venous hum. The contractions of the abdominal muscles may produce a fibrillary hum, which is due to voluntary and involuntary guarding.

Auscultatory Percussion

The patient lying prone for 5 minutes is made to assume knee-chest position so as to make the central portion of the abdomen, the most dependent part. This position makes the peritoneal fluid to follow gravity and form a puddle in the most dependent part. The diaphragm of the stethoscope is placed and held over that region by one hand. The flank is flicked constantly by other hand, so as to generate sound waves. They pass through the fluid to reach the auscultatory area. The sounds are audible through stethoscope. Such sounds disappear when the patient assumes a sitting posture.

Examination of the Rectum

The patient is asked to lie on his left side with the thigh and knee drawn up (Sim's position, after James Sims, an US surgeon). The skin of the perineum and the anal region should be inspected in a good light. The anus is viewed by drawing aside the buttocks, and the following abnormalities are looked for: anal tags, external haemorrhoids, excoriations of the skin, external opening of fissures, cracks in the mucosa (fissure-in-ano), fistulae, prolapsed rectal mucosa and ischiorectal abscess.

Then the rectal examination (per rectum, PR) is done. The right index finger covered with a finger-stall or glove lubricated with liberal amount of petroleum jelly. The pulp of the finger is placed flat against the anus, and then it is pressed firmly and slowly in a slightly backward direction. The resistance encountered by the finger during its entry gives an idea about the tone of the anal sphincter. The pulp of the finger is gently pressed into the anal canal, performing rotary movements. The examiner has to place his left hand on the patient's right hip. The patient is encouraged to relax and to strain gently. The examination is painless except in situations like anal fissure. When the finger has reached rectum, the examiner has to bring his left hand on the suprapubic region and pressure should be exerted on the sigmoid colon. The finger is moved round the rectum and its inner surface is explored. Normally it should be empty and the wall should be smooth and soft. Sometimes the finger may feel impacted fecal mass in individuals with severe constipation. There may be a hard ulcerating mass due to carcinoma of the rectum. In males, the prostate is felt anteriorly and when enlarged its two lobes project into the rectum. In women the cervix or uterus may be felt anteriorly. On withdrawing the finger, the finger-stall should be examined for the presence of mucus, pus or blood. Presence of blood indicates gut mucosal injury or neoplasm.

The rectal examination should not be done in patients with fissure or myocardial infarction.

SIX

RESPIRATORY SYSTEM

> *"A medical chest specialist is long-winded about the short-winded"*
>
> *-Kenneth T Bird*

Anatomy

The respiratory system though a continuous tract, has been divided into two parts-the upper and the lower respiratory passages, using the cricoid cartilage as the separating landmark. The nose, sinuses, mouth, throat, and larynx form the upper respiratory passages. These parts are examined while examining the head.

Lower Respiratory Tract

The trachea divides into two main bronchi—the right and the left—at carina at the level of the disc between the fourth and the fifth thoracic vertebrae. It corresponds to the lower border of the manubrium sterni in front. The roots of the lungs are situated in the interscapular region at the level of the spines of the fourth, fifth and sixth thoracic vertebrae. The right bronchus gives two side branches, called the lobar bronchi, to the upper and middle lobes, and then descends as the lower lobe bronchus. The left bronchus gives a branch—the upper lobe bronchus, and then descends as the lower lobe bronchus. These lobar bronchi divide into segmental bronchi and supply a wedge-shaped lung tissue (bronchopulmonary segments).

Each lobe and each segment have a homologue in the other lung. The segmental bronchi are ten on the right side and nine on the left. On the right side, the upper lobe bronchus divides into apical, anterior and posterior segmental bronchi, the middle into medial and lateral segmental bronchi and the lower into the apical, and four basal segmental bronchi: medial, lateral, anterior and posterior. On the left side, the upper lobe bronchus divides into two divisions. The upper division gives apicoposterior and anterior segmental bronchi, and, the lower division supplies the lingual (represents the middle lobe on the left side) as the superior and inferior segmental bronchi. The lower lobe bronchus gives apical, anterior, posterior, and lateral segmental bronchi.

Landmarks: The bony landmarks (Figs. 16a and 16b) are the sternal angle (formed by the junction of the manubrium with the body of the sternum and it corresponds with the attachment of the second costal cartilage on either side of the sternum), spine of the seventh cervical vertebra (vertebra prominence), clavicle, sternum, ribs, spine of the scapula (inferior angle overlies the

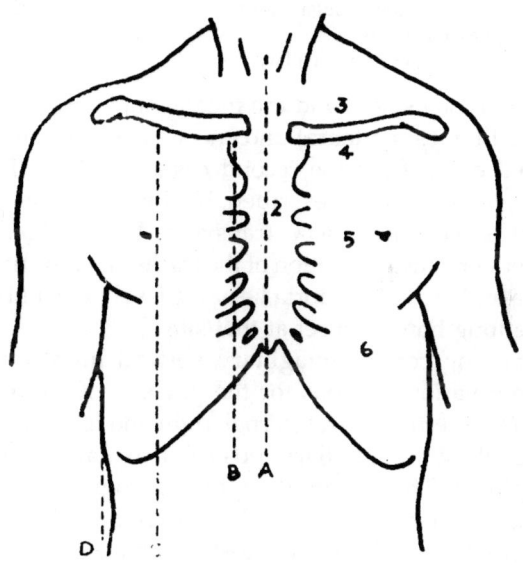

Fig. 16a Anterior view of the chest: Landmarks—

Areas:	(1) suprasternal;	(2) sternal;
	(3) supraclavicular;	(4) infraclavicular;
	(5) mammary; and	(6) inframammary
Lines:	(A) midsternal;	(B) lateral sternal;
	(C) midclavicular; and	(D) anterior-axillary.

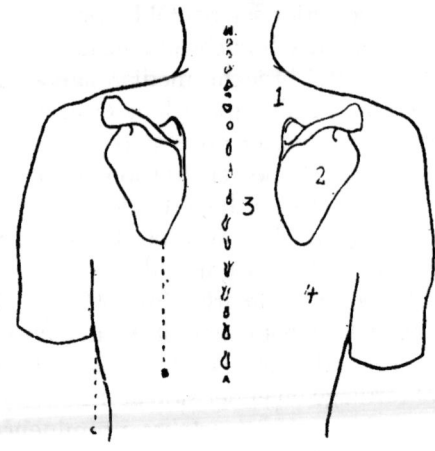

Fig. 16b Posterior view of the chest: Landmarks—
Areas: (1) suprascapular;   (2) scapular;
       (3) interscapular; and   (4) infrascapular;
Lines: (A) vertebral;   (B) scapular; and
     (C) posterior-axillary.

seventh intercostal space, and the medial angle lies on level with the second thoracic vertebra) and the vertebral spines. The ribs are counted down from the second costal cartilage. The sternal angle (angle of Louis, described by Pierre Louis, a French physician) is recognized as a transverse bony ridge. The fifth thoracic vertebra, the bifurcation of the trachea and the upper limits of the atria and arch of the aorta lie at the level of manubriosternal angle. The lung borders meet at that site.

By drawing certain imaginary vertical lines, the chest is divided into various regions for the purpose of the description. They are: mid-sternal, lateral sternal, right and left mid-clavicular, anterior axillary, mid-axillary, posterior axillary, scapular and vertebral lines. The different regions recognized are: supra-clavicular, suprasternal, clavicular, infraclavicular, mammary between the third and the sixth costal cartilages, inframammary between the sixth rib and the costal arch, sternal, axillary, infra-axillary, suprascapular, scapular (supraspinous and infraspinous), interscapular and infrascapular regions.

The abnormalities are described with reference to the lines in specific intercostal space. The nipple is not satisfactory as a landmark because of its inconstant location.

Surface anatomy: The right lung consists of three lobes and the

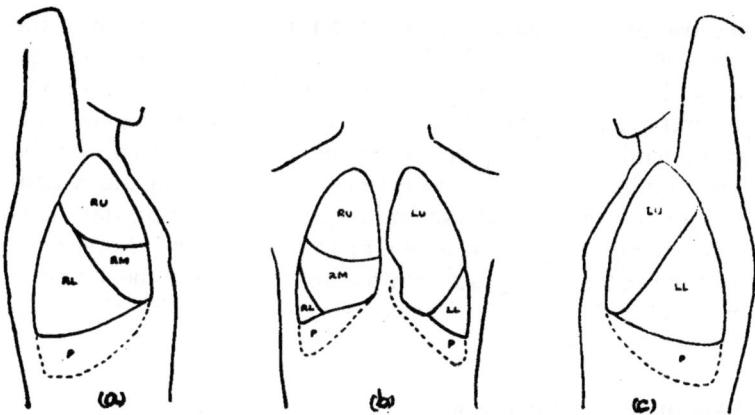

Fig. 17a (left) surface marking of right lung and pleura:
RU: right upper; RM: right middle; RL: right lower; and P: pleural
17b (centre) surface marking of the lungs and pleura (front view)
17c (right) surface marking of the left lung and pleura:
LU: left upper; LL: left lower; and P: pleura.

left two. A greater portion of the front of the chest corresponds to the upper and middle lobes on the right and the upper lobe on the left. On the back, the lower lobes occupy the area below the spine of the scapula and the apex belongs to the upper lobe. In the axilla, parts of all the lobes are closely situated. The apices of the lung rise about 2 to 3 cm above the middle of the clavicle on each side. The shoulder girdle and its musculature cover the apical and the posterior segments of the right upper lobe and the apicoposterior segment of the left upper lobe (Figs. 17a-c). The mammary region contains the middle lobe on the right side and the lingular segment on the left side.

The major interlobar (oblique) fissure corresponds to a line drawn from the spine of the second thoracic vertebra downwards and medially to the sixth costal cartilage in front. It crosses the fifth rib at the mid-axillary line. The lower lobe is situated below this line. The minor interlobar (horizontal) fissure on the right side corresponds to a horizontal line drawn from the fourth costal cartilage to the posterior axillary line where it meets the first line at the fifth rib. The region bounded by these two lines on the right side corresponds to the middle lobe. The lower border of the lung begins at the level of the sixth costal cartilage. On the left side, because of the situation of the cardia, the lower margin of the lung takes a turn laterally in an arch-like manner to reach the sixth rib. The lower margin of the lung crosses the eighth rib in the mid-axillary region, the tenth rib in the scapular line, and ends at the tenth thoracic spine. The pleural sac extends beyond the lower limits of the lung, and reaches the eight, tenth and twelfth ribs in the mid-clavicular, mid-axillary and scapular lines respectively. The cervical pleura follows closely the surface marking of the lung. Posteriorly the lower border of the lung is at the level of thoracic (T) 10 spine that descends to T 12 spine on deep inspiration.

Examination of the Chest

The chest is examined by inspection, palpation, percussion and auscultation. By these methods it is possible to recognize signs caused by changes in the physical properties of the lungs and pleura.

Inspection

To facilitate the inspection of the chest, the area is stripped of clothing up to the waist and the patient is seated in a well-lighted place on a stool. The shoulders are allowed to droop and the body has to be relaxed. In the case of a woman, the breasts are covered and the chest is examined part by part, preserving her modesty.

The chest is inspected from the front, sides and back. In addition, the upper part of the chest is inspected from above downwards by looking over shoulders while the patient is seated. In a recumbent position, the inspection of the chest is done by looking from the head of the bed over the clavicles, or from the foot of the bed towards the neck. If the patient is too ill to strip, the back may be examined by rolling him on each side, in turn.

During the inspection, it has to be ascertained whether the patient can lie down comfortably. Respiratory distress, if present, has to be observed carefully. The patient having an attack of asthma, or, in cardiac failure, prefers to sit up to increase the efficiency of the respiratory excursions. The patient adopts a position wherein the shoulders are kept in an abducted position with elbows drawn away from the chest. There may be noisy breathing. A wheezing sound may be evident during expiration in airway obstruction (asthma, chronic bronchitis). In conditions of oedema of the glottis, or laryngeal obstruction, there is obstruction to the entry of air resulting in a harsh respiration (stridor).

Normally the ribs exhibit a slope and are situated at about 45° angle in relation to the spine. The anterior ribs move upwards and outwards during inspiration. There is expansion of the chest laterally. Posteriorly the scapulae are firmly applied to the underlying chest wall. The expansion of the chest is markedly limited in conditions of air-flow limitation (during attacks of bronchial asthma, chronic bronchitis and emphysema) and accessory muscles of respiration (scalenii, sternomastoids and trapezii) will be active, and the patient appears obviously breathless. The sternomastoid muscles become taut with inspiratory contraction. There is also abnormal recession of the suprasternal and supraclavicular fossae, and lower interspaces during inspiration due to increased intrathoracic negative pressure. The patient may breathe with pursed lips in chronic obstructive pulmonary disease (COPD). The lips are held tightly opposed at the height of inspiration and they are held narrowly apart during expiration to interpose an expiratory resistance. This is perhaps to lengthen the expiratory time and to increase lung volume. The *ala nasi* may show inspiratory flaring in pneumonia and bronchial asthma.

During the inspection of the chest, the shape of the chest and the respiratory movements are to be observed carefully. The underlying respiratory diseases rarely cause any abnormality of the skin. The skin is examined for the presence of petechiae, exanthema, dilated superficial veins, supernumerary nipples, gynaecomastia, sinus, scars, distribution of hair, swellings, sternomastoid tendon, pulsations, apical impulse and lymph nodes. There may be scars secondary to operations (thoracotomy, median sternotomy, key-hole surgery), empyema drainage or branding.

Inspection of the Chest.

Shape of the chest
Movements of the chest
Rate, rhythm, type of respiration
Expansion of the chest
Position of the mediastinum
Skin

Shape of the chest: The shape of the chest is largely dependent on the build of the person. It may be short and broad in stocky individuals, or, long and narrow in asthenic individuals. Normally the chest is bilaterally symmetrical. The intercostal spaces are broader in front than behind. The transverse diameter is greater than the posteroanterior (PA) diameter in the ratio of 7:5. On cross-section the chest is elliptical. The normal ratio between PA diameter of the chest and the lateral diameter (thoracic ratio or thoracic index) is 0.7 to 0.75. The subcostal angle is less than 90° and it widens during inspiration because of the lateral expansion of the chest. In children, the chest appears cylindrical with the transverse and posteroanterior diameters being equal. With advancing age in elders, the posteroanterior diameter increases due to a slight dorsal convexity in the upper thoracic region.

The shape of the chest may alter due to the disease of the past or the present. The abnormalities may be symmetrical or asymmetrical (Fig. 18). Many of the symmetrical deformities are due to rickets and respiratory diseases suffered in childhood. The softness of the bones in childhood make the chest labile to deformities.

Symmetric Abnormalities.

Flat chest
Rachitic chest
Barrel-shaped chest

1) *Flat chest:* The postero-anterior diameter is markedly decreased resulting in an increase in the transverse diameter. The chest appears like a shield. In such a long, flat chest the scapulae may stand out prominently like wings on either side (alar chest). It was believed that such a chest is more prone to tuberculosis (phthisical chest).

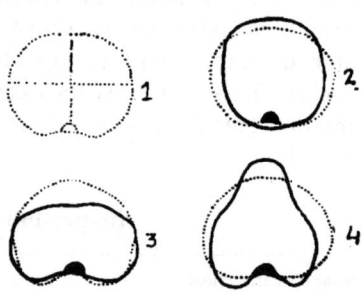

Fig. 18 Various types of the chest: (1) normal chest; (2) barrel-shaped chest; (3) flat chest; and (4) pigeon chest.

2) *Rachitic chest:* The bones are soft during childhood and they can yield to pressure resulting in various abnormalities of the chest. This phenomenon is marked in those who have suffered from rickets, nasal obstruction due to adenoids, respiratory diseases like chronic severe asthma or cardiomegaly in childhood. The deformed chest may have any of the following abnormalities:

   i) *Pigeon chest:* The sternum is bulged forwards projecting beyond the frontal plane of the thorax. It is particularly noticeable in its upper part. The ribs slope in to meet the sternum on either side, losing their curvature, and the chest appears triangular in cross-section *(pectus carinatum).*

   ii) *Funnel chest (pectus excavatum):* It is associated with funnel-like depression of the lower two-thirds of the sternum behind the frontal plane of the thorax. The costochondral junctions become prominent.

   iii) *Harrison's groove:* It appears as a horizontal groove, or constriction in the lower anterior thorax, along the line of attachment of the diaphragm on one or both sides, and the lower ribs get 'caved in'.

   iv) *Rickety rosary:* The enlargement of the successive costo-chondral junctions, give a beaded appearance.

3) *Barrel-shaped chest:* It is evident in situations of chronic airflow limitation as in emphysema and during acute severe attacks of asthma. There is distension of the lungs and the chest becomes overinflated. The anteroposterior diameter of the chest is increased. The thoracic ratio is 1:1.

The ribs are horizontal. There is retraction of intercostal spaces on inspiration and it indicates obstruction to the free inflow of air in the respiratory tract. The spine is unduly concave forwards and the sternum is prominently arched. The chest appears circular on cross-section. The subcostal angle is greater than 90° and it shows little respiratory variation. There can be an increase in the anteroposterior diameter of the chest without any obstructive airway disease as in thoracic kyphosis.

Asymmetrical chest: The asymmetry of the chest may be due to the deformity of the vertebral column, or diseases of the chest causing retraction or prominence of one side of the chest.

The vertebral column may exhibit a marked dorsal curvature (kyphosis) (Fig. 19). It may be widespread as in senile osteoporosis and ankylosing spondylitis or localized (gibbus) as in tuberculosis of the spine. The lateral curvature of the spine is referred to as scoliosis. Both deformities may exist together resulting in marked asymmetry of the chest (kyphoscoliosis). The abnormality may be developmental or secondary to neuromuscular diseases or respiratory diseases in childhood. On the side of the convexity of the vertebral column, the chest is large and the ribs are separated widely. The forward bend of the lumbar spine is referred to as lordosis.

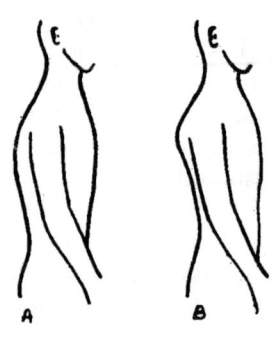

Fig. 19 Vertebral column with dorsal curvature (left) and gibbus (right).

Retraction: The chest may be flattened or even retracted on one side due to fibrosis of the lung or pleural thickening. The term, frozen chest refers to a sunken and immobile hemithorax, often secondary to greatly thickened pleura. In air flow obstruction, there is retraction of interspaces on inspiration.

Bulging: The intercostal spaces may be full, resulting in the prominence of the chest in conditions of massive pleural effusion and pneumothorax. Intercostal spaces may be bulged in emphysema. A prominent pulsatile swelling may be evident in aortic aneurysm. In empyema necessitans (pointing), a swelling may be evident in the side of the chest and exhibits an impulse on coughing. There can be localized swellings on the surface of the chest from an inflammatory process (cold abscess), or a tumour of the subcutaneous tissue or chest wall.

Movements of the Chest

Rate and depth: The normal rate of respiration is 14 to 16 per minute at rest in a normal adult. It has a definite ratio to pulse rate and it is 1:4. Respiration is referred to as 'tachypnoea' when the rate is increased and 'bradypnoea' when the rate is decreased. Cessation of respiration is called apnoea. The respiration is faster in children and slower in elderly persons. The rate is increased in acute respiratory conditions (pneumonia, pleurisy), hypoxic conditions, cardiac failure, and during excitement, exertion and fever. The depth of respiration (tidal ventilation) is about 500 ml at rest. Hyperpnoea refers to an increased depth of breathing. An increased rate and depth of respiration is noted in conditions demanding ventilation as in exercise, fever, thyrotoxicosis, ascites, hypoxic states or hypercapnoea. There is a decreased rate and depth of breathing during sleep or depression of respiratory centre (cerebral disease, narcotic poisoning).

Though the rate and depth of breathing alter together, the rate may be increased at the expense of depth as in pleurisy and fibrosis. A slow, deep respiration is encountered in depression of the respiratory centre, as in narcotic poisoning, tumours of the brain stem, airflow obstruction, and coma. The respiratory rate is counted without the knowledge of the patient. The excursion of the anterior chest wall, or of the epigastrium is counted for a minute.

Rhythm: In health, the respiration is quiet, regular in depth, and rhythmic. Inspiration is active and expiration passive. There is a short pause between inspiration and expiration. Expiration is followed by a long pause and then there is inspiration. Inspiration is longer than expiration. The rhythm becomes irregular when one is conscious of the act. The rhythm has to be assessed by looking at the patient's abdomen when the patient is unaware. The expiration is prolonged in airways obstruction. There will be a long drawn out wheeze in asthma. A prolonged inspiration is encountered in laryngeal obstruction and mediastinal growths.

Certain classical respirations with abnormal rhythm are Cheyne-Stokes breathing and Biot's breathing (Fig. 20). Cheyne-Stokes breathing described by John Cheyne, a Scottish physician, and William Stokes, an Irish physician, is a periodic form of respiration, wherein the successive respirations gradually become deeper and deeper (hyperpnoea) and then diminish until there is temporary cessation of respiration (apnoea). It is noted when a patient is asleep or unconscious. Cheyne-Stokes breathing occurs commonly in raised intracranial tension,

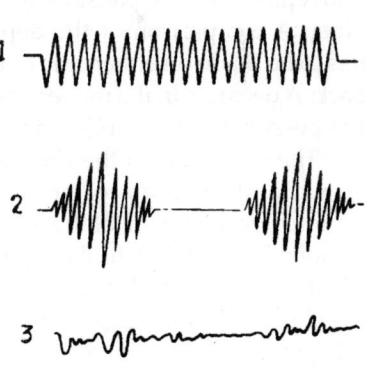

Fig. 20 Respiratory rhythms: (1) Normal breathing; (2) Cheyne-Stokes breathing; and (3) Biot's breathing.

narcotic drug poisoning of the respiratory centers, severe pneumonia, cardiac and renal failure. Biot's (described by Camille Biot, a French physician) respiration is an irregular respiration. It may become slow or rapid, shallow or deep with irregular pauses. It may be seen in meningitis.

Types of respiration: Normally, two types of respiration are encountered: thoracic (costal) and abdominal (diaphragmatic). The intercostal muscles, diaphragm and abdominal muscles take part in the respiration. In health, costal respiration is seen in women, and the abdominal in men. In abdominal respiration, the downward excursion of the diaphragm with inspiration causes free movements of the abdominal wall. Thoracic breathing is accomplished by the use of intercostal muscles. However, in health, the combinations of these breathing are encountered. Costal breathing is noted in conditions of paralysis of the diaphragm, peritonitis, ascites and diaphragmatic paralysis. Abdominal breathing is more evident in paralysis of intercostal muscles, ankylosing spondylitis, pleurisy and fibrosis of the lung.

Movements and Expansion of the Chest

Normally both sides of the chest move uniformly and synchronously. The expansion is equal and it is normally about 5 to 8 cm. During inspiration, the diaphragm moves downwards and the thoracic cage moves upwards and outwards. The terms 'movement' and 'expansion' have a different connotation to each other. A comparison of the depth (amplitude) of the movement has to be made on either side of the chest from the front, sides and back. A decrease in the movement on one side of the chest indicates the possibility of an underlying disease.

The expansion of the chest is decreased in the diseases of the airways (obstruction to the main bronchus by foreign body or tumour), parenchyma of the lung (consolidation, collapse, fibrosis, tumours), pleura (pleural effusion, pneumothorax, and thickened pleura) or unilateral phrenic nerve paralysis. The expansion of the chest is greatly decreased in conditions of airways obstruction wherein the chest may be held in a state of inspiratory position all the time.

In emphysema, there is considerable chest movement but there is little expansion. In airways obstruction, there is inspiratory indrawing of the lower intercostal spaces together with indrawing of suprasternal and supraclavicular fossae, and it is due to increased negative intrathoracic pressure. In severe upper airways obstruction (laryngeal disease or tumours of the trachea) there is indrawing of the intercostal spaces with inspiration. The movement of the apices of the lung lag behind in tuberculosis. The chest may be immobile in ankylosing spondylitis.

The breathing may be increased in rate and depth in air hunger, seen in diabetic ketoacidosis and renal failure (Kussmaul-Kiens breathing, described by Adolf Kussmaul, and Maarie Kien, German physicians). An increase in depth of breathing, may be seen in respiratory alkalosis facilitating washout of carbon dioxide. A decrease in the amplitude of the respiration is also seen in muscular weakness and depression of the respiratory centre by narcotics.

The diaphragmatic movement may be visible in the form of a wave motion in thin individuals (Litten's sign). The wave beginning at the sixth intercostal space descends down on inspiration and ascends up on expiration. This can be observed by standing at the feet of the patient in a recumbent position. Commonly, diaphragmatic excursion is assessed by observing the rise of the patient's abdominal wall with inspiration and a fall with expiration during quiet breathing. In lung hyperinflation, there is indrawing rather than flaring of anterior rib margins with inspiration and it is caused by horizontal rather than downward contraction of the diaphragm (Hoover's sign, described by Charles Hoover, a US physician). The diaphragmatic excursion is decreased or absent in pleural effusion, subdiaphragmatic abscess or phrenic nerve paralysis.

Position of the mediastinum: The position of the trachea and apex beat, are to be noted. The sternomastoid muscle may be prominent on one side indicating marked displacement of the trachea towards that side (sternomastoid or Trail's sign).

Veins: Superficial veins in the chest may become visible due to obstruction of superior vena cava (SVC) and obstruction to azygos vein. SVC obstruction above the entrance of azygos vein does not cause prominence of the veins on the chest wall. But the obstruction at the entry of azygos vein causes dilated veins on the chest. It is due to the re-routing of blood flow from jugular veins and proximal SVC through internal mammary veins to the chest wall veins to azygos and hemiazygos venous system. The venous pulses in the neck should be examined (see Chapter 7).

Palpation

The observations during the inspection are to be confirmed by palpation. Further it supplements the findings already noted during inspection. Before ascertaining the expansion of the chest, it is necessary, to palpate the swellings noted on inspection, and to feel the supraclavicular region and axilla for presence of lymph nodes, and the warmth of the skin. If the individual complains of any pain in the chest, it is necessary to elicit the region of tenderness by palpating the site with the fingers and to look at the patient's face for reaction of pain.

Tenderness over a rib may be due to a fracture, following cough or injury or it may be secondary to a malignant deposit. Tenderness may be noted over the costochondral junctions (Teitze's syndrome), intercostal muscles (intercostal fibrositis) or over the site of pleurisy and empyema. Amoebic liver abscess is also associated with tenderness over the right lower chest. A peculiar crackling sensation of air bubbles, may be felt beneath the skin in subcutaneous emphysema. It occurs due to escape of air from the lungs into the subcutaneous tissue and there is sudden equalization of pressure, when air is squeezed from an inflated to the airless component of the skin. A fluctuation has to be elicited over any abscess, and is present in cases of empyema necessitans.

During palpation, three important features are noted:
1) Expansion of the chest
2) Vibration of the chest
3) Position of the trachea and cardiac impulse

1) Expansion of the Chest

To evaluate the expansion of the chest, the chest is palpated from above downwards while the patient is breathing normally and on deep inspiration. While examining the back and apices of the lung, the examiner has to stand behind the patient and place the finger tips of both the palms on either side of the chest, so the tips of the thumbs meet in the midline, without touching, over the vertebral column. The hands are placed horizontally bracing the sides of the chest firmly. Normally the thumbs separate out and move away from the midline to an equal distance during inspiration. The movement of the thumb is decreased on the side with diminished expansion.

In bilateral disease the movement of the thumbs is decreased on either side indicating restricted expansion of the chest.

To test the movement in the infraclavicular region, the palms have to be placed below the clavicle with the tips of the fingers pointed towards the clavicle. The lift of the hands on deep inspiration is to be noted. To verify the expansion of the anterior surface of the chest, the examiner while standing in front has to place his hands over the lower anterolateral aspect of the chest along the costal margin with the thumbs pointing towards the midsternal line.

Diaphragmatic movement: The palm of one hand is placed over the epigastric region and the other palm is placed over the anterior chest wall. During inspiration both hands are lifted. In diaphragmatic paralysis, there is retraction of the epigastric region during inspiration.

Measurements: The degree of the expansion of the chest is measured by placing a measuring tape just below the nipple, with its zero mark at the middle of the sternum. In women, measurements are made either above or below the breasts. The patient is asked to breathe in and out as deeply as possible. On deep inspiration, the chest wall will expand by 5 to 8 cm in a healthy adult male. The expansion of the chest is markedly limited in conditions associated with airways obstruction (as low as 1 cm). The expansion of the hemithorax on any one side is limited in unilateral diseases of the lung or of the pleura.

2) *Vibration of the Chest*

The term *fremitus* is applied to vibration. The vibrations of the chest wall that can be appreciated are vocal, pleural friction and rhonchial fremitus.

1) *Vocal fremitus:* The vocal fremitus is a sign to detect vibrations produced by phonation that are transmitted to the palpating hand through the airways, the lungs, the pleura and the chest wall. It causes vibration of the chest wall. The patient is asked to say uniformly 'one, two' or 'ek, do, teen' or 'ninety-nine' repeatedly, and the vibrations are felt by placing the palm including the finger tips or the ulnar side of the hand on the chest. The intensity can be compared with the use of both hands placed over identical areas. The hands are moved to various regions of the chest simultaneously and the vibrations are compared. This is referred to as tactile vocal fremitus (TVF). Normally the vocal fremitus is prominent over the areas where the trachea or bronchi are closer to the chest wall (right infraclavicular region, and interscapular region).

The vocal fremitus is increased when a solidified lung (consolidation, infarction, neoplasm) or a superficial cavity is present between the bronchi and the chest wall. It is diminished or absent in airways obstruction, emphysema, collapse, fibrosis, thin-walled cavities and in conditions of pleural effusion, thickened pleura, pneumothorax, hydropneumothorax and after tracheostomy. As these vibrations are heard with the stethoscope later, there is another opportunity to verify the findings. Decrease in voice reduces intensity of vocal sounds.

2) Friction fremitus: A superficial grating sensation is felt in pleurisy over a localized area on the infra-axillary or infra-scapular region commonly. It is due to inflamed pleura rubbing against each other. It is felt during both phases of respiration and it increases on application of pressure with the hand.

3) Rhonchial fremitus: In conditions of airways obstruction, rhonchi may be felt over the chest bilaterally as coarse vibrations. These are predominantly expiratory, and can be made to disappear on coughing.

3) Position of the Trachea

The trachea is felt in the suprasternal notch (Fig. 21). Normally it is located centrally. Any evidence of deviation of the trachea has to be ascertained by its relation to the insertion of the sternomastoid muscle.

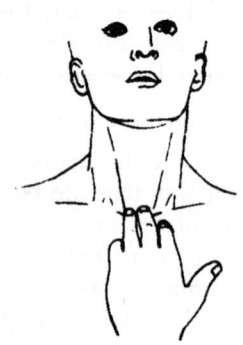

The distance between the suprasternal notch and the lower border of the cricoid cartilage is 3 to 4 fingers breadth in normal young individuals, on complete expiration. This distance decreases in patients with severe airflow limitation and in individuals with advancing age. In

Fig. 21 Position of the trachea.

former condition it is due to elevation of the sternum relative to the hilum. To note the position of the trachea from the front, the head of the patient has to be fixed with one hand while the individual is looking straight. While keeping the right index and ring fingers at the medial ends of the clavicle, the middle finger is inserted into the suprasternal notch. Normally the finger abuts directly against the trachea in the centre. When the trachea is deviated to one side, the finger slides to the other side of the trachea where the distance from the sternomastoid is greater than the opposite side (three-finger test).

When the trachea is felt from behind, the palms of the hands are placed over the apices directing the fingers towards the midline on the front, and the thumbs are approximated on the vertebral column. The index fingers are slid into the sternal notch at the level of the clavicular heads. If the trachea is deviated one finger will palpate the trachea just deep into the clavicular head of sternomastoid while the other will enter a space.

The cardiac impulse is localized with the palm and fingers. The trachea and the cardiac impulse may be pushed to the opposite side in diseases of the pleura, resulting in an increase of the volume of the chest (pleural effusion, empyema, pneumothorax, hydropneumothorax), and following single lung transplantation. In cases of the diseases of the lung (collapse, and fibrosis) causing a diminution of the volume of the lung, the trachea and the cardiac impulse are pulled to the same side. Pleural thickening and an old empyema may pull the mediastinum to the same side preventing lung re-expansion.

In conditions of the collapse, or fibrosis of the upper lobe, or a large mass in upper mediastinum, the trachea alone may be shifted to the affected side, without a shift of the cardiac impulse, indicating lateral shift of the upper mediastinum. Deviation of the cardiac impulse indicates shift of the lower mediastinum. In moderate pleural effusion the cardiac impulse may be displaced without the shift of the trachea. In minimal pleural effusion, and shallow pneumothorax, there may not be any shift of the cardiac impulse or trachea. The cardiac impulse may be displaced in diseases of the cardia and abnormalities of the bony cage (scoliosis and funnel chest). In dorsal scoliosis the mediastinum tends to deviate to the side of concavity. In pleural effusion if there is a coexistent bronchial obstruction in the upper lobe from bronchogenic carcinoma, it results in deviation of the trachea to the same side while the apical impulse moves to the opposite side.

Percussion

Percussion is a technique to produce sound waves and they vary in quality according to the density of the underlying tissues. It was first described by Leopald Auenbrugger, an Austrian physician, in 1761.

Method of percussion

When the chest is percussed, the lungs and the chest wall are set into vibration and result in a sound. Its quality depends on the amplitude, rate, pitch, duration and intensity of the vibrations. The percussion note is dampened at the change of interfaces of the media, such as air, elastic lung, fluid in the pleural cavity and chest wall and hence results in an alteration of the percussion note in diseases of the chest. Two things are observed during percussion: i) the quality of the sound produced, and ii) the resistance offered by the underlying chest wall. The character of the sound is determined by the combination of the impact sound produced by the striking finger and the vibrations coming from the chest wall.

There are two methods of percussion: direct and indirect. In direct (immediate) percussion, the finger strikes directly over the bony regions (for example, clavicle) without the intervention of any other finger (Fig. 22). Even over the clavicle a finger may be placed and percussed. The indirect (mediate) percussion is used over the chest (digitodigital percussion).

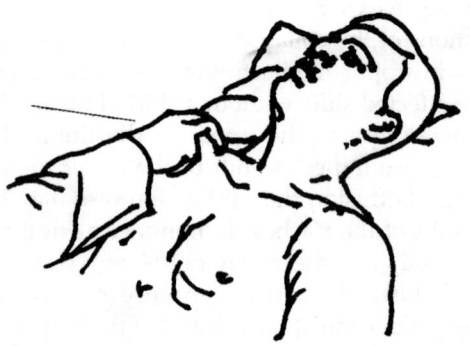

Fig. 22 Clavicular percussion.

The procedure is as follows: The left middle finger (the pleximeter) is applied flatly and firmly on the chest wall without interposing any airspace between it and the skin. The back of the middle phalanx is struck a sharp blow with the tip of the right middle finger (the plexor). The striking should not be with the fingernails. The plexor finger is so flexed that when the blow is delivered, its distal phalanx is at right angles to the metacarpal bones. The wrist should not be held stiff as the stroke is delivered with its swinging action (Fig. 23). The movement should not be from the shoulder or from the elbow. The plexor finger is raised immediately after striking once or twice. Generally light percussion is done unless the patient is obese or has a thick muscular chest. Heavy percussion is needed posteriorly due to the thick muscles and fat (Fig. 24 and 25).

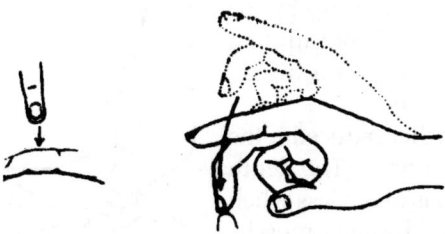

Fig. 23 Method of percussion-position of pleximeter and plexor.

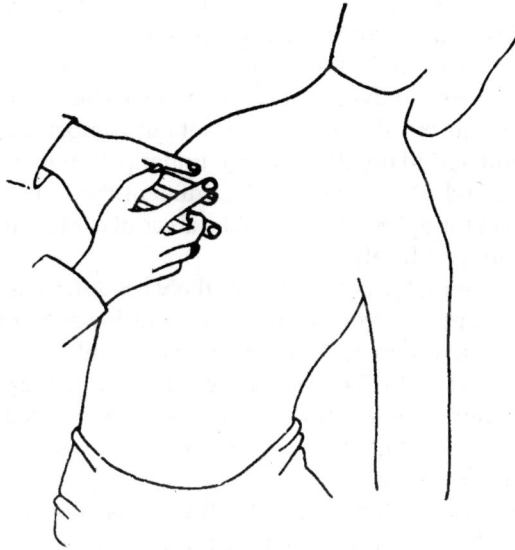

Fig. 24 Percussion of the back.

Normally, a resonant note is elicited over an aerated lung. The sounds are clear, loud and well-sustained as the aerated lung is able to produce greater amplitude (intensity) of the vibration. The chest does not offer any resistance to percussion and produces low frequency (pitch) vibrations. Normally, the vibrations of the underlying structures that are set up by the blow, spread to a depth up to a maximum of 5 cm in a highly resonant structure.

This is further reduced if the pleximeter is a bone. The depth of penetration is much less when percussed over the fat or muscle. To detect alteration in the percussion note, the lesion must be at least 2 or 3 cm in diameter.

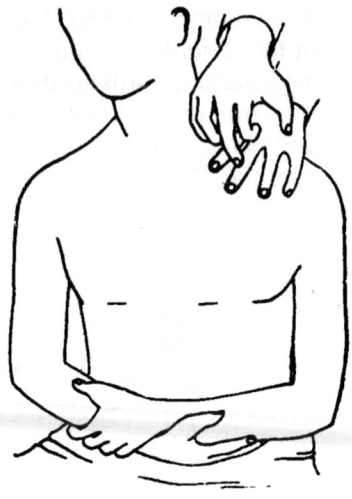

Fig. 25 Percussion of the apex.

The chest is more resonant in the infraclavicular region, and the infrascapular region where the muscles are relatively thin. There is least resonance over the scapulae.

The percussion of the chest is carried out to elicit two important points: i) to find out the percussion note in comparable areas on two sides and to find out its alteration under pathologic conditions (diagnostic), and ii) to delineate the limits of the lung resonance, particularly at the apices, bases and the areas of cardiac and hepatic dullness (topographical).

While defining the boundaries of the various organs—borders of the heart, upper border of the liver and lower border of the lungs—the percussion is done from a resonant area. The note becomes dull when the borders of the cardia or liver are reached. The transition from resonance to dullness is appreciated easily by the ear. Hence it is desirable to percuss from more resonant towards the less resonant areas.

The long axis of the pleximeter (percussed finger) has to be applied parallel to the anticipated line of dullness due to the underlying organ and moved perpendicularly to it. To define the upper border of the liver, the finger is applied in the intercostal space on the right side of the chest and percussed from above downwards in the mid-clavicular line. To define the right border of the heart the finger is applied parallel to the right border of the sternum. The left border of the heart is percussed in the region of the cardiac impulse. The cardiac and liver dullness are obliterated in hyperinflation. It may be due to asthma or emphysema. In asthma the hyperinflation is transient and in emphysema, it is permanent. In pneumothorax, depending on the site, the liver or cardiac dullness is encroached by the hyperresonant note. In perforation of the abdominal viscera, the liver dullness gets obliterated due to the presence of gas under the diaphragm. Similarly, there is obliteration of the liver dullness in atrophy of the liver and in interposition of hepatic flexure of colon under the right diaphragm and the liver.

Obliteration of Liver Dullness.

Supradiaphragmatic conditions
    Acute severe asthma
    Emphysema
    Right-sided pneumothorax
Infradiaphragmatic conditions
    Perforation of stomach or intestine
    Laparoscopy
    Atrophy of the liver
    Interposition of hepatic flexure of colon
    between diaphragm and liver

A dull note is short, high-pitched and is not loud. It is appreciated as a dull thud. The pleximeter finds little vibration. An increased vibratory sensation is appreciated in hyperresonance.

Kronig's isthmus: Normally a band of apical resonance of 4 to 6 cm in width can be demonstrated on either side over the trapezius. The resonant area is bounded medially by the dullness of the neck and laterally by the dullness of the shoulder. The area of resonance is markedly decreased in tuberculosis, as it results in retraction of the apex of the lung.

In lower borders of lung resonance is determined by percussing from above downwards. Normally the lower border of the lung extends to the sixth, eighth and tenth ribs in the mid-clavicular, mid-axillary and scapular lines respectively. The border ascends in pleural effusion, fibrosis and collapse and descends in emphysema, overinflated chest and pneumothorax. The transition is from resonance to dullness on the right side anteriorly and from resonance to tympany on the left side. The upper margin of the liver dullness begins from the fifth intercostal space anteriorly.

On the left side over the region of the upper part of the stomach, the resonant note becomes tympanitic in character. The area is an irregularly quadrilateral space bounded on the right side by the liver, on the left side by the spleen, and above by the lower edge of the heart and below by the left costal margin (Traube's space, named after Ludwig Traube, a German physician). The space can be marked by drawing perpendicular lines down from the sixth rib at the costochondral junction and the ninth rib at the anterior axillary line to the costal margin. The space is increased in collapse, and fibrosis of the lung. It is decreased in pleural effusion, pleural adhesions, pericardial effusion, enlarged spleen and liver. Preservation of Traube's space suggests that the dullness is from consolidation or atelectasis. The resonance may get impaired in consolidation of the left anterior basal segment and contiguous lingula.

Tidal percussion: To study the mobility of the hemidiaphragm it is desirable to mark out their lower margins on the back. The percussion is carried out at each lung base when the individual has exhaled with force. Then the patient is instructed to take a deep breath. The lower margin is again percussed. There will be a difference between the lung resonance on deep inspiration and on deep expiration (tidal percussion). During deep inspiration the lower border resonance moves downwards by 4 to 5 cm, approximately two posterior interspaces and is equal on both sides. The mobility is hindered in pleural adhesions, pleural effusion and in conditions associated with overinflation. In emphysema the diaphragm is low and fixed and the normal excursion is not made out. Tidal percussion is used to distinguish dull note due to pulmonary cause from that of raised diaphragm due to subdiaphragmatic lesion. In the latter the dullness becomes resonant on deep inspiration and in the former it remains dull in both phases of respiration.

Technique of percussion: Percussion is done by striking the region under examination, while the patient is sitting. He should be sitting comfortably with arms and shoulders placed symmetrically. The front and sides can be percussed easily while the patient is recumbent. In acutely ill patients the percussion of the back is difficult and it can be attempted by turning the patient on to his side.

While percussing the chest, the pleximeter finger should be kept parallel to the ribs in the intercostal spaces, and not across them. The chest is percussed on its front downwards from the apices. Direct percussion is made over each clavicle. Then the sides and the back of the chest is percussed from above downwards. The patient is asked to abduct the arms and place the palm over the scalp while percussing the axillary and infra-axillary regions. While percussing the back of the chest the patient is asked to fold the arms across the chest, so as to bring the hand over the opposite shoulders. This results in the movement of the scapulae laterally. As the interscapular region is widened, a greater area of the lung is offered for percussion. Instead of percussion from above downwards on one side and then on the other side, the corresponding areas on either side are to be compared by moving backwards and forwards from one side to the other side of the chest.

Alteration in percussion note: The normal percussion note may alter, and it can exhibit impaired resonance, dull and flat, hyperresonance or tympanitic note in either direction. A dull short and non-musical note is elicited when the lung becomes airless (consolidation) or solid (tumour) or when there is compression of the lung from an elevated diaphragm or when the fluid has interposed between the lung and the chest wall (pleural effusion and empyema), and pleural thickening. In these situations, there is interference, either with the production, or transmission of the normal resonance. Dull note of consolidation is similar to the sound and feel of percussion over the heart. The flat note of fluid is similar to the dampened percussion note elicited over the shoulder or thigh. A lesser degree of dullness is referred to as an impaired note. It is encountered in collapse and fibrosis. A definite dull note is elicited over a consolidated lobe as the chest offers greater resistance for percussion (Woody dullness). In massive pleural effusion, there is absolute dullness and it is an extreme manifestation of dullness. It is referred to as flat note (stony dullness). The level of the dullness is highest in the axillary region from which it slopes down to the front and back (Ellis S-shaped curve, after Richard Ellis, a Scottish paediatrician). The presence of pleural fluid is difficult to detect unless it is more than 300 ml in volume.

When the normal resonant note becomes louder in its pitch it is referred to as hyperresonant note. The sound is well sustained and relatively intense. The chest is more vibrant. This occurs when the amount of air is greatly increased. Such a note is elicited over pneumothorax, emphysema, large peripheral cavity and over the gas filled stomach. In the latter situation, the note is musical and is of higher pitch than that of resonant note and is referred to as tympanic. Above the level of pleural effusion and consolidation, a hyper-resonant note of a boxy quality (drum-like) may be elicited. It arises from the relaxed lung still containing air, or from the lung showing compensatory emphysema (Skodiac resonance, described by Joseph Skoda, Czech born physician).

It is necessary to familiarize with different notes by percussing different parts of the body such as lung for normal resonance, lower abdomen for hyperresonance, liver for dullness and thigh for stony dullness.

Shifting dullness: The upper border of the dullness is horizontal in conditions of hydropneumothorax or pyopneumothorax, unlike pleural effusion, where it is highest in the axillary region. In the presence of air and fluid, the fluid can be made to shift its position by altering the position of the patient. It is demonstrated as follows: The upper border of the dullness is made out by percussing downwards either anteriorly or on the sides of the chest while the patient is sitting. Then the patient is asked to lie down on his back or on his sides without moving the pleximeter finger. The new position allows the fluid to move down and away from the chest wall. If the pleximeter finger is percussed now, a resonant note is elicited. Such a note is also elicited in the area which was originally dull for percussion.

Myoidema or myotatic irritability: When a light tap is given directly on the sternum, a transitory localized swelling appears due to the contraction of the unduly irritable pectoral muscles in conditions associated with cachexia.

Though percussion is diagnostic of many underlying pathologic conditions, the note may not show any change in lesions situated quite deeply (more than 5 cm) of size smaller than 2 cm in diameter. Normally, an alteration of the percussion note signifies an underlying abnormality. Still many diseases exist without any alteration in the percussion note.

Coin sound: In the presence of pneumothorax or a giant bulla, clear bell-like sounds are heard when the front of the chest is percussed with coins. The coin acts as pleximeter and plexor instead of the fingers. The examiner listens with the stethoscope at the back of the chest, while the coin (a rupee) placed on the front of the chest is struck with the edge of another coin. Normally,

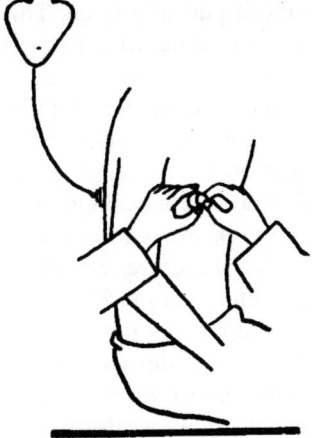

Fig. 26 Coin test.

a flat clicking sound is heard. The air-containing lung dampens the sound making its transmission poor (Fig. 26).

Auscultation

Auscultation refers to the act of listening to sounds produced within the body. It is accomplished by use of binaural stethoscope. It consists of a bell or diaphragm connected with rubber tubing to the metal frame ending in ear-pieces. This facilitates clear transmission of sounds from the patient to the ear of the examiner. The ear-pieces must fit properly and comfortably. Low-pitched sounds are better heard with the bell that is kept lightly on the skin and the high-pitched sounds on application of firm pressure from the diaphragm.

The Chest is Auscultated to Note.

the air entry,
the characteristics of breath sounds,
presence of additional (adventitious) sounds, and
the character of the vocal resonance

The chest piece of the stethoscope is to be applied accurately and firmly over the chest. It should not be allowed to move on the surface of the skin and too much pressure should not be applied. The patient must be relaxed and asked to breathe at a regular depth keeping the mouth partially open. The various regions of the chest are auscultated systematically from the apex downwards on either side, anteriorly and posteriorly, and compared. Identical regions on both sides must be compared. Upper lobes are examined by placing the chest piece in the infraclavicular and suprascapular regions; the lower lobes on the back in the region bounded by 7th and 10th ribs. Auscultation in the axilla gives an access to parts of all lobes. The topography of the segments offer a 'listening post'. The sounds produced by shivering, contact of hair on the chest wall, and movement of the chest pieces on the surface of the skin are likely to produce extraneous sounds and have to be excluded. The patient may be made to sit sideways so that he does not breathe or cough on the examiner's face.

Air entry: The air entry may be normal, decreased or absent. The normal air entry is appreciated by auscultation of various regions of the chest and is recognised by experience. The presence of breath sounds indicate ventilation of lung underlying the stethoscope. A local reduction in their intensity suggests decreased air entry to a particular lobe or segment. The sound transmission is also affected by pleural effusion or pneumothorax. The air entry is decreased in early stages of consolidation, collapse, fibrosis, thickened pleura, pleural effusion, pneumothorax and airway obstruction. Complete absence of air entry is noted in massive pleural effusion, pneumothorax and occlusion of a bronchus.

Mechanism of breath sounds: Breath sounds are closely related with the dynamic events of breathing. Normally, the airflow is turbulent in the glottis, trachea and main bronchi, lobar bronchi, and probably segmental bronchi. The turbulence is dependent on the flow rate of air. The flow rate is sufficient in the large airways. The velocity of airflow gets progressively diminished towards the periphery as the bronchi divide and subdivide. However it is still turbulent in the intermediate airways. Towards the periphery the gas stream splits into layers and forms vortices. The flow becomes laminar beyond the fifteenth generation of bronchi and it moves at a very slow velocity.

The breath sounds are likely to be produced only in the larger airways where the flow conditions are conducive for their oscillation. The breath sounds are continuous with no definite pitch. They exhibit random variation in amplitude. The sounds are produced in the upper airways, trachea and main bronchi by turbulent airflow, exhibiting rapid changes of gas pressure associated with random collision of gas molecules. The intermediate airways with their repeated branchings create turbulent eddies of gas flow and also contribute to the production of breath sounds. Small airways transmit sounds, but it is doubtful that breath sounds are produced in them. Since the airflow is slower in these smaller airways, they lack the necessary turbulence to produce sound.

Breath sounds over the upper respiratory tract contribute frequencies from 200 to 800 Hz and the lower respiratory tract from 200 to 400 Hz. At the trachea the breath sounds are harsh, loud and high-pitched, and are heard in both inspiration and expiration. The breath sounds audible over the chest have to pass through the lobar and segmental bronchi and across the peripheral airways, alveoli, pleura and chest wall. The lung behaves like a low-pass filter with a steep cut off of frequencies above 200 Hz. They allow low-pitched sounds to pass but filter higher pitched sounds. As the sound passes peripherally, the caliber of airways becomes too small for the transmission of the sound. The air-filled alveoli are poor transmitters of the sound. There is loss of sound and a change in its character.

The inspiratory sound is low-pitched and the expiratory sound high-pitched. After their passage through the peripheral airways and alveoli the breath sounds become soft and get attenuated and are confined to inspiration with a soft early expiratory component, as the high-pitched sounds are selectively filtered. Turbulence is generated during inspiration and it is carried towards the periphery. The flow rate falls during expiration. As there is a difference in the flow rate at different regions of the lung, the intensity of breath sounds exhibits variation. At the apex of the lung in the upright position the breath sounds are more intense at the beginning of inspiration, whereas at the base during the middle of inspiration. The most peripheral airways and alveoli do not contribute anything for the production of breath sounds.

While listening to the breath sounds, their intensity (loud or soft), quality (rustling, breezy, tubular), duration and pitch (frequency) of inspiration and expiration (high or low) relative to one another are looked into.

The normal breath sounds heard over a normal lung vary a great deal in their intensity. The intensity (amplitude) of breath sounds on the chest depends on the flow variations in the underlying lobar and segmental bronchi, and the transmitting properties of the lung and the chest wall. When a segment or a lobe of the lung becomes solid from consolidation the tracheal (or laryngeal) breath sounds are heard as bronchial breathing, since the higher frequencies are transmitted through the patent bronchi without any change in their character. The sounds will have the same quality as those heard over the trachea. The transmission of sounds from the trachea is affected when the bronchus is occluded, leading to breath sounds not being heard. Breath sounds are also absent over a pleural effusion, or pneumothorax as the fluid, or air in the pleural cavity forms relatively complete acoustic barrier and sounds get attenuated or absent at the pleural surface. In widespread airways obstruction due to chronic bronchitis and emphysema, the breath sounds are faint. It is due to regional differences in the flow rate and the filter effect at the pleural surface. The loss of elastic recoil of the lung makes the expiration prolonged.

Breath Sounds

Vesicular breath sounds: The normal breath sounds (vesicular) are heard over the chest as a breezy rustling sound, indicating the penetration of the air into the normal lung tissue and its expulsion. The inspiratory phase is fairly intense, longer and of high-pitch (Fig. 27). The expiratory phase is shorter with its length being equal to a third of the length of inspiration. The inspiration is harsher than the expiration. Its intensity is greater than that of expiration. There is no gap between the inspiration and the expiration. Vesicular breath sounds are heard over the greater part of the normal lung, except over the trachea and the region where major

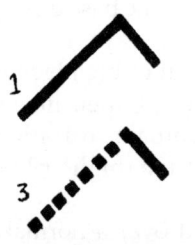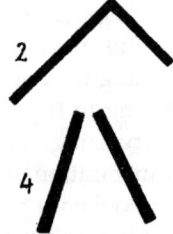

Fig. 27 Breath sounds:
(1) vesicular   (2) bronchovesicular
(3) cog-wheel   (4) bronchial.

bronchi are situated near the surface of the chest wall. The term 'vesicular' is a misnomer since no sound is generated within the alveoli. It is preferable to call as 'normal breathing' (breath sounds).

Points to be noted on Auscultation of the Chest.

Breath sounds
    Vesicular
    Bronchovesicular
    Bronchial
        Tubular
        Cavernous
        Amphoric
Adventitious sounds
    Wheezes
    Crackles
    Stridor
    Pleural rub
Vocal resonance
    Whispering pectoriloquy
    Bronchophony
    Aegophony

Disease states can alter either generation or the transmission of breath sounds or both. They affect one or more of these characteristics of breath sounds.

The vesicular breath sounds are diminished in their intensity (amplitude) from interference of sounds transmission to the periphery or from low flow rate. There is decreased transmission of breath sounds due to bronchial obstruction of a main stem bronchus (mucus plugs, foreign bodies or neoplasm) or by fluid (pleural effusion, empyema, haemothorax) or air (pneumothorax) in the pleural space. The breath sounds are diminished in their intensity in pleurisy, thickened pleura, bronchopneumonia, collapse, fibrosis, emphysema, and are absent in pneumothorax, thickened pleura, hydropneumothorax and massive pleural effusion. A low flow rate seen in hypoventilation of central nervous system or muscular disease is associated with diminished breath sounds. Breath sounds are absent in surgical or congenital absence of the lung. The sounds may be heard with a greater intensity in situations of hyperventilation (increased gas flow rates) or from processes that interfere with the sound filtering ability of the alveoli (lobar pneumonia).

Cog-wheel breathing: In children the breath sounds are harsher than in adults (puerile breathing). In nervous individuals and in conditions of pleural adhesions, the breath sounds, instead of being steady, appear jerky and the inspiratory phase appears broken (cog-wheel breathing). The expiratory phase is prolonged in asthma and emphysema. The pitch of breath sounds is altered, by diseases that modify the filtering capability of the alveoli.

Bronchial breath sounds: The passage of air through the larynx, trachea and major bronchi result in the laryngeal (tracheal or bronchial) breath sounds. The presence of such sounds over the chest speaks of the underlying pathologic lesion. Bronchial breath sounds are heard when the normal dampening effect of the air-containing alveoli is lost. The sounds are transmitted through the solidified lung without any change (for example, consolidation). Airless upper lobes irrespective of bronchial patency transmit the bronchial sounds as their mediastinal surface is in contact with the trachea. As such a direct path of transmission exists to the lower lobes and the sounds reach only if the bronchus is patent. The existence of bronchial breathing can be appreciated easily if one listens over the trachea and makes a comparison of the sound. The tracheal breathing is louder and of a lower pitch than bronchial breathing.

The bronchial breath sounds show great variation from normal breathing and they are loud, harsh, high-pitched and snorting type of sounds. The duration of expiration is as long or longer than that of inspiration and the pitch of the expiratory sound is high or higher than that of inspiration, and it has a more sibilant (hissing) character than the inspiratory one. There is a short silent gap between inspiration and expiration, as the inspiratory sound becomes inaudible shortly before the end of inspiration.

Type of bronchial breath sounds: The quality of the sound may be hollow or tubular. The breathing may be high-pitched or low-pitched. It is referred to as tubular breathing when the pitch is high and is heard over an area of consolidation of the lung as in lobar pneumonia. Consolidated lung transmits sounds better than aerated and ventilated lung. It is referred to as cavernous breathing when its pitch is low and is heard over cavities. Amphoric breath sound is a variant of bronchial breathing and can be mimicked by blowing across the mouth of a jar. A number of high-pitched sounds overlap the fundamental low-pitched sounds. Amphoric breathing has a hollow reverberatory quality. It may be audible over an open pneumothorax and over a large thin-walled cavity communicating with a bronchus as the laryngeal sounds are conducted through the resonating chamber of space.

Bronchovesicular breath sounds: An intermediate type of breathing referred to as bronchovesicular breathing having features of both vesicular and bronchial breathing may be heard. The inspiratory phase is similar to that heard in vesicular breathing. The length and pitch of the expiratory phase is similar to that of bronchial breathing. There is a short gap between inspiration and expiration. Such breathing is heard over the right second space anteriorly and over the right interscapular region, where the trachea and bronchi come near the surface. It is heard over the lung in early stages of consolidation, asthma and emphysema. Breath sounds are soften and more difficult to hear in diffuse airways obstruction. The duration of expiration is prolonged to a variable degree.

Adventitious (Added) Sounds

Adventitious sounds are sounds audible in disease but not present in the normal person. Their presence is usually a sign of disease. They are superimposed on the breath sounds that may be normal or abnormal. The adventitious sounds are louder than underlying breath sounds. They may arise in the lung or in the pleura. Those arising from the lungs are broadly classified as rhonchi (wheeze, continuous sounds), and crackles (crepitations, rales, discontinuous or interrupted sounds). Pleural rub arises from the pleura.

Rhonchi or Wheezes

Rhonchi or wheezes are continuous, dry, musical sounds produced by an acoustic mechanism similar to that of a simple uncoupled oscillating reed or violin. The airways narrowed to the point of closure, make their opposing walls to come in close contact, and oscillate like a reed of a musical instrument. The walls are set in oscillation by the turbulent air flow within their lumen. The gas flow velocity increases as the airway is narrowed.

Commonly the physical conditions required to produce wheeze are unstable. The bronchi are narrowed by contraction of bronchial smooth muscles, by oedema of the mucosa or by viscid secretions in their lumen. Narrowing is also due to dynamic compression. Rhonchi are more conspicuous during expiration, than inspiration, as the bronchi are further narrowed during that phase. It reflects the oscillation of airway walls that occurs when there is airflow limitation, or intralumnal obstruction of airway.

Wheezes are characteristic of widespread air flow limitation (bronchitis and asthma) and are heard bilaterally over the chest. They may be palpable as rhonchial fremitus. They may be inspiratory or expiratory, short or long, single or multiple. They vary frequently in intensity and character from time to time and may disappear totally. Rhonchi are bipolar in origin and the sound is produced as air makes its entry and exit through the area of obstruction. Paradoxically, the wheeze may be absent in severe widespread air flow obstruction as the minimal airflow fails to oscillate the airways to the point of closure. The pitch is determined by the tightness of the closure, and by the mechanical properties of the solid structures set into vibration.

Rhonchi may be high—or low-pitched, depending upon the rate of flow past the obstruction and the mass of the obstructed bronchus. It was believed that obstruction of smaller bronchi results in high-pitched rhonchi as whistling or squeaking sounds (sibilant rhonchi). Those arising from the obstruction of larger bronchi are low-pitched and have a snoring quality (sonorous). The pitch may rise and fall during the respiratory cycle in parallel with variations in the tightness of compression. Simultaneous onset (polyphonic, polyphasic) wheezes are noted in bronchial asthma. Tight expiratory dynamic compression in asthma is associated with a high-pitched wheeze. They are heard easily over the trachea.

A wheeze is transmitted widely with varying relative intensity to different points on the chest wall. They may be inspiratory, expiratory or both, with the component notes beginning and ending at different times. Polyphasic wheezing is encountered in narrowing of many small airways. A wheeze in those cases is confined to expiration where successive harmonically unrelated musical notes begin and end simultaneously. They are produced by dynamic compression of the central bronchi.

Rhonchi may be heard over a localized area on the chest due to a localized obstruction of airway. Bronchi can be narrowed by a plug of mucus, intrabronchial tumour, foreign body, or cicatricial stenosis. There can be pressure on bronchi from glands or growth. These are referred to as low-pitched monophasic (single musical notes) fixed wheezes. Often they are audible in inspiration. They do not alter at site or timing even after coughing.

Stridor

A loud musical sound of constant pitch is called stridor and is heard in laryngeal or in tracheal obstruction (a narrowed upper airway). The term should not be confused with noisy breathing. The pitch is lower than that of a wheeze, and is jerky and it is as loud in inspiration as in expiration. The crowing sounds are accompanied by supraclavicular inspiratory retraction.

Crackles (Crepitations, Rales)

Crackles are discontinuous, interrupted explosive, non-musical crackling or bubbling sounds produced in the proximal and distal airways or sometimes in the cavities. These added sounds are thought to result from the sudden reopening of a succession of small airways. Energy for their generation is developed by an increased pressure gradient across the closed segment or by traction on the segment by the expanding lung. Their intensity is related to the size of the opening airways. They may be heard in either phases of respiratory cycles. These sounds have a wide spectrum of frequencies between 300 and 2000 Hz. They may be fine or coarse, high-pitched or low-pitched, faint or loud, scanty or profuse, and regular or irregular. Crepitations are also produced by bubbling of air through secretions in the larger airways.

Fine crackles: They are also referred to as fine crepitations, fine rales or fine Velcro-like sounds. They are most often heard during inspiration. However, they are also accompanied by expiratory crackles. Fine crackles are soft, high-pitched and have a shorter duration than coarse crackles. These sounds can be simulated by rubbing a lock of hair between the thumb and the finger close to the ear. They may be heard either in the early or late inspiratory phase of respiration.

Early inspiratory crackles are characteristically heard in conditions of diffuse airflow limitation due to chronic bronchitis, emphysema or bronchiectasis. They are attributed to early opening of proximal and larger airways, prematurely closed during previous expiration. The number of crackles are few and they do not repeat the same pattern from breath to breath. They are cleared or changed dramatically after coughing. They are transmitted to the mouth, and are audible at the open mouth.

Late inspiratory crackles originate in the peripheral airways. They are profuse in number and are not transmitted to the mouth. They begin in mid-inspiration and continue to the end of inspiration and are characteristically heard in restrictive lung diseases (interstitial pulmonary fibrosis, idiopathic pulmonary fibrosis, pulmonary oedema, congestive heart failure) and consolidation. In interstitial fibrosis, crackles are profuse at the lung bases in the upright posture and become less prominent or absent on bending forwards when lung bases are not dependent. In restrictive lung diseases, the peripheral airways close early in expiration and do not open until the next inspiration. The crackles coincide with the late opening of the peripheral airways. They do not alter from breath to breath but appear in the same sequence. They are not transmitted to the mouth. They are not altered by coughing or by deep breath.

Coarse crackles: They are low-pitched and loud adventitious sounds. They appear ?s bubbling sounds. They arise in bronchiectasis from the bubbling of respired air through the retained secretions in bronchi of various sizes or in the cavities from bursting of small or large air bubbles or during the resolution stage of pneumonia. They begin early in inspiration, and continue to mid-inspiratory phase and then fade, and again they are heard in expiration. The site of origin is proximal airways. They may vary from breath to breath and get modified by coughing.

Post-tussive crackles: Crackles may be made audible or intensified on taking a deep inspiration after coughing and they are known as post-tussive (latent) crepitations. They are heard over minimal lesions of tuberculosis or cavities.

Pleural Rub

Normally the visceral and parietal pleura glide over one another during respiration without producing any sound.

The inflamed and roughened pleural surfaces due to pleurisy, rub against each other during respiration, to produce the pleural rub. It is heard in both phases of respiration, each time in the same part or phase of the respiratory cycle, as a superficial to-and-fro grating type of sound and is heard close to the ear. It may be coarse or fine. It is a low-pitched, repeatedly interrupted sound like leather surfaces creaking together. A similar sound can be produced, by holding the thumb and forefinger near the ear and rubbing them against each other with force. On application of firm pressure by the stethoscope over the affected region, the sound is heard with greater intensity. This does not happen in the case of crepitations. Pleural rub is heard frequently over the axilla and inflammatory region as the movement of the pleura is maximum in those regions. Sometimes the rib is heard over a widespread area. It does not alter on coughing unlike crepitations. It disappears on holding the breath. The rub can be felt over the affected area and there may be local tenderness. The breath sounds are not audible clearly in that region.

When the pleural rub has developed along the edge of the left lung in close contact with the heart, it assumes the rhythm of cardiac pulsations. It is called pleuropericardial rub. However, it disappears on holding the breath unlike a pericardial rub.

Succussion Splash (Hippocratic Succussion)

A splashing sound is heard over the chest in cases of hydro or pyopneumonthorax while the chest is jerked to-and-fro. The stethoscope is placed near the interface of fluid and air, determined by percussion and the patient is shaken suddenly. It mimicks the sound heard when a coconut is shaken. The splashing sound can also be heard in conditions of herniation of the stomach or of the intestine, into the thorax through the diaphragm and over a large cavity containing fluid and air in the lung. A splashing sound may be heard after meals due to the presence of fluid and air in the stomach, and in gastric outlet obstruction.

Clicking Sounds

A loud crunching or a clicking sound usually to the left of the sternum synchronous with the cardiac sound and audible even when the breath is held, may occur in mediastinal emphysema or a shallow pneumothorax (Hamman's sign, named after Louis Hamman, a US physician) on the left side. In the latter condition, the sounds are often louder at the expiration and when the patient leans over to the left. The sounds are produced either by the impact of cardia on the mediastinal surface of the lung, or by sudden displacement of trapped air in the mediastinal pleura by the direct impact on the heart. Occasionally such a clicking sound may occur due to the heart beat causing a wave in a small effusion complicating a pneumothorax. Sometimes there is an inefficient junction between the cartilage of the eight or ninth rib and the costal margins. Rarely trauma or pregnancy may cause slipping of such a displaced costal cartilage and produce a painful clicking sound. The sound may be induced by breathing or movement.

Post-tussive Suction

A sucking noise is sometimes heard immediately after coughing over a cavity in the lung. In these instances the walls of the cavity are not rigid, but are thin walled and collapsible and communicate with a bronchus. The sound is produced by the rush of air into the cavity, from which the air has been expelled by coughing.

Vocal Resonance

The voice sounds can be heard over the chest. The low frequency sounds up to 200 Hz are transmitted while those above 200 Hz are attenuated. Hence the speech is heard as a low-pitched rumble and indistinct, and an attempt is made to note the intensity and character of the vocal resonance. The patient is asked to repeat the words 'one', 'two' or 'ninety-nine' again and again. The chest is listened to and the sounds are compared over corresponding areas on either side from above downwards in front and back. Normally the sounds are heard indistinctly. The intensity depends on the loudness and depth of the voice of the patient, and on the conductivity of the lungs. Vocal resonance of normal intensity gives an impression of its production at the chest-piece of a stethoscope. Vocal resonance enables one to hear the high-pitched resonant sounds by the stethoscope which are not easily palpable. Vocal resonance varies in a similar way as the vocal fremitus.

The vocal resonance is increased when the sounds appear louder than normal and nearer to the ear, than to the chest-piece of a stethoscope. It is encountered over areas of consolidation, superficial cavity, tumours and collapsed upper lobe with displacement of the trachea to that side. It is decreased in collapse, pleural effusion, pneumothorax, thickened pleura and overinflated chest.

If the transmitted voice is heard with greater intensity simulating the voice heard over the trachea or bronchi coming near the surface at the interscapular region and the right apex, it is referred to as bronchophony and generally it exists together with bronchial breathing. When spoken words are clearly audible, it is referred to as spoken pectoriloquy. It gives an impression that the voice is nearer to the ear and spoken right into the listener's ears. This is considered an extreme degree of increased vocal resonance. In such instances the patient is asked to whisper the words and the chest is listened to. The syllables of the whispered sounds, if distinctly heard, are called 'whispering pectoriloquy'. Here the abducted vocal cords do not oscillate and voice sounds are produced by a turbulent flow of air through the trachea, glottis and pharynx. They are high-pitched, and may be heard over an area of consolidation, over a big cavity communicating with a patent bronchus, and at the upper border of a pleural effusion. Whispering pectoriloquy may be present over the spine in the interscapular region indicating enlargement of lymph nodes (D'Espine's sign, after Adolfe D'Espine, a French physician).

The spoken voice on auscultation, when it exhibits a high-pitched nasal quality resembling a jerky bleating of a goat, is called aegophony (goat voice). It is due to a selective transmission of high-pitched voice sounds. When the patient says 'eeee', it is audible over an area of compressed lung tissue above the level of a pleural effusion, or, in some cases over an area of consolidation, where the low-pitched sounds are intercepted.

Physical Signs of Various Pathologic Conditions Affecting the Respiratory System.

Consolidation: Diminished movements of the chest on the affected side, increased VF, dullness, tubular breathing, crackles, increased VR, bronchophony and whispering pectoriloquy and egophony, no shift of the trachea and apical impulse (for example, lobar pneumonia).

Collapse: Diminished movement of the chest on the affected side with shift of the trachea and apical impulse towards it, decreased VF, impaired or dull percussion note, decreased VR, diminished or absent breath sounds, no adventitious sounds (for example, obstruction to a major bronchus).

Fibrosis: Diminished movements and flattening of the chest on the affected side with shift of the trachea and apical impulse towards it, normal or increased VF, impaired or dull percussion note, bronchial breathing, coarse crepitations, normal or increased VR.

Pleural effusion: Diminished movements with prominence of the intercostal spaces on the affected side, and shift of the apical impulse and trachea to the opposite side, diminished or absent VF, stony dull (flat) percussion note rising in the axilla, diminished or absent VR, absence of breath sounds, sometimes presence of a pleural rub (for example, tuberculosis, pneumonia, pulmonary infarction, malignancy of the lung).

Pneumothorax: Diminished movements with prominence of the intercostal spaces on the affected side with shift of the trachea and apical impulse to the opposite side, diminished of absent VF, hyperresonant percussion note, positive coin test, diminished or absent VR, absence of breath sounds, sometimes presence of amphoric breath sounds (tuberculosis, rupture of emphysematous bulla).

Hydropneumothorax: Diminished movements with prominence of the intercostal spaces, on the affected side with shift of the trachea and apical impulse to the opposite side, diminished or absent VF, percussion note dull below with horizontal upper limit and hyperresonance above, presence of shifting dullness, positive coin test, decreased or absent VR, absence of breath sounds, sometimes presence of amphoric breath sounds, and presence of succussion splash.

Cavity (large communicating): Diminished movements of the chest, increased VF, impaired, dull, hyperresonant or cracked pot resonance on percussion, absence of shift of the trachea and apical impulse, bronchial or cavernous breathing, post-tussive suction, crepitations and increased VR.

Overinflated chest (emphysema, during attacks of asthma): Bilateral signs, overinflated chest assuming a barrel shape, diminished expansion of the chest being held in a state of inspiration, indrawing of lower anterior ribs, Hoover's sign, accessory muscles of respiration active, trachea in the center, diminished VF, hyperresonant note with obliteration of the cardiac and liver dullness, decreased VR, wheezing present, distantly audible heart sounds.

Bronchitis: Diminished movements of the chest bilaterally, no shift of the trachea or apical impulse, no alteration in the percussion note, prolonged expiration, high-pitched rhonchi and coarse crackles.

Interstitial lung disease: diminished movements of the chest, resonant chest, normal VF and VR, vesicular breath sounds, crackles that vary with posture.

SEVEN

CARDIOVASCULAR SYSTEM

> *"Of all the ailments which blow out life's little candle, heart disease is the chief"*
>
> *William Boyd*

Anatomy

The examination of the cardiovascular system includes the examination of the cardia, peripheral arterial and venous systems.

The heart is situated obliquely in the chest, and two-thirds of it lies to the left of the midline. The right ventricle forms a greater portion of the front of the heart and its inferior margin forms the lower border of the heart, which extends from the lateral border of the sternum at the level of the seventh costal cartilage to the apex. The left ventricle is seen as a narrow strip in the front and it forms the apex. The left border extends from the apex to the left second intercostal space within the parasternal line. A greater part of the atrium is situated posteriorly, and the left auricular appendage reaches the highest point in the thorax and is situated behind the second intercostal space. The right atrium is present on the right side forming the right cardiac border. The boundary can be drawn in the form of a curved line joining the points on the right lateral border of the sternum at the levels of union of the third and seventh costal cartilages. The anterior aspect of the chest overlying the cardia is referred to as the precordium.

The important bony landmarks and the imaginary vertical lines have been referred to in the examination of the respiratory system. Before the actual examination of the cardia, the pulse, blood pressure and neck veins are to be examined.

Arterial Pulse

A pulse is felt by compressing an artery against a bone. Normally the pulse is felt in the radial artery at the wrist with the tips of the ring, middle and index fingers placed in that order. The forearm is kept pronated and the wrist slightly flexed (For routine purposes it is sufficient to feel the radial pulse on one side). In cardiovascular disorders the radial, dorsalis pedis and the carotid pulsations should be felt and compared on both sides to confirm symmetry.

Symmetry: The carotid pulse should be felt in all neurologic conditions. The common site of occlusion is the beginning of the internal carotid artery. The occlusion may occur by arteriosclerosis or arteritis. Impairment of one or both carotid pulsations may arise from aortic arch syndrome, dissecting aneurysm of the aorta and from aortic intimal thickening seen in supravalvular aortic stenosis. As it is difficult to define the carotid pulse in those situations, it should be auscultated for the presence of systolic bruit. Its presence indicates an incomplete occlusion of the artery.

The pulse may be unequal on either side of the upper limbs

Inequality of Pulse on Either Side of the Upper Limbs.

Aberrant course of the arteries
Aortic aneurysm
Aortic arch syndrome
Proximal coarctation
Dissecting aneurysm
Tumours pressing on the vessels
Cervical rib
Sclaenus anticus syndrome
Supravalvular aortic stenosis
Thromboembolic phenomenon

Normally the femoral pulses occur slightly earlier than the radial pulses. The pulse may be felt normally in the upper limb, and it is feeble and delayed in the lower limbs, and in situations such as coarctation of the aorta, dissecting aneurysm, and thromboembolism. The arterial occlusion leads to a diminution or absence of the pulsation in the limbs. The level of the obstruction in the arteries can be ascertained by feeling the pulsations at the proximal sites in the course of the artery as follows.

Location of Sites to Feel Arterial Pulsations.

Arteries	sites where pulsations are felt
brachial	just above the elbow held in hyperextension
common carotid and external carotid	in the neck medial to the sternomastoid,
temporal	in front of the ear
abdominal aorta	in the epigastric region
femoral	at the inguinal ligament
popliteal	in the popliteal fossa with knee kept flexed
posterior tibial	1 cm behind the medial malleolus
dorsalis pedis	on the dorsum of the foot on either side

While examining the pulse the following features are observed (Fig. 28 and 29):

rate,
rhythm,
quality (volume and form),
the condition of the vessel wall and
presence or absence of radiofemoral delay

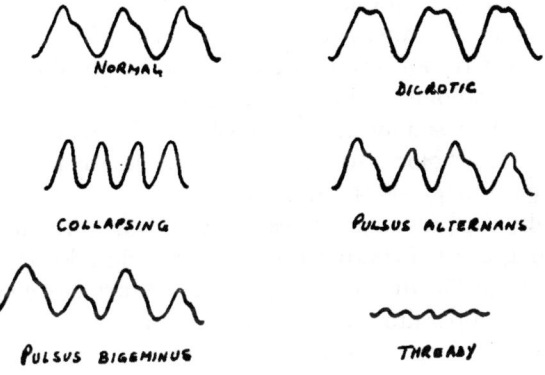

Fig. 28   Arterial pulse waves.

Rate: The normal resting pulse rate varies from 70 to 80 per minute. The rate is variable in the same individual under different circumstances. Normally the pulse is counted for a minute and expressed as beats per minute. The counting of the pulse is not done as soon as the examination is begun. Nervousness increases the pulse rate. Hence the counting is done only when the initial nervousness is over.

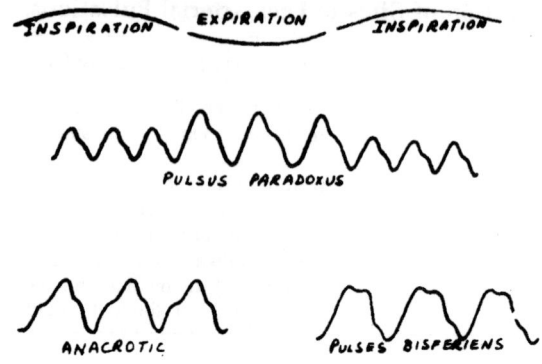

Fig. 29 Arterial pulse waves.

Tachycardia: The pulse rate is increased (tachycardia) during and immediately after exercise, anxiety, nervousness, in febrile conditions, thyrotoxicosis, anaemia, after haemorrhage, hypovolaemia, peripheral circulatory failure, cardiac failure, myocarditis, acidotic states, paroxysmal supraventricular tachycardia, ventricular tachycardia, atrial fibrillation, atrial flutter and ventricular tachycardia.

Bradycardia: The rate, when slow with a rate less than 60 per minute is referred to as bradycardia. It may be physiologic as in athletes or pathologic as in myxoedema, obstructive jaundice, digoxin toxicity, raised intracranial tension with vagal stimulation and complete heart block. Young children and elderly persons may have high or slow pulse rate respectively.

Normally the pulse rate increases by 10 beats per minute for every half degree rise in body temperature (centigrade). It is called relative bradycardia when the rise in pulse is much less compared to the rise of temperature. It is noted in the first week of enteric fever, influenza, Dengue fever and meningococcal meningitis.

Pulse deficit: When the pulse is irregular, not all beats may be transmitted to the wrist. In atrial fibrillation, there is a difference between the pulse and the heart rate. It is because some of the ventricular contractions are too weak to generate sufficient pressure to open the aortic valves or to initiate a pulse wave in the aorta. The heart rate is high when compared to that of the pulse rate. The heart rate should be counted by auscultation at the apex. The pulse rate if less than (more than 10 beats) that of the heart rate is referred to as pulse deficit. A similar situation may be noted in multiple premature contractions of ectopic origin.

Atrial Fibrillation.

Irregularly irregular pulse
Irregular volume
Pulse deficit
Varying intensity S_1
Absence of 'a' waves in the neck

Rhythm: The rhythm of the pulse has to be described as regular or irregular. If it is irregular whether it is regularly or irregularly irregular. Normally the pulse is felt in a rhythmical manner; it comes on regularly at constant intervals.

Arrhythmia: In sinus arrhythmia, the pulse quickens during inspiration and slows down during expiration. It is commonly noted in children and young adults. It may be demonstrated in them on taking a deep breath. In atrial fibrillation, the pulse is irregularly irregular without any dominant rhythm. The force is irregular wherein the length of the preceding pause does not give guidance to the strength of the succeeding beat. A weak beat may follow a long pause and *vice versa*.

In premature contractions arising in the atria, AV node or ventricle (often referred to as extra systoles) the irregularity may appear at regular or irregular intervals, on a regular pulse rhythm. The extra beats occur prematurely and are weaker than normal ones. It is followed by a longer pause before the next normal impulse. Sometimes the extra systoles are too weak to produce a wave, thus resulting in an impression of a dropped beat. When the rate is slow, extra systoles are recognized by the presence of a small pulse followed by a long pause and then a big pulse.

In intermittent heart block the beats are dropped occasionally in an otherwise regular rhythm. There is no sequence like small beat then a wide pause followed by a large strong beat. The premature beats can be made to diminish or disappear by exercise unlike in atrial fibrillation where the irregularity persists. In the presence of a cardiac disease, exercise is not allowed to verify this finding.

Pulsus bigeminus: The pulse is referred to as *pulsus bigeminus* (bigeminal pulse) when two beats come in couples. Bigeminal rhythm is caused by alternating normal and premature contractions, that result in their alternate strong and weak beats. The second beat appears weaker, and is followed by a pause. The rhythm is not regular. It is noted in partial heart block, digitalis, quinidine and beta-adrenergic blockers toxicity. *Pulsus trigeminus* refers to a regular repetition of three beats followed by a pause, and *pulsus quadrigeminus* refers to a regular repetition of four beats followed by a pause.

Quality (Volume): The blood is pumped into the aorta by the left ventricle under pressure and it causes distension of the ascending aorta. The pressure is transmitted as a wave over the entire circulatory system. The amplitude of the movement of the vessel wall during the passage of the pulse wave is referred to as the volume and it gives an idea about the pulse pressure that is dependent on the stroke volume and the compliance of the arteries. Normally carotid pulsation is not visible. However, a large volume pulse causes pulsation in the neck (Corrigan's sign). Aneurysm or kinking of carotid artery makes the carotid pulsation visible. Arterial pulsations are graded 0-4 with grade 3 representing the magnitude of the normal pulsation.

The volume of the pulse is large (grade 4) in hyperdynamic circulatory states as they are associated with an increased stroke volume, and peripheral vasodilatation and in aortic regurgitation. Hypertension is also associated with a big volume pulse. The volume of the pulse is low (grade 1 and 2) in conditions of diminished stroke output (cardiac failure, shock, mitral stenosis, aortic stenosis). Low volume pulse is also encountered in pericardial effusion, constrictive pericarditis, pulmonary stenosis, and obstructive cardiomyopathy. The local arterial obstruction causes diminution of the volume of the pulse in one limb. The volume of pulse is diminished in lower limbs than in the upper in coarctation of the aorta or peripheral atherosclerosis. Further the pulse is also delayed as it is transmitted to the lower limbs *via* the collateral vessels (radio-femoral delay). The volume of the pulse is irregular in atrial fibrillation in addition to its irregularity in rhythm.

Character: The form (shape) of the pulse wave can be recorded graphically. It can be recognized easily by palpating a large vessel like the carotid artery. It is the pulse very near to the heart and it is least subjected to damping or distortion in the arterial tree. Carotid pulses should not felt simultaneously. The right carotid should be felt with the left thumb and the left carotid with the right thumb. The thumb has to be pressed backwards at the medial border of the sternomastoid muscle at the level of the thyroid cartilage. The character of the pulse wave has great diagnostic significance as it gives a rough indication of stroke volume. Normally the pulse wave has a smooth quick upstroke, a momentary summit and a smooth quick down stroke.

Collapsing pulse: In aortic regurgitation, severe mitral regurgitation, hypertrophic obstructive cardiomyopathy (idiopathic hypertrophic subaortic stenosis), patent ductus arteriosus, rupture of sinus of Valsalva, aquired arteriovenous fistula, and hyperdynamic circulatory states such as anaemia, and thyrotoxicosis, there is a rapid or quick rise and fall with a momentary peak. The rapid upstroke is due to a large stroke volume vigorously ejected and the fall is due to regurgitation of blood back into the left ventricle during early diastole and to decreased systemic vascular resistance. This is referred to as a 'waterhammer' pulse (collapsing pulse). It is appreciated when the arm of the patient is raised above the level of the head. The flexor surface of the wrist held by the palm of the hand with the fingers encircling it. The pulse is felt with the palm. 'Waterhammer' is a hermetically sealed glass tube containing water in a vacuum. When it is inverted the water falls down quickly giving a knock to the hand. The collapsing pulse gives a similar sensation. Large volume pulse is apparent as pulsation of the neck in patients with significant aortic regurgitation (AR, Corrigan's sign). Advanced AR may produce an up-and-down bobbing of the head ('yes-yes' sign) with each heart beat. A large volume pulse may not be collapsing and it is noted in bradycardia requiring a large stroke volume.

Significance of Arterial Pulse.

Abnormal pulse	clinical significance
Pulsus bisferience	aortic stenosis and aortic regurgitation
Pulsus alternans	left ventricular systolic dysfunction
Pulsus paradoxus	constrictive pericarditis, cardiac tamponade
Collapsing pulse	aortic regurgitation
Pulsus parvus et tardus	severe aortic valvular stenosis

Pulsus parvus et tardus: In aortic valve stenosis, there is a slow upstroke due to slow ejection of blood from the left ventricle and a downstroke. The upstroke may be associated with a notch (anacrotic pulse). The peak appears sustained (plateau pulse). The pulse is of small volume. It is referred to as pulsus parvus or pulsus tardus. It is identified by palpating the carotid pulse.

Pulsus bisferiens: Pulsus bisferiens is characterized by two systolic peaks. The first peak is due to the transmission of the left ventricular pressure in early systole (systolic or percussion wave), and the second peak is due to a recoil of the vascular bed (tidal wave). Though the latter occurs normally in diastole as dicrotic wave, the tidal wave occurs in late diastole when the left ventricle empties rapidly or is obstructed from emptying completely. There is a slow upstroke and a collapsing pulse giving a feel of double humps (double systolic impulse). It is felt best in the carotid artery, and is diagnostic of aortic stenosis and aortic regurgitation, hypertrophic obstructive cardiomyopathy, and some cases of aortic regurgitation.

Pulsus alternans: The successive beats of the ventricle may be strong and weak in an alternating manner. This occurs from an alternate strong and weak ventricular contraction of left ventricular myocardium. The premature beats are generally weak. The rhythm is regular. The varying amplitude of the alternate pulses is appreciated best in the femoral artery and is referred to as pulsus alternans (alternating pulse).

Though the beats occur in regular succession, the low volume pulse is separated from the succeeding high volume pulse by a shorter interval compared to that of the preceding high pulse. Pulsus alternans is one of the earliest and most subtle signs of left ventricular systolic dysfunction (and a reduced ejection fraction). It is seen in patients with hypertensive heart disease, coronary artery disease, aortic valvular disease and dilated cardiomyopathy. In such a situation, all the fibres of the myocardium are incapable of contracting during each heart beat. Rarely the condition may be noted in paroxysmal tachycardia without any defect in myocardium. Often it is palpated transiently after premature ventricular contractions and may be sustained when there is significant LV systolic dysfunction. Pulsus alternans may be brought out or accentuated in the sitting or upright position (due to a decrease in venous return). The patient should hold his breath so that respiration has no effect on pulse volume. The suspicion of this type of pulse is confirmed by a sphygmomanometer as the condition is associated with an alteration in the intensity of the heart sounds (cardiac alternans).

In pulsus alternans, when the arm cuff pressure is raised above systolic pressure level and then deflated very slowly, the sounds are heard in a regular fashion and their rate is half the number of beats felt at the radial artery as the alternate strong beats are only audible. On further deflation of the cuff, the sounds double in their number as the weaker beats also are heard. In milder cases, as the cuff pressure is decreased slowly at the systolic pressure level, all sound are heard distal to the cuff, but they alternate in their intensity. The systolic blood pressure may vary from beat to beat.

Pulsus paradoxus: Normally there is some decline in the systolic pressure (5 to 10 mm Hg), or pulse volume with inspiration due to a diminished left ventricular stroke output and the transmission of the negative decreased intrathoracic pressure to the great vessels. There is an exaggerated inspiratory fall (>10 mm Hg) in systolic pressure during quiet breathing in pulsus paradoxus. The term paradoxical pulse is a misnomer because it is an exaggeration of a normal phenomenon. There is decrease in pulse amplitude or disappearance of pulse on inspiration.

Pulsus paradoxus is an exaggeration of the normal respiratory variation in the arterial pulse. Inspiration prevents the heart filling by splinting it between expanding lungs and within the pericardium. There is an increased systemic venous return and increased right ventricular volume. It causes an impediment to left ventricular filling, hence fall in the left ventricular stroke volume at the height of inspiration from the increased intra-pericardial pressure. There can also be pooling of blood in the dilated pulmonary veins causing reduction in the flow of blood into the left atrium. While examining for a pulsus paradoxus, the patient should breathe as normally as possible and should not be made to breathe deeply. If the pulse can be felt to wane with inspiration in all accessible arteries, and if the cardiac rhythm is regular, then a paradoxical pulse is said to be present. It is noted in pericardial effusion, chronic constrictive pericarditis, cardiac tamponade, severe asthma, COPD, mediastinal tumour, tracheal obstruction and occasionally in restrictive cardiomyopathy, endocardial fibrosis, pulmonary embolism and hypovolumic cardiac failure.

As a paradoxus, the heart sounds are audible over the precordial region at a time when radial pulse is not felt. It indicates cardiac tamponade in massive pericardial effusion. The inspiratory fall of blood pressure in pulsus paradoxus can be quantified using a sphygmomanometer. The blood pressure cuff is inflated until no sounds are audible through the stethoscope over the brachial artery, and then it is slowly deflated until sounds are heard in expiration only. The deflation is continued further until the sounds are heard throughout the respiratory cycle. The pulsus paradoxus is considered present, if the difference between these two pressure levels exceeds 10 mm Hg. A reversed pulsus paradoxus refers to a rise in arterial systolic and diastolic pressure during inspiration. It is noted in patients with congenital subaortic stenosis and in those receiving intermittent positive pressure breathing for left ventricular failure. The rise of blood pressure during inspiration appears to result from increased stroke output from the left ventricle.

Anacrotic pulse: Anacrotic pulse refers to a pulse having a slow upstroke and a small amplitude giving the picture of a dome. There is an extra impulse during the upstroke. The dicrotic notch is small and delayed.

Dicrotic pulse: When the early diastolic dicrotic wave of the arterial pulse is exaggerated it may be palpable at the wrist or in the carotids. Thus the finger tips perceive a double arterial impulse-first, the normal systolic impulse and second, the exaggerated dicrotic wave. It is present in febrile conditions, particularly in typhoid fever and in cardiomyopathy (non-obstructive).

Tension: To assess the tension, firm pressure is applied by the ring finger at the distal end of the pulse, so as to prevent the pulse coming from the collateral ulnar artery. Further pressure is exerted by the index finger and the pulse is felt with the middle finger. The pressure necessary to obliterate the pulse by the index finger is noted. The pulse of low tension can be easily compressed and that of high tension with great difficulty. The tension corresponds to the diastolic pressure. The recording of the blood pressure is preferred to this method.

Conditions of the vessel wall: The pulse is made to disappear at the radial artery by applying sufficient pressure over the brachial artery by the thumb. Then the radial artery is rolled beneath the fingers against the underlying bone. Generally the arterial wall is not felt in young individuals. It may appear hard from arteriosclerosis in elderly persons.

The loss of elasticity of the wall due to the medial arteriosclerosis with advancing age renders the brachial artery tortuous and the pulsations are visible in the lower third of the upper arm (locomotor brachial).

Capillary pulse: It is appreciated in the regions adjoining the poorly vascular and richly vascular areas of the capillary systems.

The common site selected is the nail bed. With each heart beat a forward and backward movement of the margin between red and white areas is noted in aortic incompetence. It can also be demonstrated by pressing a glass slide against the everted lip.

Suzman's sign: In coarctation of the aorta, the superficial arteries may appear dilated and tortuous from the anastomosis and are seen in the interscapular and infrascapular regions. They are made prominent by asking the patient to bend forward with the arms hanging down by the sides.

Radio-femoral delay: There will be symmetrical reduction and delay of the femoral pulse compared with the radial pulse in coarctation of the aorta. It is also assessed as brachio-femoral lag.

The description of the arterial pulse in health will be as follows: Pulse 72/min, regular in rhythm, equal in volume, normal in character and arterial wall not thickened.

Blood Pressure

The arterial blood pressure is the lateral pressure or force exerted by the blood on a unit area of the blood vessel wall. Normally the blood pressure shows fluctuation from moment to moment during the course of the cardiac cycle and has a diurnal variation. The systolic and diastolic blood pressures refer to the highest and the lowest pressures in the cardiac cycle.

The arterial blood pressure is determined by a variety of factors such as cardiac output and peripheral vascular resistance. In addition, the volume of blood in the arterial system, viscosity of the blood and elasticity of the arterial walls have influence on the blood pressure. The stroke volume of the heart and the stiffness of the vessels receiving the stroke volume control systolic blood pressure and the diastolic pressure is maintained by vascular tone controlling the peripheral resistance, and an intact aortic valve.

Instrument: Though a rough idea of the blood pressure (BP) can be obtained by knowing the degree of digital compression required to obliterate an artery, it is measured accurately with a sphygmomanometer introduced in 1896 by Riva-Rocci, an Italian Physician.

Blood pressure is measured by sphygmomanometer and the instrument may be mercury-gravity or anaeroid in type. Each consists of a pressure manometer, a compression cuff consisting of an inflatable rubber bladder enclosed within an inelastic covering, and a pressure source consisting of a rubber hand bulb and pressure control valve. Mercury-gravity type of manometer is routinely preferred as it gives accurate readings. It does not require recalibration. If anaeroid manometer is used, it should be made sure that the indicator needle is to zero area on the dial before inflating the cuff.

The compression cuff must be of the correct width for the diameter of the person's arm. For an average adult, it should be of 12.5 cm width and 30 cm length. It is applied snugly to the upper arm, 2.5 cm above the bend in the cubital fossa. The length of the pneumatic bag bladder should encompass at least one half of the circumference of the arm. The centre of the cuff bladder should be over the brachial artery. An undersized cuff causes falsely high readings, and an oversized cuff results in falsely low readings.

The blood pressure is recorded by palpatory and auscultatory methods. Systolic BP can also be estimated by oscillatory method, looking at the fluctuation of the mercury column. The blood pressure is recorded in the right arm with the patient in a sitting or lying position. All clothing should be removed from the arm. The arm is abducted, slightly flexed and supported on a smooth, firm surface, at a level with the heart. The manometer is kept at the same level as the observer's eye. The deflated compression cuff is wrapped evenly and snugly around the arm 2 to 3 cm above the bend in the cubital fossa.

Palpatory method: The compression cuff is inflated until the radial pulse disappears. Then it is deflated slowly at a rate of 2 to 3 mm Hg per heart beat and the reappearance of the pulsation in the radial artery is noted. It corresponds to the systolic blood pressure. It is produced by transmission of the left ventricular systolic pressure.

Auscultatory method: The blood pressure is determined by auscultatory method. The chest piece of the stethoscope is placed lightly over the brachial artery just under the distal edge of the cuff and listened to the sounds. It must be noted that the sounds are loudest in the centre of the cuff. The sounds are produced by the oscillation of the artery wall under a partially constricting BP cuff. The sounds occur only when the cuff pressures are between the systolic and diastolic levels. The cuff is inflated to a pressure of 10 mm Hg above the level of the systolic blood pressure noted by the palpatory method. Then the cuff is slowly deflated at the rate of 5 to 10 mm Hg per second.

The appearance of clear taping sounds (Phase I) indicates the peak systolic pressure, and are noted during the propagation of the pulse wave. While the deflation is continued, the sounds become less distinct and then become loud and sharp (Phase II and III). The sounds are due to the turbulent flow of blood through the artery that is partially constricted under the cuff. Then the sounds suddenly become muffled (Phase IV) and later inaudible (Phase V). Korotkoff, a Russian Physician described the sounds of Phase I, II, III and V in 1905. Erlanger in 1921 added the fourth phase. These sounds are not transmitted heart sounds. There may be difficulty to hear Korotkoff sounds in aortic stenosis (due to slow rate of rise in the pulse wave), poor blood flow to the limbs or a small pulse pressure. The sounds may be made audible by asking the patient to open and close his fist about 10 times, either before or during cuff inflation.

The measurement of the diastolic blood pressure is done at the time of muffling (American Heart Association Criteria) or at the time of disappearance of the sounds. In the former situation, the diastolic pressure is higher by 8-10 mm Hg compared to phase V. When the diastolic blood pressure is reached, there is a sudden decrease in the maximum oscillation of the mercury column. Though the point of disappearance of the sound is more consistent, in aortic regurgitation and arteriovenous fistula or in hyperkinetic circulatory states, the point of muffling is taken as the diastolic pressure.

The blood pressure is recorded when the patient is resting quietly for at least 5 minutes before the measurement is taken. In nervous individuals, the initial reading is often very high. In such individuals a second reading, after reassurance is desirable. Casual blood pressure is the record of the blood pressure taken at random. The reading will be high as the pressure is affected by various physical, mental and emotional factors (exertion, emotion, anxiety, after food and change of posture). These factors are minimized by adequate rest. After complete relaxation, the reading will be lower than the casual reading. It is referred to as the basal blood pressure. The blood pressure is higher while sitting than while lying. It is still higher while standing. In conditions of hemiplegia, the blood pressure is recorded over the non-paralysed limb. A wider cuff is necessary such as a thigh cuff in obese patients. Smaller cuff sizes are available for children and thin individuals.

Hypertension: Normally the blood pressure shows fluctuation from moment-to-moment and has a diurnal variation. In adults, the systolic blood pressure is 120 mm Hg (range 100–140 mm Hg) and diastolic blood pressure 80 mm Hg (range 60–90 mm Hg). Generally the blood pressure readings are rounded off to nearest 5 or zero digit rather than the nearest 2. The blood pressure is dependent on the peripheral resistance and cardiac output. An increase in these factors results in high blood pressure (hypertension). The systolic blood pressure is subjected to great variations. An increase of cardiac output alone results in systolic hypertension (hyperthyroidism, anaemia, arteriovenous fistula, complete heart block and arteriosclerosis). In aortic stenosis, the blood pressure is maintained by an increase in peripheral resistance, even though stroke volume falls. In aortic regurgitation, systolic pressure is high due to an increased stroke volume; however the diastolic pressure is less than normal because of a fall in peripheral resistance. The diastolic blood pressure signifies the constant load felt on the walls of the arterial system. The duration of diastolic run-off into the periphery and the elasticity of the aorta also influence the diastolic pressure. In true hypertension the diastolic level will be high. Systolic hypertension is also an important factor in increasing mortality from the coronary artery disease. When the systolic reading exceeds 140 mm and diastolic 90 mm Hg, the condition is referred to as hypertension.

Hypertension could be Essential or has the Following Causes.

1. Renal: acute and chronic nephritis, pyelonephritis, polycystic kidney
2. Vascular: coarctation of the aorta, renal artery stenosis, diabetic glomerulosclerosis, polyarteritis nodosa
3. Endocrine: Cushing's syndrome, pheochromocytoma, Conn's syndrome
4. Toxaemias of pregnancy
5. Medication: history of intake of oral contraceptives, steroidal and non-steroidal anti-inflammatory drugs, nasal decongestants
6. Sleep-apnoea syndrome

Pulse pressure: Difference between systolic and diastolic blood pressures is referred to as pulse pressure. Normally it is 40 mm (range from 30 to 60), thus making the ratio between the systolic, diastolic and pulse pressure, 3: 2: 1. Pulse pressure is increased in fever, thyrotoxicosis, hypertension, aortic incompetence, AV fistula, and PDA. It is decreased in mitral stenosis, aortic stenosis, pericardial effusion and hypotension.

Cardiac Diagnosis on the Basis of Pulse Pressure.

Pulse pressure	clinical significance
Wide	aortic regurgitation, AV fistula, inelastic aorta in elderly
Narrow	severe heart failure, shock, aortic stenosis

Pseudohypertension: There can be misleading high systolic, diastolic or mean blood pressure measured with a cuff compared with the pressure measurement directly by intra arterial needle. Such a situation may be encountered in medial sclerosis of the brachial arteries (that resists compression by a BP cuff). Pseudo-hypertension should be suspected when the BP is elevated dispro-portionately to the clinical findings or a palpable radial artery after the radial pulse has been eliminated by inflation of the cuff above systolic pressure.

Hypotension: When the systolic blood pressure is below 90 mm Hg consistently, it is referred to as hypotension. The diastolic blood pressure may be 50 or 60 mm Hg in such situations. The low blood pressure may be constitutional, acute (peripheral circulatory failure, myocarditis, myocardial infarction, pericardial effusion, vasovagal attack, postural hypotension and toxic states) or chronic (Addison's disease, Simmond's disease, after Morris Simmond, a German physician, and cachexia).

Silent gap (auscultatory gap): This may be evident in some patients with high blood pressure. During deflation of the cuff, the sounds may disappear suddenly and make their reappearance after a varying length of time at a much lower level of blood pressure. Thus a silence separates the sounds. The sounds may first appear at 200 mm Hg systolic pressure and disappear from 180 to 160 mm Hg and finally disappear at 110 mm Hg (diastolic pressure). If the cuff is not inflated sufficiently in the beginning, the level of reappearance of the sound may be recorded erroneously as the systolic blood pressure. This error can be overcome by noting the blood pressure by the palpatory method before auscultation is carried out. Auscultatory gap can be prevented by making the patient to clench his or her fist 10 times and inflating the cuff rapidly. The cause of this phenomenon is undetermined and it appears to be related to arterial stiffness from atherosclerotic plaques.

Recording of blood pressure in the legs: In some instances the recording of blood pressure in the legs is necessary. The patient is asked to lie with his face downwards and the thigh cuff (wider and longer than the arm cuff, 18 cm) is applied above the knee. The sounds are heard over the popliteal artery by keeping the chest piece in the popliteal fossa. Normally the popliteal pressure is either similar or 20 mm Hg higher than in the arms. The usual arm cuff when used on the thigh, gives high readings. To get comparable results the ordinary cuff may be applied over the lower half of the leg and auscultated over the posterior tibial or dorsalis pedis artery. Foot pressures are normally higher than arm pressure. In coarctation of the aorta, pseudo coarctation due to a buckling of an elongated thoracic aorta, or atherosclerotic obstructive disease of the terminal part of the aorta or of the iliac arteries, the systolic pressure in the leg is much lower than in the arm. The systolic pressure is much higher in the legs than in the arms in aortic incompetence and it is referred to as positive Hill sign.

BP difference in the arms: Normally there is not much difference in the blood pressure readings in both arms. There can be higher blood pressure in one arm than in the other. A higher blood pressure is noted in conditions associated with interference with blood flow in the subclavian or innominate arteries by aneurysm, thrombosis, embolism, pressure by tumours or cervical rib and aortic arch syndrome. BP may be higher on the right due to supravalvular aortic stenosis. BP may be lower in one arm than the other in subclavian steal syndrome presenting with vertebrobasilar insufficiency. It is necessary to measure blood pressure in the recumbent and the standing positions in patients on antihypertensive therapy and in suspicion of postural hypotension. Normally there is a fall in cardiac output on standing and it results in a fall in the systolic pressure by a few millimeters of mercury. In postural (orthostatic) hypotension and syncope there is a precipitous fall in the blood pressure when the patient stands erect.

Cardiac irregularities: The recording of blood pressure is also useful in recognizing some of the cardiac irregularities like pulsus alterans, pulsus paradoxus and atrial fibrillation. In pulsus alternans, there is alternate fluctuation in pulse pressure. When the arm cuff is deflated slowly, the sounds are heard in a regular fashion and their rate is half the number of beats felt at the radial artery. When the cuff is deflated further, the sounds become loud and are followed by a soft sound each time. Now the number corresponds to the pulse rate.

In pulsus paradoxus, there is an inspiratory fall of blood pressure. The blood pressure cuff is inflated until no sounds are audible with the stethoscope over the brachial artery, and then it is slowly deflated until sounds are heard in expiration only. Then deflation is continued further until the sounds are heard throughout the respiratory cycle. Pulsus paradoxus is considered present when the systolic blood pressure falls more than 10 mm Hg during inspiration.

In atrial fibrillation, majority of the sounds are heard together in succession at the commencement of the systolic blood pressure. Similarly a majority of the sounds get muffled when the diastolic level is reached.

Veins

The veins are examined at various sites. The examination of the veins in the neck gives valuable information about the pressure and volume changes in the right atrium and the cardiac rhythm.

The presence of veins is looked for over the chest and abdomen that can appear conspicuous due to the obstruction to the venous return either in the superior or inferior vena cava. The veins are examined in the legs for the evidence of varicosity or thrombophlebitis.

Veins in the neck: As the neck veins communicate directly with the right atrium, the study of their pulsations and pressure reflects accurately the pressure in the right atrium and its variation during the cardiac cycle. The alternate filling and emptying of the vein with blood results in the venous pulse. It is caused by the fluctuations in the pressure and volume within the right atrium during the cardiac cycle. The venous pulse (pressure, pulse waves) is studied by the examination of the external and internal jugular veins. The external jugular vein is superficial and the internal jugular vein is situated deep to the sternomastoid muscle. The inspection of the external jugular vein is made to note distension and that of internal jugular vein for its pulsations.

Examination: The absence of valves and its more direct route to right atrium make the internal jugular vein better than the external jugular vein for estimation of pressure and assessment of wave form. Further external jugular vein does not empty into the superior vena cava directly and it may erroneously show engorgement due to obstruction by the fascial and muscle layers through which it passes or to kinking at the base of the neck. Normally the right internal jugular vein is selected for inspection as the left internal jugular vein may show a rise in jugular venous pressure (JVP) from partial obstruction of left innominate vein by an unfolding of aorta especially in elderly patients.

It is necessary to delineate the internal jugular vein which lies beneath the sternomastoid muscle. Normally the height of a column of blood in the jugular vein is about the level of the manubrium sterni in any position of a person. It represents the zero position in the venous system when the patient is resting with the head in the same plane as the chest without flexion of the neck. The jugular pulse should not be more than 1 or 2 cm above the level of manubrium sterni. If the level ascends over 4 cm it is considered abnormal. When the patient is supine with the head elevated to 45°, the level of the blood in the jugular veins reaches to about one-third of the neck and the level corresponds with that of the sternal angle of Louis (junction of the manubrium sterni with the body of the sternum) and thus to the right atrium.

The venous pressure is studied by placing the head, neck and upper part of the chest of the recumbent patient over the pillows at an angle of about 45° from the horizontal position in a tangentially directed light. Normally, the venous pulsations are not visible in a healthy person when he sits upright. The neck muscles must be relaxed when the patient is placed at a 45° angle, and that position allows the filling of the neck veins in a plane horizontal to the sternal angle (Fig. 30). The neck should not be flexed. It is preferable to examine the patient lying with the trunk at an angle of 45° from the horizontal position. The mean hydrostatic pressure in the right atrium is recognized, by using the jugular vein as a manometer. For this purpose the internal

CARDIOVASCULAR SYSTEM

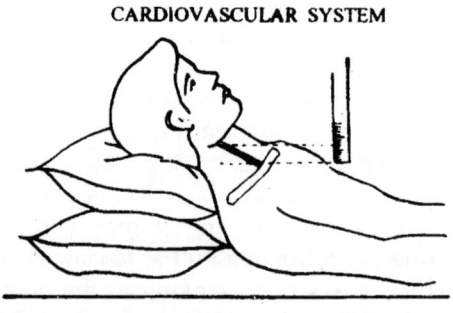

Fig. 30 Venous pressure measurement.

jugular vein on the right side is selected, as the external jugular vein may demonstrate a false elevation due to the compression at the thoracic inlet. A measuring scale is placed vertically at the level of the sternal angle. Then a pencil is placed horizontally from the top level of pulsation to the scale. The vertical distance between the sternal angle and the top level of venous pulsation at the end of a quiet expiration corresponds to the right ventricular filling pressure and is expressed in cm of water. The sternal angle is approximately 5 cm higher than the mid right atrium and it is used as a reference point to measure the height of JVP. By adding 5 cm to the vertical distance measured in cm from the sternal angle, the JVP is accurately estimated. It is important to inspect the veins on either side of the neck. If the venous pressure is generally elevated, the neck veins should be distended on both sides.

Occasionally in an elderly patient, one may find distension of the left jugular vein only. This is due to kinking of the left innominate vein as it passes in front of a dilated aortic arch and is usually associated with hypertension or atherosclerosis. The left innominate vein may also be compressed by the aneurysm of the aortic arch. Rarely bilateral innominate veins may be compressed resulting in bilateral elevation of venous pressure. Deep inspiration produces a dramatic fall in the pressure and such a change does not occur in superior vena cava obstruction in the mediastinum. Rarely the venous pressure may be very high, and the pulsations may be visible as high as the angle of the mandible when the patient sits upright.

Pulsations in the neck: The visible pulsations in the neck may be arterial or venous and the venous pulsations have to be differentiated from those of the common carotid artery. The venous pulsations are more lateral while the arterial are medial. The arterial pulsations are prominent in the erect posture. Venous pulsations are best seen when the patient turns his head slightly away from the examiner, thereby relaxing the neck muscles. An upper level of venous pulsation can be made out and it alters with respiration, posture and / or abdominal pressure. The height descends with inspiration due to the reduction in the intrathoracic pressure and drainage of the blood towards the heart, and then rises with expiration. Rarely the veins can undergo further distension on inspiration (Kussmaul's sign). It is a sign of decreased right ventricular compliance as seen in patients with right-sided heart failure, constrictive pericarditis, tricuspid stenosis, or right ventricular infarction. This sign is not visible in patients with cardiac tamponade. They can collapse during diastole as in pericardial effusion and constrictive pericarditis. The venous pressure rises rapidly again as the ventricles are stiff and cannot be distended. The rapid fall and rise of jugular pressure is referred to as Friederich's sign, named after Nikolaus Friederich, a German physician.

The veins are made more prominent on assumption of the recumbent posture. Respiration and posture have no effect on carotid pulsation. The venous pulsations can be obliterated by application of light pressure at the supraclavicular region. The pulsations become more prominent and the level ascends on application of pressure over the abdomen (hepatojugular reflux). The venous pulse becomes more prominent when the patient assumes the recumbent position and will become less prominent in the erect position. The external jugular vein may be made to distend further by application of pressure at its root.

The venous pulsation exhibits a wavy pattern with three distinct positive waves during each cardiac cycle and is better seen than felt. The arterial pulsation exhibits a single sharp wave. It can be seen and felt easily and has a thrusting character. The venous pulse exhibits an inward motion towards the midline and the arterial pulse shows an outward movement.

Jugular venous pressure: The venous pressure is increased in congestive heart failure of any aetiology and it is one of the earliest signs of right-sided heart failure. It is elevated in constrictive pericarditis, tricuspid stenosis, right ventricular infarct, or cardiac tamponade . Though superior vena caval obstruction is associated with a raised jugular venous pressure, the veins are non-pulsatile. The venous pressure is slightly elevated in situations of an increased blood volume such as anaemia, pregnancy, acute nephritis and in sodium and water overload. The raised intrathoracic pressure and intra-abdominal pressure as noted in massive pleural effusion and large ascites respectively may be associated with raised jugular venous pressure.

Jugular venous pulse: The internal jugular vein shows three positive waves (crests), *a, c* and *v* and two negative waves (troughs), *x* and *y* (Fig. 31). The summits of the waves correspond to presystole, systole and diastole respectively. Ordinarily only '*a*' and '*v*' waves are visible to the eye of the examiner. The first and second heart sound should be used as reference points. The heart should be listened to while inspecting the neck veins. The '*a*' wave is due to the right atrial contraction and it is the highest of the venous waves. It precedes the carotid pulsation. It can be made out by palpating the left carotid artery while the pulsation of the right jugular vein in inspected. The first heart sound occurs on the descending limb of the '*a*' wave.

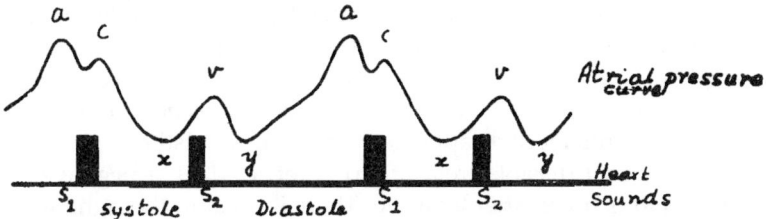

Fig. 31 Jugular venous pulse.

When examining the right jugular pulsations the patient's chin should be slightly elevated and turned to the left thus exposing the right supraclavicular fossa. The right-sided neck veins are situated directly above the right atrium, and the pulsations reflect the pressure changes in the right atrium, better than the left-sided veins. Forceful contraction of the right atrium is associated with prominent '*a*' waves and is seen in pulmonary hypertension from any cause such as left ventricular failure, mitral stenosis, pulmonary embolism, COPD or in conditions with significantly diminished RV diastolic compliance, right ventricular hypertrophy, severe pulmonary stenosis, tricuspid stenosis, pulmonary hypertension, cardiomyopathy and myxoma of the right atrium.

Conditions Associated with Large '*a*' Waves.

Pulmonary hypertension
Right ventricular hypertrophy
Pulmonary stenosis
Tricuspid stenosis
Cardiomyopathy
Right atrial myxoma

In complete heart block, the carotid pulsations occur at a slow rate irregularly while regular '*a*' waves are recognized in the neck. However, '*a*' waves of large amplitude, often called 'cannon waves' are noted from time to time irregularly, when the right atrium contracts against a closed tricuspid valve during ventricular systole. The carotid pulsations occur at a slower independent rate. Such intermittent giant waves are noted in AV dissociation, and may occur with premature ventricular contractions, ventricular tachycardia, supraventricular tachycardia, and complete heart block and with electronic RV pacing.

Most often the 'a' wave is dominant. The 'a' wave disappears in atrial fibrillation due to the absence of atrial contraction as a single unit. In atrial flutter the wave is replaced by rapid smaller oscillations that occur at approximately 300 times per minute. The 'a' wave completely disappears with atrial standstill.

The atrial diastole (relaxation) is reflected by a negative 'x' wave and is noted after 'a' wave. There is a fall in the right atrial pressure and 'x' descent is prominent in constrictive pericarditis with pericardial effusion. The normally negative 'x' wave may get reversed in tricuspid regurgitation, when a positive wave occurs during ventricular systole. The 'c' wave is inscribed as a small positive wave in 'x' descent. The 'c' wave heralds the onset of the ventricular systole. It begins at the end of the first heart sound. In the right atrium, it occurs from a tricuspid valve closure due to the rising right ventricular pressure. It used to be thought that in the neck, the 'c' wave is largely produced by the underlying carotid arterial pulsation. It does not appear to be correct. The 'c' wave is small in size and brief in duration. It is rarely seen normally. The 'a' to 'c' wave interval is increased when the P-R interval is increased. It helps in identification of 'a' wave more readily.

The 'v' wave is due to passive filling and it is due to filling of the right atrium from the venous return, and from rising pressure while the tricuspid valve remains closed. It occurs in the latter part of the ventricular systole. The 'v' wave occurs simultaneously with carotid pulsation. The 'v' wave coincides with the second heart sound, and is prominent in conditions of hyper-dynamic states which hasten circulation time and accelerate filling of the right atrium.

The 'v' waves are prominent in tricuspid regurgitation due to the regurgitation of the blood into the right atrium during ventricular systole (Fig. 32). The large systolic expansion of the internal jugular vein may cause the patient's head to move from side to side ('no-no sign'). In severe tricuspid regurgitation, the

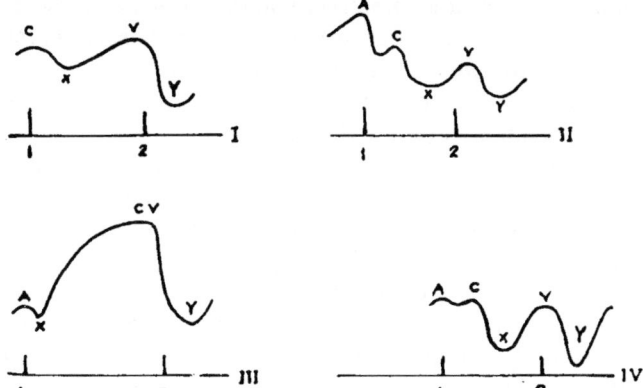

Fig. 32 Different jugular venous wave forms: I. atrial fibrillation; II. Giant '*a*' wave; III tricuspid regurgitation; IV. constrictive pericarditis.

ear lobes appear moving with systole, as the large '*v*' waves cause them to 'dance' with each pulsation. Prominent '*v*' waves may also be noted in ASD.

In atrial fibrillation '*c-v*' wave may be the only visible wave in the neck. Following the '*v*' wave, there is the negative '*y*' wave inscribed as the tricuspid valve opens, allowing entry of blood into the right atrium into the right ventricle rapidly, thus lowering the pressure in the right atrium. The '*y*' descent is steep in tricuspid regurgitation and chronic constrictive pericarditis. The '*y*' descent is markedly slow in tricuspid stenosis. The jugular pulses exhibit their negative phase during ventricular ejection. The negative waves '*x*' and '*y*' are more prominent during inspiration.

Hepatojugular reflux: An early right heart failure can be recognized by eliciting hepatojugular reflux. While the patient is placed at a 45° angle, and breathing normally, firm sustained pressure is exerted with the palm of the hand for 10 seconds or more over the right upper abdomen, or elsewhere in the abdomen (abdominojugular test) if there is tenderness in the right upper abdomen while carefully looking the jugular venous pulsations. Normally there is a brief rise and decline in the mean JVP. If the reflux is positive there is distension of the neck veins, and the level of the venous pulsation moves up. It suggests an elevated pulmonary capillary wedge pressure (PCWP) in patients with right and left heart failure. RV infarction will produce a positive response without elevation of PCWP. Occasionally, the patient may stop breathing from pain due to pressure on the tender, congested liver and cause distension of cervical veins. It may erroneously be labeled as positive reflux. Hence the patient is advised to breathe normally during this procedure. The reflux confirms the venous nature of pulsations noted in the neck.

Venous hum: An hyperdynamic circulatory state such as anaemia, thyrotoxicosis, or uraemia with low haematocrit, and sometimes congestive heart failure with blood flowing very rapidly through the great veins to the heart or partial obstruction to the continuous flow due to the kinking of one of the large veins in the neck, creates a turbulence of blood either by confluence of flow through the internal jugular and subclavian veins or by an anterior angulation of the internal jugular vein by the transverse process of the atlas, and results in a continuous roaring murmur referred as 'venous hum' (*Bruit de diable*). It is heard like a continuous roar or like 'the sound of the sea'. The diastolic component is often higher pitched and louder than the systole. In children it may simulate the continuous murmur of PDA. The circulation time is faster than normal.

The venous hum is heard by placing the bell of the stethoscope very lightly over the internal jugular vein on the right side of the neck, above the clavicle either medial to the sternomastoid or between its insertion, when the person is in the seated position, and turning the neck up and away from the area of auscultation or listening through the stethoscope when the patient is lying down or by stopping the venous return (by application of pressure on the ipsilateral internal jugular vein above the area of auscultation). The right jugular vein is selected as it is larger than left and nearly 66 per cent of intracranial venous drainage passes through it. It increases in its intensity on inspiration, and on pulling back the head so as to stretch the neck veins. It is a low- or medium-pitched murmur and is heard loudly during diastole. It becomes less prominent or disappears by relieving the venous obstruction (by turning the neck on to the side of the auscultation, or listening when the patient is lying down) or by stopping the venous return (by application of pressure on the vein above the area of auscultation). Rapid flow of blood in the cervical veins produces a continuous roar in the region below the left clavicle, and it may be misinterpreted as being due to a patent ductus arteriosus. However, a venous hum lacks the late systolic accentuation characteristic of the murmur of a patent ductus.

A venous hum is common in inguinal region in normal persons in the supine position.

Inspection and Palpation of the Cardia

These two methods of physical examination may be combined together while examining the cardia. The patient is stripped to the waist and is examined in good light, both in the erect and recumbent postures. The examiner may be seated, either facing the patient, or on his right side. On completion of the inspection, the palm of the hand may be placed over the precordium to obtain further information on cardiac impulse.

After noting the size and shape of the chest (described in the inspection of the chest), the shape of the precordium, cardiac impulse (location, extent, force and character), thrills, pulsations in the neck and epigastrium (described in the examination of the neck and the abdomen) and other pulsations have to be carefully examined.

Shape of the Precordium

The prominence or retraction of the precordial region may occur from skeletal deformities (kyphoscoliosis, as part of rachitic chest) or from diseases of the lung and pleura. The bulging of the ribs and intercostal spaces may occur from hypertrophy of the left ventricle. There is also involvement of the sternum in the right ventricular enlargement. This is common in those who have cardiac disease from childhood, as the bones are soft and resilient. In pericardial effusion, there may be a bulging of the intercostal spaces without pulsations. The aortic aneurysm, there may be a prominent swelling and pulsation. The bulging is appreciated by looking at the chest while standing at the foot end of the bed.

The Cardiac Impulse

The cardiac thrust is greatest normally at the site of the apical impulse (apex beat), and the latter's position and character should be determined. The apical impulse is the lowermost, outermost point of the cardiac pulsation. It is produced by the isovolumetric contraction of the left ventricle, left ventricular and septal forces and very rarely dilated, hypertrophied right ventricle. The normal apical impulse is appreciated as a brief outward movement in early systole. It lifts the chest wall before retracting medially. Apex beat is visible and distinctly palpable 9 cm (7.5–10.5 cm from the midsternal line or 1.25 cm medial to the midclavicular line in the left fifth intercostal space. It is well circumscribed and usually covers a small area (2–2.25 cm in diameter). The time interval during which the normal apex beat is felt is shorter than the duration of the ventricular systole. It may be displaced upwards or downwards depending on the stature or build of the patient. It may be present in the fourth interspace in people with a short, broad chest or in the sixth interspace in people with a long narrow chest.

Internal to the apical thrust, there can be an area of systolic retraction caused by movement of the right ventricle. The apical impulse is felt with the patient first lying flat and then sitting in the erect posture. It will be displaced to the left if the patient is lying on his left side. It is appreciated by placing the palm of the right hand firmly over the apex beat and over the base of the heart, and then it is localized, by placing the pulps of the tips of the index and middle fingers lightly over the cardiac thrust. Normally, the apical impulse gently raises the palpating fingers. The apex beat involves a small area in the left ventricular enlargement and a wide area in the right ventricular enlargement (Fig. 33)

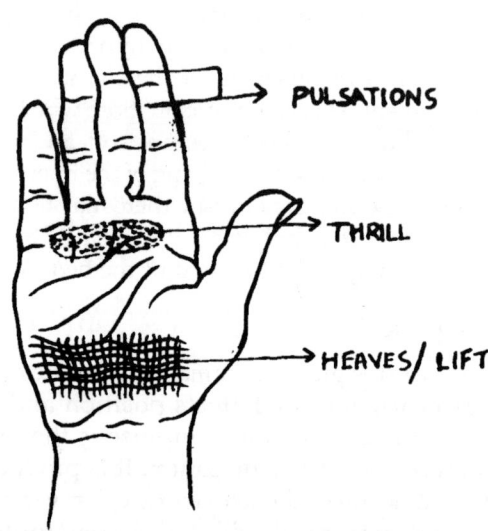

Fig. 33 Palpation for pulsations, thrills, and heaves.

The apical impulse may be displaced due to diseases of the heart, or due to the diseases affecting the lungs, pleura, thoracic cage and abdomen. The conditions like pleural effusion, pneumothorax or hydropneumothorax and pulmonary fibrosis or collapse can shift the apical impulse. Pleural conditions like pleural effusion and pneumothorax will 'push' the apical impulse to the opposite side, whereas the lung conditions like fibrosis and collapse will 'pull' it to the same side. Deformities of the thoracic cage like scoliosis, kyphoscoliosis and pectus excavatum (depressed sternum) can displace the apical impulse further laterally. In scoliosis with convexity to the left, tends to shift the apex to the right while the opposite occurs in scoliosis with right-sided convexity. In kyphosis there is a downward shift of the apex beat. In a funnel chest the apex tends to displace to the left. The conditions associated with a raised diaphragm like pregnancy, obesity or ascites are able to displace the apical impulse upwards or to the left.

The apex beat may be felt on the right side instead of the left in dextrocardia. Such an abnormality will not be missed if it is made a practice to place the hand on each side of the chest in turn. This becomes especially important when apex beat is not felt in its normal position. The diseases affecting the heart may result in hypertrophy or dilatation or both and may shift the cardiac impulse. In the left ventricular hypertrophy due to obstruction to the outflow system as in valvular aortic stenosis, systemic hypertension (pressure overload, resistant load), and cardio-myopathy the apex is heaving (forceful, slow, and sustained lift throughout systole) and is displaced outwards towards the axilla. In the left ventricular dilatation, from an increased filling of the ventricle as in aortic or mitral regurgitation (volume overload), the apical impulse is diffuse and active but less sustained due to rapid ejection of blood from the ventricles and is felt downward that is in the 6th or 7th space (thrusting apex beat). In combined hypertrophy and dilatation, the apical impulse is forceful and the force is sustained (heaving) and is situated downwards and outwards.

The enlargement of the right ventricle produces a lift in the left parasternal region known as parasternal heave, which can be seen when observed tangentially (mild), or felt by placing the ulnar border of the hand, firmly over the precordium just to the left of the sternum (moderate to severe). The heave may be of 3 grades.

The palpating hand may feel pulsations without any lift (grade I), lift without application of any pressure (grade II) and lift even after application of pressure (grade III).

The pulsations of enlarged left atrium may produce a parasternal heave and it occurs before the apical impulse or carotid pulsation. In a gross enlargement of the right ventricle, the apical impulse may be formed by the right ventricle, and is diffuse and wavy in such an instance (right ventricular type). It causes outward displacement of the apical impulse. Snapping or tapping apical impulse is felt due to a palpable first heart sound in mitral stenosis. There is a vibratory knock without any lift of the fingers due to movement of the anterior cusp of the mitral valve.

In conditions associated with hyperdynamic circulation the impulse may be forcefully felt over a diffuse area. It is sudden and does not last long.

The apical impulse may be bifid or double. Two apical pulsations with each heart beat are felt due to an outward movement during systole from LV dilatation or hypertrophy and a palpable presystolic (S_4) or early diastolic component (S_3). The diastolic impulse may be noted during early diastole (ventricular gallop, S_3) or presystole (atrial gallop, S_4). The palpable atrial impulse in hypertrophic obstructive cardiomyopathy may give rise to bifid apex. Similar impulse may be felt in the left ventricular aneurysm due to the accentuated outward movement in late systole. Bifid apex is also noted in complete LBBB. There may be retraction of the apex with each heart beat from mediastinopericarditis. There is dense adhesion of the heart and pericardium with the chest wall. Hypertrophic obstructive cardiomyopathy can produce a presystolic, along with a double-systolic outward thrust, resulting in a characterstic 3-component apical impulse ('tripple ripple').

The apical impulse may not be felt in individuals having a thick chest wall (thick muscle or fat), large breasts, an overinflated chest, pericardial or pleural effusions, or when the impulse underlies a rib.

Other Pulsations

The pulsations should be carefully studied in; 1) sternoclavicular area, 2) aortic area, 3) pulmonic area, 4) right ventricular area, 5) apical area, 6) epigastric area, and 7) ectopic areas.

Normally, in adults, little or no pulsations are felt, by the hand over the base of the heart or great vessels. Pulsation in the second left intercostal space may be seen normally in children. The swelling from an aneurysm of the aorta exhibits expansile pulsations. The pulsations may be to the right of the sternum in aneurysm of an ascending aorta. In aneurysm of the aortic arch, there will be less distinct pulsations under the manubrium sterni. Pulsations may be seen in the region of the right sternoclavicular joint from the right-sided aortic arch and from a tortuous innominate artery. Prominent systolic pulsations in the suprasternal notch may be due to unfolding, or aneurysm of the arch of the aorta.

Slight pulsations may be visible in the pulmonary area, from increased pressure in pulmonary artery (pulmonary hypertension secondary to mitral stenosis or primary pulmonary hypertension), or an increased flow (atrial septal defect, ASD), or a combination of both in pulmonary artery. The pulsations are slow, sustained and forceful in pulmonary hypertension and they are vigorous and less sustained in ASD. Post-stenotic dilatation of the pulmonary artery in pulmonary stenosis may produce a palpable sustained pulsation.

Left parasternal pulsations may be produced by the right ventricular hypertrophy, and they can appear as transmitted pulsations from an enlarged left atrium due to severe mitral regurgitation. An enlarged right atrium secondary to severe tricuspid incompetence may cause a right parasternal impulse occasionally. An ectopic systolic pulsation may be seen, or felt in the third and fourth intercostal spaces midway between the pulmonary area and the apex. This may be noted in some patients following an acute myocardial infarction, and it indicates a dyskinetic segment of myocardium expanding paradoxically during systole. It suggests the presence of LV aneurysm. There can be pulsations overlying the scapula from the anastomotic channels in coarctation of the aorta and are felt over the posterior chest wall.

Atrial and ventricular gallop sounds could be palpable at times as double or triple or quadruple apical impulses. Epigastric pulsations are noted in the right ventricular hypertrophy. Pulsations in the suprasternal notch are noted in unfolding of the aorta and in aneurysm of the arch of the aorta.

Thrills

A thrill is a purring or vibratory sensation imparted to the distal palm (metacarpals) of the palpating hand when placed lightly over the chest. It is the palpable equivalent of a cardiac murmur grade 4 or more. The same factors that produce the murmur, therefore are responsible for the thrill also. Presence of a thrill implies that the murmur is organic. It must be remembered that a long thrill is never felt in the absence of a loud murmur.

The site, extent and its timing in relation to the cardiac cycle have to be noted. The thrill can be made prominent by altering the posture (left lateral position for thrills in mitral area; sitting and leaning forward for aortic thrills), by manoeuvers increasing the flow of the blood (exercise) or by holding the breath in expiration enabling the heart to come close to the chest wall by retraction of the lung.

Presence of a thrill indicates an organic heart disease and gives localization of the disease in the heart but in no way it indicates the severity of the lesion. Exceptions to this may occasionally occur. The thrill is produced when there is an obstruction to the flow of blood from the chambers of the heart through a narrowed valve, and when there is an abnormal blood flow through an incompetent valve or congenital deformity. Thrill is appreciated with the flat of the hand rather than with the fingers.

Systolic Thrill.

Location	abnormality
Right second intercostal space	valvular aortic stenosis
Left second intercostal space	pulmonary stenosis
Apex	mitral regurgitation
Lower left sternal border	VSD, tricuspid regurgitation

The thrill is timed with the apical impulse, as systolic or diastolic in time. It is referred to as systolic when it coincides with the apical impulse, and occurs during the outward movement of apex. The thrill is diastolic when it occurs during retraction of the apex and precedes the apical impulse. The thrill may be timed with the systolic pulsations of the carotid artery in the neck. The thrills in the basal regions may radiate in an upward direction either towards the right or left side of the neck. The thrills are commonly systolic at the base of the heart. A powerful systolic thrill is felt over the second right interspace in aortic stenosis and in aneurysm of the great vessels at the root of the neck. A systolic thrill in the pulmonary area may be due to pulmonary stenosis, ASD, or PDA.

The diastolic thrill in the mitral area is indicative of mitral stenosis. Mitral regurgitation may be associated with a systolic thrill at the apex. A continuous thrill felt during systole and diastole in the same region may be due to PDA or arteriovenous (AV) aneurysm. Rarely highly vascular mediastinal tumours or enlarged overactive thyroid gland may mimic as continuous thrill. A systolic thrill in the third intercostal space suggests an infundibular pulmonary stenosis and a systolic thrill in the fourth or fifth left parasternal region indicates VSD and rarely tricuspid regurgitation. A diastolic thrill due to aortic regurgitation is unusual. A rupture of aortic valve may produce it. A systolic thrill may be felt over a pulsating aneurysm or on an arteriovenous shunt.

A pericardial friction rub imparting a superficial scratchy sensation to the palpating fingers may be felt in conditions of dry pericarditis. It is synchronous with each heart beat.

Palpable heart sounds: The accentuated heart sounds may be felt by the palpating hand as shocks. A loud snappy first sound at the apex may be felt in mitral stenosis. The pulmonary component of the second sound may be felt as a diastolic shock at the base when there is pulmonary hypertension. In systemic hypertension and syphilitic aortitis, the loud second sound may be felt in the aortic area. The third heart sound felt at the apex, or slightly inside is diagnostic of a gallop rhythm, characteristic of the left ventricular failure. An atrial impulse may be felt at the apex in some patients with ischaemic heart disease, and it occurs in late diastole as an audible atrial gallop (S_4).

Percussion

It is possible to get a rough estimate of the size and shape of the cardia by percussion. However it has been discredited as it can be determined with greater accuracy by using radiology and echocardiography.

It is preferable to have the patient supine to determine the location of the borders of cardiac dullness. Percussion is to be done from resonant (lung) towards the dull (heart, sternum) area. The left border of the cardia is defined by percussing the fifth, fourth and third intercostal spaces, beginning laterally in the infra-axillary region. Then the pleximeter finger is moved towards the sternum and placed either parallel, or at right angles to the sternum while standing to the left or to the right of the patient respectively. When the left border of the heart is approached the resonant note becomes dull. Generally, it is found a centimetre medial to the midclavicular line or 7–9 cms lateral to the mid-sternal line. The left border is 2 to 4 cm from the mid-sternal line in the third left interspace, from which point it extends downwards and outwards to the apex. The left border of the heart extends beyond the normal limits in the left ventricular enlargement, pericardial effusion and in the shift of the heart to the left. In the left ventricular enlargement, the dullness extends up to the point beyond the known confines of the apex beat. The dullness in the second and the third interspaces may extend from the normal limits in conditions with enlargement of the left atrium or pulmonary artery.

The right border of the cardia is made up of the right auricle. Though the dullness extends 1 cm to the right of the sternum at the level of the third and the fourth intercostal spaces, generally it is masked by the resonant note of the adjacent lung and sternum. These regions become dull in conditions associated with enlargement of the right atrium (tricuspid stenosis, and Ebstein's anomaly, after Wilhelm Ebstein, a German physician), aneurysm of the ascending aorta, pericardial effusion and shift of the heart to the right side. In pericardial effusion, the fifth right interspace close to the sternum exhibits a dull noise. To define the right border, first the upper border of the liver dullness is delineated, by percussing from above downwards. Then the percussion is done in a space above that and the pleximeter finger is moved towards the sternum either parallel or at right angles to the sternum. The inferior border of the heart is demarcated, by a line joining the lower point of the right and left border of the cardia.

In aortic aneurysm, the supracardiac dullness is widened and the dullness extends to the right (ascending aorta) or to the left (arch of the aorta) of the sternum at the level of the second interspace. A band of dullness may extend laterally from the manubrium in substernal goiter. In pericardial effusion, the cardiac dullness extends beyond the normal limits on either side, and it is stony dull in character. Often it gives a globular shape with its border and below. The sternum gives a dull note on direct percussion in pericardial effusion, large aortic aneurysm and mediastinal tumour. Normally sternum acts like a 'sounding board'.

In conditions of ascites, obesity and advanced pregnancy, the diaphragm is pushed upwards causing the heart to lie more horizontally, so as to increase the cardiac dullness. In emphysema, the area of cardiac dullness gets diminished or obliterated. In individuals with thick chest wall or obesity, the percussion gives less accurate information about the location of cardiac border.

Auscultation

The binaural stethoscope is used to listen to the heart sounds, breath sounds, intestinal sounds and other adventitious sounds. The modern stethoscope has evolved from Laennec's (introduced in 1819 by Laennec, French physician) cylinder to the present form. The ear-pieces should fit into the ears properly and comfortably. The axis of the ear-pieces should be parallel to the long axis of the external auditory canals. The chest piece consists of two parts-the bell and the diaphragm-of diameters 2.5 and 3.75 cm respectively. A valve facilitates to change over either to bell or diaphragm.

The bell has to be applied lightly (except S_4 that requires firm pressure) on the skin just enough to prevent room-noise leak, to listen to the low-pitched (vibrations from a sound in producing structures acting on either ear, frequency) sounds (diastolic filling sound S_3, and S_4) and to the mitral and tricuspid diastolic murmurs. The diaphragm should be applied firmly against the skin to listen high-pitched sounds (S_1 and S_2, and non-ejection clicks) and murmurs (aortic and pulmonary diastolic murmurs, and mitral and tricuspid regurgitant murmurs, and the pericardial rub). The tube connecting the metal frame to the chest pieces should be of 30 cm in length with an internal diameter of 4.6 mm. It should be of either vinyl or thick walled rubber.

The auscultation should be carried out in a quiet room to appreciate the sounds better. The examiner must stand on the right side of the patient. The patient must not be shivering; otherwise the muscle noises are heard. The breathing may be stopped for a few seconds while listening to the heart sounds. The auscultation may be done in sitting, supine, and left lateral recumbent positions.

The cardia is auscultated in four classical areas over the precordial region. These areas are the mitral, tricuspid, pulmonary (better called left second interspace) and aortic (better called right second interspace) areas. The latter two areas are the basal areas. Though these areas do not correspond to the anatomic locations of the valves named after them, the sounds and murmurs arising from them are best heard at these areas (Fig 34).

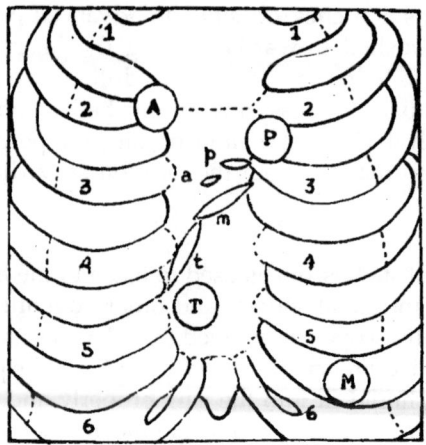

Fig. 34 Precordium: position of the valves an auscultatory areas:
Valves: tricuspid (t); mitral (m); aortic (a) and pulmonary (p)
Areas: tricuspid (T); mitral (M); aortic (A) and pulmonary (P).

The auscultation should not be limited to these areas as the sounds and murmurs heard from particular area do not necessarily come from that particular valve; for example, aortic systolic murmur is frequently better audible at the apex, and aortic diastolic murmur in the left third interspace.

Area	site of auscultation
Mitral	apex beat
Tricuspid	just to the left of the lower end of the sternum
Pulmonary	left of the sternum in the second intercostal space, however pulmonary events can be best heard anywhere along left sternal border
Aortic	right of the sternum in the second intercostal space, however aortic events may be heard anywhere in a line from the second right interspace to the apex

If one restricts the auscultation to the four classical areas, it leaves many gaps in the areas of auscultation of the cardia. Generally the auscultation of the heart is begun at the apex and then the chest piece is moved in a systematic manner from the apex to the lower left sternal border and then by 'inching' upwards along the left sternal border in the fourth and third interspaces to the base of the heart-the pulmonary and later aortic areas. Each area is examined with both chest pieces. Other important areas of auscultation are; the third left interspace lateral to the sternum (second aortic, neo-aortic or Erb's area) to hear the early diastolic murmur of aortic regurgitation, the fourth interspace left of the sternum for the pansystolic murmur of ventricular septal defect (VSD), and the area below the medial end of the left clavicle to hear the continuous murmur of patent ductus arteriosus.

The sounds and murmurs can be made more prominent by adapting different postures; the lying position to listen diastolic filling sounds, left lateral position for the murmurs at the apex, and sitting and leaning forwards and holding the breath at the end of the expiratory phase for the basal murmurs. In conditions of emphysema, the cardiac sounds are distant and can be heard better by listening over the xiphoid or upper epigastric region. Respiration will have a significant effect on the heart sounds. Inspiration accentuates the heart sounds and murmurs arising from the right side of the heart.

The rate and rhythm of the heart sounds, the quality and intensity of the first and second heart sounds at the different areas, the presence of murmurs and other added sounds (third and fourth heart sounds, opening snap, and ejection click) should be carefully listened to. The timing of the sounds in done either with the apical impulse or carotid pulsations. Proper identification and timing of heart sounds and murmurs in the cardiac cycle plays an important part in auscultation. Normally the second heart sound (S_2) is louder than the first heart sound (S_1) at the aortic area. Keeping S_2 in mind, the stethoscope is to be moved down along the left sternal border to the apex. Extrasounds and murmurs that occur before S_2 are labeled as systolic and after S_2 as diastolic. The heart rate has to be counted for a minute when there is irregularity in the rhythm.

Heart Sounds

The haemodynamic events taking place during the opening and closure of the cardiac valves and filling of the ventricles, result in the occurrence of the heart sounds. They are classified as valvular (opening and closing sounds) and muscular (filling sounds). The sounds are valvular opening sounds (ejection clicks and opening snaps), valvular closing sounds (first and second heart sounds, S_1 and S_2) and valvular filling sound (3rd and 4th heart sounds, S_3 and S_4-physiologic or pathologic) (Figs. 35a and 35b). There can be prosthetic valve sounds.

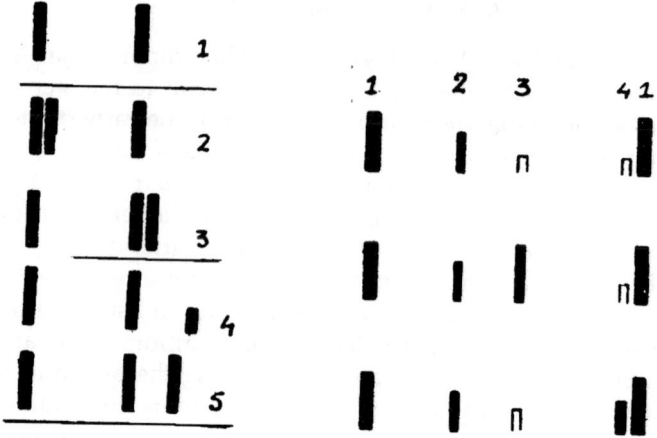

Fig. 35a Heart sounds (1) normal; (2) split first sound; (3) split second sound; (4) split second sound; (4) third heart sound, and (5) opening snap.

Fig. 35b Heart sounds (third and fourth sounds inaudible): protodiastolic gallop with audible III sound; presystolic gallop with audible IV sound.

Normally, two heart sounds are heard at a short interval of time over the cardia. The interval following the second sound is relatively long and the sequence appears at 'lub-dup-pause'. The systole begins with S_1 (lub) and the diastole with S_2 (sup). S_1 is dull and prolonged. It is heard best in the mitral and tricuspid regions. S_2 is short and sharp. It is heard best in the basal region. In an over-inflated chest (emphysema, asthma), a thick chest, obesity and pericardial effusion the heart sounds are diminished in intensity and they are loud and clear in young persons, thin chest (thin covering of muscle or fat) individuals or after exercise.

First Heart Sound

Although the atrial, muscular, valvular and vascular components of the first heart sound can be demonstrated by special recording methods, the first heart sound is appreciated due to the closure of the atrioventricular valves (the mitral and tricuspid valves, in that order). It heralds the beginning of ventricular systole. It occurs at a time of, or shortly after the beginning of pressure rise in the left ventricle. The major component heard at the bedside is due to mitral valve closure. It occurs with the onset of the apical impulse. The diaphragm of the stethoscope should be used when listening to the first heart sound. The first heart sound can be timed by keeping a finger over the apical impulse while listening to the heart. The rise of the finger and lifting of the diaphragm of the stethoscope by the cardiac impulse coincides with the first heart sound. The carotid pulsation occurs 1/10 second after the first heart sound. The sound is louder and of a longer duration than the second sound at the apex. It is low-pitched. The left and right ventricular contractions occur almost simultaneously. Usually the mitral valve closes slightly before the tricuspid valve. The time interval is so short that it is not possible to distinguish them while listening (sounds separated by an interval more than 0.02 seconds are only appreciated).

Splitting of the first heart sound: Splitting of the first sound may be noted as 'l-lub' over the lower end of the sternum on its left side in the right bundle branch block, due to delay in the onset of the right ventricular systole, but not in the left bundle branch block, as it does not result in the late onset of the left ventricular contraction. In normal individuals, splitting of the first heart sound may be noted at the apex, and it has not much significance.

However, the addition of another sound is usually caused by a combination of the first sound with a preceding atrial sound or subsequent ejection click. Presystolic triple rhythm precedes S1 by a wider gap. It is softer and of lower pitch in quality. The ejection click exhibits a sharper and higher pitched sound.

Intensity of the first heart sound: The intensity of the first heart sound depends chiefly on three factors: 1) position of the AV valve at the onset of the ventricular systole, 2) structure of the leaflets of the valves themselves (normal or thickened), and 3) the rate of pressure rise and tension development in the ventricle (force of ventricular contraction).

Increased intensity: The first heart sound is loud and abrupt in rheumatic mitral stenosis, due to delayed, high-velocity closure of a stiff, but mobile mitral valve. It is heard over the whole of the precordium. The fibrosed valve cusps are drawn into the left ventricle due to shortened cardiac tendinae in mitral stenosis during ventricular late diastole. There is decreased ventricular filling. The valves close abruptly when ventricle contracts rapidly and forcibly.

The first heart sound is loud in hyperkinetic circulatory states with strong left ventricular contraction, increased rate of left ventricular pressure development, and short atrioventricular conduction time (short PR interval). The first heart sound is loud in anaemia, fever, pregnancy, thyrotoxicosis, valvular aortic stenosis and idiopathic hypertrophic subaortic stenosis. The left ventricle contracts rapidly and forcibly causing an abrupt closure of AV valve. In tachycardia, diastole is short causing diminished ventricular filling. The ventricle closes rapidly to cause a loud first sound. It is loud following exercise, inhalation of amyl nitrite or isoprenaline administration. The sound is loud in papillary muscle dysfunction, ventricular aneurysm and left atrial myxoma.

Decreased intensity: The intensity of the sound is decreased greatly in conditions associated with low cardiac output, with decreased left ventricular function and decreased rate of left ventricular pressure development (hypothyroidism, acute myocardial infarction, dilated cardiomyopathy, shock, severe congestive heart failure, calcified mitral valve, mitral regurgitation, acute severe aortic incompetence and first degree A-V block (with prolonged PR interval). The intensity of first heart sound is diminished when the mitral valve is calcified and immobile. In mitral regurgitation, S_1 is soft as the valve does not close properly. Severe hypokinesis of the left ventricle causes diminution of the force of the left ventricle and of the intensity of the first heart sound.

Variable intensity: The intensity of the first heart sound varies from beat to beat when the relationship between atrial and ventricular systole is not constant as in ventricular tachycardia or complete heart block. The diagnosis of complete heart block is easier in the presence of bradycardia and constantly changing first heart sound. The sound is loud when the PR interval is short.The explosive sound is known as 'cannon sound'. It is not synchronous with the cannon waves, where the associated first heart sound is muffled. The sound becomes soft when the PR interval is long. Similarly in atrial fibrillation and atrial flutter S_1 varies from beat to beat due to a disordered sequence of atrial and ventricular contractions. It causes variation in ventricular filling and force of contraction.

Second Heart Sound

The closure of the aortic and pulmonary valves in that order results in the second heart sound (S_2) and it occurs at the end of the systole. It is short and high-pitched. These sounds are heard best when the diaphragm of the stethoscope placed over the aortic or pulmonary area. The second sound is normally louder than the first sound in these areas. The components of the second heart sound are to be listened in the pulmonary area. The pulmonary valve normally closes later than the aortic valve due to the lower pressure in the right ventricle and longer right ventricular ejection time than that occurring on the left side of the heart. Hence the two components can be recognised in the form of the split second heart sound in the pulmonary area ($A_2 P_2$), with aortic component preceding pulmonary component. Though it is a normal phenomenon, it is not well appreciated unless A_2 and P_2 are separated by an interval greater than 0.03 seconds. P_2 is shorter and has a lower intensity than A_2. An attempt has to be made to appreciate splitting during normal quiet respiration.

Accentuated sound: The conditions leading to systemic and pulmonary hypertension are associated with an accentuated second heart sound. The aortic component of the second sound is accentuated in the aortic area in systemic hypertension. Pulmonary hypertension is associated with loud pulmonary component of the second sound in the pulmonary area. Dilatation of the pulmonary artery without involvement of valve cusps in also associated with a loud second sound. Generally the pulmonary valve closure sounds appear louder than the aortic valve closure sounds. This because the right ventricle and pulmonary artery enlarge anteriorly as a result of hypertension and the pulmonary valve and pulmonary root are closer to the sternum than the aortic valve and the aortic root. Loud aortic valve closure sounds heard in systemic hypertension, at time, become ringing or tambour-like. In aortic aneurysm a tambour-like closure sound (S_2A) is audible. Aortic second sound is also loud in hyperdynamic circulatory states. A_2 is muffled in aortic stenosis and in systemic hypotension. In aortic stenosis, the valve is relatively immobile. Low blood flow in cardiac failure makes S_2 soft. P_2 is muffled in severe pulmonary stenosis and it may be absent in Fallot's tetrology.

Pulmonary component: The pulmonary component (P_2) is heard in the pulmonary area only, unlike the aortic component (A_2) which is transmitted to the neck and over to the apex. Normally P_2 is barely heard at the apex. Significant pulmonary hypertension and the right ventricular enlargement are suspected when P_2 is heard at the apex. P_2 is clearly audible in normal children or young adults. The splitting is accentuated during deep inspiration as it prolongs the right ventricular ejection in order to eject the increased venous return occurring during that phase of respiration and consequent delay in the pulmonary valve closure. In addition, there is a diminished left ventricular filling and stroke volume causing early aortic valve closure. It is referred to as normal or physiologic splitting (Fig. 36). The dynamic changes in the impedence characteristic of the pulmonary vessels also contribute to the normal physiologic splitting. The splitting gets narrowed in expiration as the disparity in ejection times of the two ventricles is minimized. The splitting is best appreciated at the base, especially the pulmonary area. The movement of P_2 is greater than that of A_2.

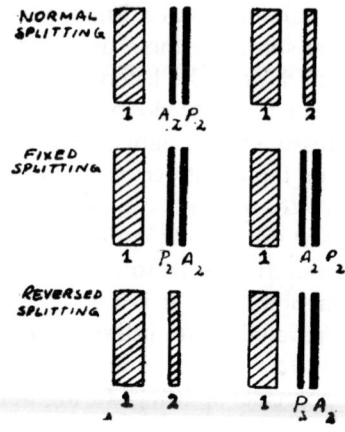

Fig. 36 Splitting of the second sound.

Wide splitting

Pathologic splitting of S_2 may occur either as abnormally wide split or as a reversed split. Wide splitting occurs when there is a delay in the closure of the pulmonary valve. It can occur from the delayed activation of the right ventricle (right bundle branch block), or from prolonged right ventricular systolic ejection due to the right ventricular outflow obstruction (pulmonary stenosis with an intact ventricular septum). RBBB delays right ventricular emptying resulting in delayed pulmonary valve closure. S_2 is widely split during expiration and it further increases during inspiration as there is prolonged right ventricular ejection. Pulmonary stenosis causes obstruction to the right ventricular emptying and there is prolongation of the right ventricular ejection. It delays the pulmonary valve closure sound and its intensity may be diminished. In ventricular septal defect and severe mitral regurgitation, there is a selective reduction in the left ventricular ejection time and premature closure of the aortic valve, causing a wide splitting. These conditions have a regurgitant or shunt pathway having a low resistance.

Fixed split

The splitting of the second heart sound is wide and fixed exhibiting no expiratory variations in ASD. There is a delay in pulmonary valve closure due to increased right ventricular stroke volume and longer ejection time from left-to-right shunting of blood. It causes a wide separation of the components of the second sound. Both atria behave as a single chamber due to free communication. During inspiration there is an increase in systemic venous return and decrease in the volume of shunted blood. The reverse happens during expiration. Thus the total right ventricular inflow volume is fixed relative to the volume of inflow into the left heart. Abnormally a large quantity of blood enters the right ventricle during both phases of respiration and the right ventricular systole is prolonged during inspiration and expiration. Thus the split appears fixed and widely split. The splitting may not remain fixed when significant pulmonary hypertension supervenes in ASD. Rarely fixed split may be encountered in massive pulmonary embolism resulting in a severe right heart failure, cardiomyopathy causing impaired right ventricular function and sometimes in idiopathic dilatation of pulmonary artery.

Paradoxical split

Delayed closure of the aortic component may cause splitting to become narrow. If the delay is sufficiently prolonged, there is a reversal of sequence of the closure sounds. The pulmonary closure sound precedes the aortic closure sound. It is referred to as 'reversed' or 'paradoxical splitting'. It is indicative of cardio-vascular abnormality. In this situation the splitting is noted during expiration and it disappears or narrows during inspiration, because of delay in the pulmonary valve closure sound and the right ventricular systole is prolonged during inspiration.

The condition is noted in an electrical delay in the excitation of the left ventricule (left bundle branch block), mechanical obstruction to the left ventricular outflow (congenital valvular aortic stenosis, hypertrophic subaortic stenosis), a selective volume overload of the left ventricle (PDA), and in poor myocardial function (myocardial infarction). Rarely severe hypertension may be associated with paradoxical splitting due to prolonged left ventricular ejection time.

Narrow splitting

The splitting becomes arrowed with an increased resistance

in the pulmonary vascular bed. There is a progressive shortening of the right ventricular systolic ejection. The two components of S_2 get narrowed and can only be appreciated during inspiration (Eisenmenger complex, named after Victor Eisenmenger, a German physician).

Single second sound

The second sound may appear single. It may be as a result of the absence of one of the components or fusion of both components or separation of the components by a narrow gap of less than 0.03 seconds. Such a sound becomes significant when it is audible over the pulmonary area. It may be encountered in gross pulmonary valve stenosis (absence of pulmonary component) and aortic stenosis (absence of aortic component).

The Third and Fourth Heart Sounds

Two low-pitched sounds may be audible in diastole in addition to the high-pitched first and second heart sounds. They are heard as soft 'thudding' noises immediately before the first heart sound (fourth heart sound) or after the second heart sound (third heart sound). The presence of a third or fourth heart sound produces a cadence of having three beats (lub-dup-lub) rather than the normal two beats (lup-dub). It should be noted that splitting of the first or second heart sounds, ejection click and opening snap do not take part in the production of the triple rhythm.

The ventricular filling is marked at two periods during diastole. Initially there is rapid flow over a short period in early diastole on opening of the atrioventricular valves. The fall in atrial pressure is reflected by a marked 'y' descent in the venous pulse. Nearly 0.06 to 0.10 seconds after opening of the atrioventricular valves there is a sudden reduction in the rate of ventricular filling. The second peak of increased flow occurs in late diastole on contraction of the atria. Sometimes the ventricular filling during the two peaks may result in extra heart sounds referred to as the third (S_3) and the fourth (S_4) heart sounds respectively.

Third Heart Sound

The third heart sound is produced by the mitral and tricuspid valvular and left and right ventricular muscular movement during transition from the rapid early diastolic flow to the longer slow rate of passive distension of the ventricle. This gallop sound is low-pitched occurring early in the diastole about 0.15 sec after the aortic closure sound. It corresponds to the 'v' wave of the jugular pulse. It may be produced from either the left or right ventricle. In the former, it is heard at the apex of the heart from the bell of the stethoscope, with the patient in the left lateral position. When it is arising from the right ventricle the sound is best heard at the lower left sternal border and gets accentuated in inspiration. It is normally associated with a RV heave, a large jugular 'v' wave and rapid heart rate. However, S_3 increases in its loudness both during inspiration and expiration. A third heart sound may be audible in children, healthy young adults and pregnant women during the last trimester. The physiologic S_3 gets exaggerated from an increased blood flow through the mitral valve as in VSD, PDA and mitral regurgitation.

S_3 has pathologic significance in elderly persons and its presence implies cardiac decompensation; hence, is sometimes referred to as a sound of 'distress'. There is no difference in timing, quality, and loudness between the physiological and pathological S_3. Pathological S_3 is associated with raised left atrial pressure, a noncompliant heart and a large ventricle associated with a poor ejection fraction. A left ventricular gallop sound implies presence of left ventricular dysfunction and the right ventricular gallop implies right ventricular dysfunction.

The left ventricular S_3 is heard in the left ventricular failure from myocardial infarction, hypertension and cardiomyopathy. A benign third heart sound may be heard in conditions associated with increased ventricular filling early in diastole as in anaemia, thyrotoxicosis, complete heart block, VSD and mitral regurgitation. In these situations the gallop sound is due to an accelerated blood flow into the ventricle rather than ventricular dysfunction.

The right ventricular S_3 is heard best over the right ventricule just to left of the mid-sternal area and at the left sternal edge. It increases in intensity during inspiration. It is noted in pulmonary hypertension, massive pulmonary embolism, and in the right ventricular failure. A benign right ventricular gallop sound may be audible in a secondum type of ASD where the sound is due to an accelerated blood flow rather than right ventricular dysfunction. S_3 has to be distinguished from opening snap. Opening snap is a high-frequency, short, sharp click best heard with the diaphragm near the left sternal border, and is associated with a short loud S_1.

It separates further from the A_2 when the patient stands. S_3 is low-pitched and it heard as a thud. It is audible with the bell near the apex. It may or may not have loud S_1, S_3 does not change its distance from A_2 on standing.

Fourth Heart Sound

The fourth heart sound occurs from the vibrations generated by the surge of ventricular filling that accompanies vigorous contraction of the atria (atrial systole). The atrial gallop sound occurs just before the first heart sound. Any condition in which the ventricle has decreased distensibility generates a strong atrial contraction. It may be associated with augmented ventricular filling as in severe anaemia, thyrotoxicosis, heart block, severe mitral regurgitation, and large arteriovenous fistula or with an increased ventricular end-diastolic pressure as in aortic or pulmonary stenosis, systemic or pulmonary hypertension, cardiomyopathy and coronary artery disease. In the latter situations it signifies poor compliant ventricle. The sound is often referred to as a sound of 'cardiac stress'. The sound may be audible in normal elderly individuals. The sound is felt more easily than it is heard.

In the electrocardiogram P wave indirectly produces S_4, and the QRS is responsible for the S_1 and S_2 occurs at the end of T. Thus the rhythm of S_4, S_1 and S_2 is the same as that of P, QRS and of T. Physiological S_4 is rarely audible as it is too soft and too low-pitched. It is often close to the S_1 to be separated from it by the ear.

The fourth heart sound is noted in situations of vigorous contraction of atria. The vibrations set in motion by the entry of the blood into the ventricle which is not easily distensible, results in a soft low-pitched sound. It is of a short duration and heard in late diastole and just before the first heart sound. It is heard from the same sites and with the same manoeuvers as in the case of the third heart sound. It is heard only in patients in sinus rhythm and disappears in atrial fibrillation. S_4 is audible in mitral regurgitation secondary to papillary muscle dysfunction or LV dilatation due to fibrosis or ischaemia, or ruptured chordae tendinae. S_4 is not audible in mitral stenosis or tricuspid stenosis, as there is failure of translation of atrial contraction into an increased late diastolic filling of the ventricles. S_4 is not heard when there is a decreased venous return. S_4 is not heard in constriction or tamponade. The left sided S_4 is audible at the apex and is louder on expiration.

The right sided S_4 is loud at the lower sternal edge and is accentuated on inspiration, and is associated with a prominent 'a' wave in the jugular venous pulse.

The presence of S_4 in patients with aortic stenosis or pulmonary stenosis implies a severe degree of stenosis.

Extra Sounds

Opening of the heart valve, unlike its closure, is normally silent. An extra sound may occur during systole (aortic and pulmonary ejection click) or diastole (opening snap, S_3 and S_4, gallops and pericardial knock).

Ejection click: A sharp high-pitched sound may be heard in early systole immediately after the first heart sound as an audible signal of opening of abnormal heart valves. It is produced by sudden opening of a deformed but pliant and non-calcified AV valve cusps during rapid ventricular ejection phase. The ejected blood causes rapid distension of the aorta or pulmonary artery and produces an extra sound. It is considered as systolic buckling of the abnormal aortic or pulmonary valve leaflets. The click is best heard using the diaphragm of the stethoscope. It may simulate splitting of the first heart sound.

Aortic ejection clicks are heard in dilatation of the aortic root, aneurysm of ascending aorta, congenital bicuspid aortic stenosis and hypertension. Pulmonary ejection clicks occur in pulmonary valvular stenosis, pulmonary hypertension from any cause, dilatation of pulmonary artery and in hyperthyroidism. The presence of the click implies the mobility of the concerned semilunar valve and it disappears when it becomes calcified and immobile.

Aortic ejection clicks are best heard in the aortic area, along the left sternal border and at the apex, and are preceded by a loud first heart sound. Aortic clicks usually do not change with respiration. On the other hand, the pulmonary ejection clicks are best heard in the pulmonary area and radiate poorly. They change strikingly in intensity, becoming loud and sharp on inspiration. An aortic ejection click may be associated with aortic regurgitation and a pulmonary click may be associated with a secondum atrial septal defect.

'Mid-systolic' click: The clicks occur in early, mid- or late part of the systole. The mid-systolic click occurs in association with sudden prolapse of either one or both-more usually posterior and

less commonly anterior-leaflets of the mitral valve into the left atrium during ventricular systole. It is noted in the presence of congenitally deformed mitral valve or in myxomatous degeneration of mitral valve (mitral valve prolapse syndrome).

The clicks coincide with the time of maximal prolapse. Often they are followed by a late systolic murmur of mitral regurgitation. Unlike the third heart sound, the mid-systolic clicks are high-pitched. They are best heard with the diaphragm of the stethoscope placed at the apex. The click is noted earlier in systole when the patient stands.

Opening Snap

Nearly 0.02 to 0.04 seconds after closure of the aortic valve, atrial and ventricular pressures equalize. A small atrio-ventricular pressure gradient develops across the closed mitral valve as there is continued fall in ventricular pressure. It causes the valve cusps that had been bowed towards the atrium, to move in a downward direction rapidly into the ventricle along with the fibrous annulus surrounding the atrio-ventricular valves during ventricular isometric relaxation, and separate. Normally, the opening of the mitral and tricuspid valves is silent. In the presence of mitral stenosis, rarely in tricuspid stenosis, the events associated with the opening of the valve leaflets and the beginning of ventricular filling may be associated with a characteristic high-pitched, short snapping sound, referred to as the opening snap (OS). It coincides with a transient slowing or momentary cessation of the valve movement near the end of its excursion into the ventricle. The movement of the valve cusps is probably interrupted due to tensing of a shortened *chordae tendinae* or limitation in the movement of the leaflets due to a scar tissue. Their kinetic energy is translated into sound vibrations. The presence of an opening snap implies that the valve leaflets are pliable. When the mitral valve cusps are severely calcified or fused, there is reduction in the opening velocity of the mitral valve and they fail to buckle from the inward rush of blood from the left atrium into the left ventricle during diastole, and it is associated with disappearance of the opening snap. OS may not be audible when the mitral stenosis is minimal.

The mitral opening snap is heard best with the diaphragm of the stethoscope placed medial to the apex, between the apex and the lower left sternal border as an extra sound in the early part of the diastole 0.04 to 0.12 seconds after the second heart sound. The sound is also heard over the entire precordial area. In such an instance the sound may be confused with the split second sound. However the split sounds are similar in character and are close to each other. Opening snap does not vary with respiration.

The duration of A_2–OS interval is inversely related to the severity of mitral stenosis. The stenotic valve causes marked obstruction to the ventricle filling and there is an elevation in the atrial pressure, so as to curtail the period of ventricular isovolumetric relaxation. Thus, in severe and tight mitral stenosis, the opening snap is close to the aortic valve closure and A_2–OS interval is narrowed. The time interval between A_2 and OS is about 0.12 seconds when the left atrial pressure is only slightly elevated above normal, about 0.08 seconds, when the left atrial pressure is moderately elevated above normal, and about 0.04 seconds when left atrial pressure is markedly elevated.

In tricuspid stenosis, the opening snap is heard at the lower end of the left sternum and gets intensified during inspiration. Rarely, the opening snap is heard in situations associated with increased ventricular flow as in thyrotoxicosis and ventricular septal defect.

Diastolic Gallop Rhythms

The physiologically not well heard normal third and fourth heart sounds may become louder and be well heard, and thus indicate a pathologic state of the ventricular myocardium. Being ventricular filling sounds they are heard in early diastolic (S_3) and presystolic (S_4) filling of the ventricles. When the heart rate is rapid, the addition of a S_3, S_4, or both to the normal first and second heart sounds, produces a cadence, resembling that of a galloping horse (gallop rhythm, gallop sound, gallop). The presence of S_4 is often referred to as ventricular gallop or protodistolic gallop and S_4 as atrial gallop or presystolic gallop. The presence of extra heart sound should be labeled as 'gallop' and is indicative of ventricular failure. In the presence of tachycardia with both extra sounds, the time between S_3 and S_4 decreases due to shortening of diastole. They may even occur simultaneously and fuse into a loud mid-diastolic sound called summation gallop. The summation sound is nearly always loud. By carotid sinus massage, heart rate is slowed. It causes disappearance of gallop.

The gallop rhythm has to be distinguished from the triple rhythm by the presence of features of heart disease and tachycardia. These sounds are to be looked carefully when the patient is supine and holding his breath at the end expiration. Their presence signifies grave prognosis.

Pericardial knock

The pericardial knock has been recognized as a valuable diagnostic clue of constrictive pericarditis. It appears as a low-pitched extra sound early in diastole and if present, occurs 0.09 to 0.12 seconds after the aortic closure. Generally it occurs later than the opening snap but earlier than S_3. Its pitch and intensity are greater than S_3. Its location is variable. The knock coincides with an abrupt stoppage to ventricular filling in early diastole from restrictions imposed on expansion of ventricular volume by the rigid pericardium. It is loudest at the left sternal border, and is heard best with the diaphragm of the stethoscope. Pericardial knock is not present in tamponade, but is usually present in patients with effusive-constrictive type of pericarditis.

Tumour 'Plop'

A right or left atrial myxoma may produce a low-pitched early diastolic sound known as a 'tumour plop' when its prolapse through the mitral (or tricuspid) valve in diastole is abruptly stopped by its stalk. It occurs 0.08 to 0.13 seconds after the aortic closure sound and may be mistaken for S_3 or the opening snap. The sound occurs after an opening snap but before the third heart sound. The condition is associated with a mild diastolic rumble. These auscultatory evidences are not constant and are noted intermittently in different positions of the patient. The diastolic rumble increases in its intensity when the patient is seated.

Extracardiac sounds

Pericardial friction rub: Pericardial friction sound or rub is diagnostic of acute pericarditis of any aetiology. It is produced by the movement of the inflamed layers of pericardium, over one another, in the presence of an exudate. The pericardial rub is a to-and-fro high-pitched sound having a superficial scratchy or grating character. It often sounds like two pieces of sand paper rubbed against one another. It is a 'tripartite' producing a sound-like 'che-che-che' occurring at three intervals of the cardiac cycle (one in systole and two in diastole) when the heart moves relative to the pericardial sac-at the time of ventricular systole, during rapid ventricular filling in early diastole, and at the time of atrial systole. Of the three major rub components, the systolic component is almost always present followed by atrial systolic thus the rub is heard during the ventricular and atrial systole, out of step with the cardiac sounds. Though rub can be heard over any part of the precordium with the diaphragm of the stethoscope, the most frequent site is the left sternal border at about third or fourth left interspace. It may be restricted to a small area or heard extensively over precordium. Pericardial rub is louder during inspiration. The intensity of the rub is variable from day to day, and from hour to hour and it may be palpable. The friction rub is heard transiently during the course of acute myocardial infarction.

The rub increases in its loudness when the patient sitting upright bends forwards and when pressure of the chest piece is increased. It may still be audible even after the appearance of the pericardial effusion as some parts of the visceral and parietal pericardial surfaces remain in contact. When there is involvement of overlying pleura in the inflammation, the rubbing of pleura against the anterior layer of pericardium produces the noise as a pleuro-pericardial friction rub.

Prosthetic sounds

Mechanical replacement of heart valves produces loud clicks due to opening and closing of the valves. These sounds may get muffled or disappear if the valve movement is restricted by a thrombus or vegetation.

Pacemaker sounds

There can be a pacing sound just before the first heart sound, synchronous with the pacing impulse. The sound appears to be due to contraction of intercostal muscles or diaphragm.

Mediastinal crunch

A series of systolic knocks or crunching sounds associated with the heart beat may be heard on the left of the sternum in the case of a left sided shallow pneumothorax (noisy pneumothorax). It is better audible during expiration with the patient leaning to the left. A shallow pneumothorax at the left lung apex can result in air pockets on the medial aspect of the lung. The contraction of the left ventricle against these air bubbles may produce sounds at the apex that are synchronous with systole or diastole. It may be noted in young males.

Metallic tinkle

A metallic tinkle that is synchronous with systole may be heard in hydropneumopericardium (a mixture of fluid and air in the pericardial sac). A large amount of air if introduced into the pericardium to replace the fluid removed, can produce a churning, splashing sound and it is called 'mill-wheel' murmur.

Hamman's sign

Mediastinal emphysema can produce soft or loud crackles and churning sounds with each cardiac contractions. Such a crunching may be produced by a dilated lower oesophagus or gastric dilatation or bullous emphysema of the lingual lobe. The sign is named after Louis Hamman, a US physician.

Murmurs

Normally, the blood flow is laminar in character and is silent. The flow can become turbulent with an increase in its velocity. It results in the production of vibrations at or near a valve, or of an abnormal communication within the heart, or as bruits at the site of arterial stenosis (Fig. 37). Generally, the turbulence of the flow is facilitated by an alteration in the size of the tube-constriction or dilatation— or by the presence of a vibrating flap in the lumen or decreased viscosity of the blood. The murmurs are referred to as organic (significant or guilty) when they arise from the damaged heart and as functional (innocent, insignificant, haemic or flow) when they are produced by the rapid flow of the blood through normal valves.

The haemic murmurs are faint and systolic in time. Increased flow across the pulmonary valve due to vigorous myocardial contraction with its associated increased stroke output leads to such murmurs. They are increased by exercise and are commonly

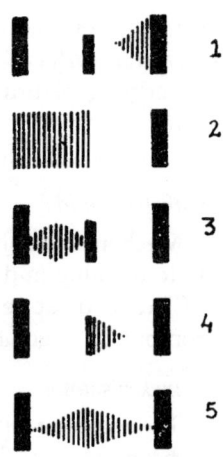

Fig. 37 Murmurs: (1) mid-diastolic and pre-systolic with loud first heart sound; (2) pansystolic with muffled first sound; (3) mid-systolic; (4) early diastolic; and (5) continuous.

found over the pulmonary area and to a lesser extent over the cardiac apex. They are ejection in type being noted at an interval after the first heart sound and disappear before the second heart sound. However, systolic murmurs of significance may be noted even in the absence of valve damage. Papillary muscle-chordae tendinae dysfunction may result in a murmur of mitral regurgitation without involving the mitral valve. Similarly the left ventricular dilatation from hypertension or aortic valvular disease may produce systolic murmur without any involvement of the mitral valve.

In health, the cardiac valves prevent the backward flow (regurgitation) of the blood by their closure. They do not obstruct the forward flow when they are open. During the systole, the mitral and tricuspid valves are closed, thus preventing the regurgitation of the blood into the atrium. The aortic and pulmonary valves are opened allowing the forward flow of the blood without any impediment. During diastole, the aortic and pulmonary valves close, preventing the regurgitation of the blood into the ventricles and the mitral, and the tricuspid valves open allowing the entry of the blood from the atria to the ventricles.

In conditions of valvular insufficiency (incompetence), the valves do not close completely and allow the blood to regurgitate back. The backward flow of the blood through an incompetent valve, septal defect or patent ductus arteriosus sets the valves and the wall of the heart into vibrations resulting in a murmur. Similarly, impediment to a forward flow of blood, through a stenosed or an irregular valve and into a dilated vessel or chamber results in a murmur. A murmur is also produced from an increased flow through normal or abnormal valves.

While Describing a Murmur the Following Features have to be noted Carefully.

Timing
Sitel
Loudness
Pitch
Duration
Character
Configuration
Transmission
Relation to respiration
Effect of posture
Effect of physical manoeuvres
Alterations with irregular rhythm
Onset
Effect of pharamacological agents

1) Timing: The location of the murmur in the cardiac cycle should be taken. The precise time of onset and time of cessation of a murmur depends on the instant in the cardiac cycle at which an adequate pressure difference between two chambers arises and disappears. At normal cardiac rate, the systole is considerably shorter than the diastole. The duration of both phases of cardiac cycle approach each other in tachycardia. The systolic or diastolic murmurs occur either with systole or diastole respectively. The murmur may be continuous throughout the systole and the diastole. There is a lift of the fingers with each systole of the heart corresponding with the first heart sound. The carotid artery has to be palpated when the apex beat cannot be felt. Its pulsations follow that of the contraction of the ventricles by 0.1 second.

The second heart sound is loud at the base and it is taken as a reference point to locate the murmur in the cardiac cycle. In the presence of extrasystoles, the beat immediately following a compensatory pause should be identified and it will be the first heart sound.

2) Site: Generally the murmur is heard with a great intensity near the site of its origin. Depending on the valve, the murmur is heard at the site where the valve sound is heard best normally. The murmurs arising from the pulmonary and tricuspid valves are generally localized in their area of the precordium and the area overlying the corresponding valves. The murmur of aortic or mitral origin can radiate to a wide area. The aortic systolic murmur may be heard at the apex of the heart with the same intensity as in the right second intercostal space. It radiates to the carotid arteries. The murmur of severe mitral regurgitation is heard most often loudest at the cardiac apex. It may radiate to the left sternal border and base of the heart when the posterior mitral leaflet is predominantly involved or to the axilla and back when the anterior leaflet is more severely affected.

3) Loudness: Loudness of a murmur reflects the degree of turbulence. It relates to the volume and velocity of flow and not the severity of the heart lesion. Depending on the intensity of loudness, systolic murmurs are classified into six grades (introduced by Freeman and Levine in 1933, and modified by Levine and Harvey in 1959): Grade I: very faint murmur audible only after the listener has 'tuned in'; Grade II: faint murmur heard immediately upon placing the stethoscope on the chest; grade V: very loud murmur which cannot be heard with the stethoscope removed from the chest wall, but can be heard with the rim of the chest piece touching the skin; Grade VI: loudest murmur audible with the stethoscope removed from the chest wall. Grade III and IV are intermediate. The grade III murmur is not accompanied by a thrill. The grade IV murmur is accompanied by a thrill. The loudness of the murmur does not reflect the extent of the underlying damage to the valve or wall.

Systolic murmurs are also classified as either mid-systolic ejection murmurs heard in obstruction to pulmonary or aortic valve outflow tracts or pansystolic regurgitant murmurs heard in mitral or tricuspid regurgitation or ventricular septal defect. A pansystolic murmur begins with the first heart sound and continues through to the second heart sound. The intensity of a pansystolic murmur is uniform. Ejection murmurs having a diamond or kite or spindle-shaped configuration reach a peak in midsystole or late systole, and then diminish before the second heart sound. It implies more severe stenosis if the intensity peaks later during systole.

Diastolic murmurs used to be graded as grade I (very soft); Grade II (soft); Grade III (moderate) and Grade IV (loud or associated with palpable thrill).

It is not possible to make conclusions on the intensity of the murmur. A small defect in ventricular septum may be associated with a loud murmur and severe aortic regurgitation may be associated with a soft murmur.

4) Pitch: The murmur may be of a high, medium or low-pitch. It is dependent on the velocity of the flow. An increase in the velocity results in a high-pitched murmur. A decrease in the velocity results in a low-pitched murmur.

The intensity of rough systolic murmur of aortic origin assumes a higher pitch towards the cardiac apex and the intensity of the murmur decreases abruptly at the apex as the murmur does not radiate laterally beyond the apex. The intensity of the murmur of aortic valve stenosis increases during ventricular systole following the long diastolic pause produced by a premature ventricular contraction.

The intensity of the murmur is dependent on the stroke volume and the force of ventricular contraction. It may be faint or loud. The murmur becomes markedly diminished or even disappears when the left ventricular contractility is severely diminished. In the presence of pulsus alternans the murmur may alternate in intensity. The intensity of systolic murmur peaks early in systole in aortic valve sclerosis.

The systolic murmur of mitral regurgitation begins immediately after the first heart sound and lasts throughout systole. It may diminish in intensity in late systole as the left atrium fills with blood.

5) *Duration:* The length of the murmur may be short (early systolic, early diastolic, late systolic), medium (mid-systolic, mild-diastolic) or long (pansystolic). Late systolic murmurs are due to mitral valve prolapse, non-rheumatic mitral regurgitation, or hypertrophic cardiomyopathy with obstruction. The murmur begins in the latter part of systole and continues up to and through the aortic component of the second heart sound.

Diastolic murmur may be early diastolic, mid-diastolic or late diastolic (pre systolic). Early diastolic murmur begins at the second heart sound (aortic and pulmonary regurgitation). Mid-diastolic murmur of mitral or tricuspid valve stenosis, begins after a short gap following the second heart sound. Pre systolic murmur ends in loud first heart sound (mitral valve stenosis).

6) *Character:* The loudness of the murmur may be increasing or decreasing in intensity during its course. The obstructive murmurs resulting from obstruction to the flow of the blood are loud and rough; the regurgitant murmurs from the leak of the blood backwards are soft and blowing. Functional and haemic murmurs are soft in character. Depending on the quality of the murmurs they are described with terms such as blowing, rumbling, squeaking, musical or harsh. The mitral diastolic murmur is crescendo in character whereas the aortic diastolic murmur is diminuendo in character.

7) *Configuration:* The configuration of a murmur may be crescendo, decrescendo, cresecendo-decrescendo (diamond-shaped, or kite-shaped) or plateau. The mitral diastolic murmur is crescendo in character whereas the aortic diastolic murmur is decrescendo (diminuendo) in character. The basal ejection systolic murmurs have a crescendo-decrescendo configuration. The pansystolic regurgitant murmurs exhibit a plateau configuration.

8) *Transmission:* An attempt has to be made to note whether the murmur is circumscribed or conducted to other parts of the chest wall. The murmur is transmitted (conducted) in the direction of the blood flow. Aortic and mitral murmurs may radiate over a wide area. The high-velocity systolic murmurs of aortic stenosis and mitral regurgitation are directed towards the neck and the axilla respectively.

Aortic systolic murmur may be heard along the left sternal border and at the cardiac apex, and it may be conducted to the neck and the suprasternal notch. Early diastolic murmur of aortic regurgitation is heard along the left sternal border. The murmur of mitral regurgitation may radiate from the cardiac apex to the left sternal border and base of the heart when the posterior mitral leaflet is predominantly involved or to the axilla and often to the inferior angle of the left scapula when the anterior leaflet is more severely affected. As the distance of auscultation increases from the site of origin of the murmur, the intensity of the murmur decreases.

In situations of rupture of chords to the anterior leaflet of the mitral valve, mitral leaflet hoses the blood posteriorly allowing the murmur to radiate posteriorly to the back and it may be heard up and down the spine. The rupture of chords to the posterior leaflet allows the posterior valve leaflet to hose the blood anteriorly allowing the murmur to radiate anteriorly so as to be heard over the precordial region including pulmonary and aortic areas. Often these abnormalities are associated with rupture of the chordae to both leaflets.

9) Relation to respiration: The murmurs arising in the mitral or aortic valves are better heard at the end of expiration and the murmurs arising in the tricuspid or pulmonary valves are better heard at the end of inspiration. During inspiration, intrathoracic pressure decreases with increased systemic venous return to the right ventricle. There is an increase in right ventricular stroke output and ejection time. It leads to accentuation of the sounds and murmurs of right ventricular origin. As more blood is retained in the lungs during inspiration due to the increase in the capacity of the lungs the stroke output of the left ventricle gets decreased. The sounds and murmurs of the left ventricle are attenuated. The reverse occurs during expiration. The physiologic changes in cardiac haemodynamics during the respiratory cycle are responsible for the varying intensity of the murmurs during inspiration and expiration. However, these features are not apparent in the presence of congestive heart failure.

All right-sided heart sounds and murmurs (except pulmonary ejection sound) increase in intensity with inspiration. Systolic and diastolic murmurs of the tricuspid valve disease become louder during inspiration. The aortic diastolic murmur is heard better when the individual has held the breath in end expiration in a sitting and leaning forward position. The late systolic murmur of mitral valve prolapse is accentuated due to inspiratory reduction in the left ventricular size. The mid-systolic click occurs early. Similarly systolic murmur of idiopathic hypertrophic subaortic stenosis gets accentuated.

The cardio-respiratory murmurs disappear at the height of inspiration and expiration. They are better heard in mid-inspiratory and mid-expiratory phases. The innocent murmurs often disappear at the height of inspiration.

10) Effect of posture: The murmurs are auscultated when the patient is recumbent or in an upright (sitting or standing) posture. The alteration of posture causes a transient elevation of heart rate and cardiac output. The diastolic murmur of mitral stenosis is heard best with the bell of the stethoscope, when the patient is recumbent in the left lateral position. Left lateral decubitus increases the systolic murmur of mitral regurgitation, mitral valve prolapse and Austin-Flint murmur. The diastolic murmur of aortic regurgitation is heard better with the diaphragm of the stethoscope, and when the patient is sitting up and leaning forward.

There is an increase in venous return while lying down from the standing or sitting posture. There is an increase in stroke volume initially of the right followed by the left ventricle resulting in accentuation of systolic murmurs. The effect can be further increased by passive leg raising. Similar phenomenon is also noted when the patient adopts squatting position from standing. Squatting increases both venous return and systolic arterial resistance, thus ventricular after load. It increases most murmurs except those due to hypertrophic cardiomyopathy and mitral regurgitation due to prolapsed mitral valve. Those murmurs are diminished on lying down due to an increase in left ventricular end diastolic volume and reduced obstruction.

Sitting or standing increases systolic murmur of hypertrophic cardiomyopathy, and late systolic murmur of MVP, the systolic click moves closer to the S_1 and murmur becomes longer and often louder. This is due to decrease in the left ventricular volume. Squatting decreases systolic murmur of hypertrophic cardio-myopathy, and in MVP the systolic click moves closer to the S_2 and murmur becomes shorter and softer (Fig. 38) Functional murmurs disappear in a sitting posture. Venous hum is better audible in an erect position.

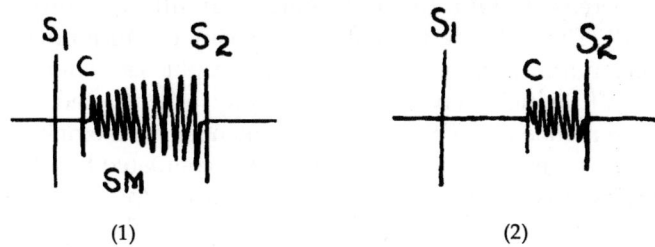

(1)   (2)

Fig. 38 Effect of standing (1) and squatting (2) on mid-systolic click and late-systolic (murmur) of mitral valve prolapse.

Effect of Posture.

Abnormality	auscultatory sign	standing	squatting
Hypertrophic obstructive cardiomyopathy	systolic murmur	increases	decreases
mitral valve prolapse	mid-systolic click	earlier onset closere to S_1	later onset closere to S_2
	late systolic murmur	longer, louder	shorter, softer

There is alteration in the murmur of atrial myxoma as myxoma gets displaced in upright and lateral positions. Functional murmurs disappear in a sitting posture. Venous hum is better audible in an erect position and when the chin is tilted upwards. The hum is abolished by recumbency.

11) Effect of physical manoeuvres (dynamic auscultation): The faint murmurs can be made audible with exercise, as there is an increase in the rate of blood flow. A few sit-ups prior to auscultation accentuate faint murmurs. An ambulatory patient may walk up and down the room ten times to achieve a greater increase in the cardiac output. Isometric hand-grip exercise (squeeze both empty fists simultaneously for half a minute) or transient arterial occlusion of both arms with 2 blood pressure cuffs increases systemic vascular resistance, arterial pressure, heart rate and cardiac output. The murmurs of mitral regurgitation, mitral stenosis, VSD and aortic regurgitation increase in their intensity. There is a decrease in the intensity of systolic murmurs of aortic stenosis and hypertrophic cardiomyopathy.

Valsalva's manoeuvre: When the supine patient strains against examiner's hand placed on mid-abdomen for 15 seconds (forced expiration against a closed glottis after full inspiration) there is an increase in intrathoracic pressure, fall in systemic venous return and decreased right and left ventricular filling (ventricular preload). There is a decrease in the intensity of murmurs except systolic murmurs associated with hypertrophic cardiomyopathy and MVP, which may be paradoxically accentuated during Valsalva manoeuvre. On release of the manoeuvre the right-sided murmurs return to normal intensity earlier compared to left-sided murmurs. It is due to an early venous return to the right heart.

12) *Alteration with irregular cardiac rhythm:* The intensity of systolic murmur of the valvular aortic stenosis becomes louder after the pause following a long RR interval as in atrial fibrillation or premature ventricular beats. However, the holosystolic murmur of mitral regurgitation tends to be of constant loudness irrespective of the rhythm. In contrast, murmurs due to aortic valve regurgitation or a VSD do not alter much during the beat following a prolonged diastole.

13) *Onset:* Recent onset of a heart murmur may suggest infective endocarditis such as acute mitral regurgitation or acute aortic regurgitation, or a serious complication in a patient with acute myocardial infarction (acute VSD, mitral regurgitation).

14) *Pharmacologic interventions:* Inhalation of amyl nitrite increases systolic murmurs of valvular aortic stenosis and hypertrophic obstructive cardiomyopathy, and decreases the murmurs of mitral regurgitation, VSD and aortic regurgitation.

Systolic Murmurs

Based on the mode of origin, systolic murmurs are classified into the following varieties: mid-systolic ejection murmur, pansystolic regurgitant murmur, and late systolic murmur. They are heard best with the diaphragm of the stethoscope.

Heart Sounds and Murmurs over the Precordium.

Location	sounds and murmurs
Second right intercostal space	sounds and murmurs of aortic valve and aorta
Second left intercostal space	sounds and murmurs of pulmonary valve and pulmonary artery
mid left sternal border	diastolic murmur of aortic regurgitation
lower left sternal border	I heart sound, systolic clicks, right-sided S_4 and S_3 gallops, tricuspid valve sounds and murmurs,
VSD	murmur
apex	left-sided S_4 and S_3 gallops, murmur of mitral
valve	origin, aortic ejection sound and murmur

The organic systolic murmur has to be distinguished from the functional systolic murmur. The latter is a soft ejection murmur occupying early systole. It is heard in conditions associated with hyperkinetic circulatory states such as severe anaemia, thyrotoxicosis, beri beri, peripheral AV fistula, pregnancy, fever, exercise, or cardiac dilatation. Such a murmur may he heard in association with skeletal abnormalities such as kyphoscoliosis, or pectus excavatum. The haemic murmur is heard in the pulmonary area or the cardiac apex or sometimes in the left parasternal region, and is localized. The murmur is short, blowing with a uniform pitch. It is noted in the recumbent position in full expiration. It is absent in upright position. The murmur is not accompanied by a thrill.

Ejection Murmur

Ejection systolic murmurs are produced by the forward flow of blood across aortic or pulmonary outflow tracts. They can occur as a result of a forward flow of blood across a stenosed region (aortic or pulmonary valve stenosis), increased flow across a normal valve or outflow tract (aortic insufficiency, thyrotoxicosis, ASD) or forward flow of blood into a dilated pulmonary artery or aorta. The murmurs are mid-systolic, medium-pitched with the intensity ascending and descending (crescendo-decrescendo) in a diamond-shaped configuration. An interval exists between the first sound and the beginning of the murmur (isometric contraction time); similarly, a gap exists between the end of the murmur and the second sound. The murmur produced in the right ventricular outflow obstruction ends before the pulmonary component of the second sound and the ejection systolic murmur produced in the left ventricular outflow obstruction ends before the aortic component of the second sound.

As the intensity of the systolic ejection murmur is directly proportional to the velocity of the blood flow, there is variability of murmur as each beat changes in the stroke volume. In situations associated with increased stroke volume of the ventricle and increased flow of blood across the valve, the systolic murmur reaches its peak early and then fades out quickly ('kite-shaped' murmur). The systolic ejection murmurs vary with changes in the length of the cardiac cycle and stroke volume unlike regurgitant murmurs.

Aortic systolic murmur (Bruit de scie): The murmur is heard in the congenital deformity of aortic valve (cone-shaped unicuspid valve with abnormal features from infancy, bicuspid or asymmetric tricuspid valves with progressive fibrosis and calcification with thickening and decreased mobility over years), rheumatic heart disease, or a calcified valve, dilatation of the ascending aorta (hypertension, atherosclerosis and aortic aneurysm) and increased left ventricular stroke output as in hyperkinetic circulatory states and aortic regurgitation. The murmur of aortic valve stenosis is usually heard best in the second right intercostal space adjacent to the sternum (aortic area). It may be audible along the left sternal border and at the cardiac apex (Fig. 39). It is conducted to the carotid vessels above and to the apex below. At the apex the murmur has a higher pitch and is musical in character. However the murmur does not radiate laterally beyond the apex. The murmur decreases in intensity during inspiration.

The murmur retains its diamond configuration. The murmur exhibits an accentuation at the early systolic phase as the rate of ejection is high at that stage. The intensity of the murmur depends on the stroke volume. The murmur decreases in its intensity or disappears when there is marked diminution of the left ventricular contractility. In the presence of pulsus alternans the murmur may alternate in its intensity. The murmur may become spindle-shaped exhibiting the peak intensity of the murmur during the later part of systole. It implies severe stenosis. It is associated with a

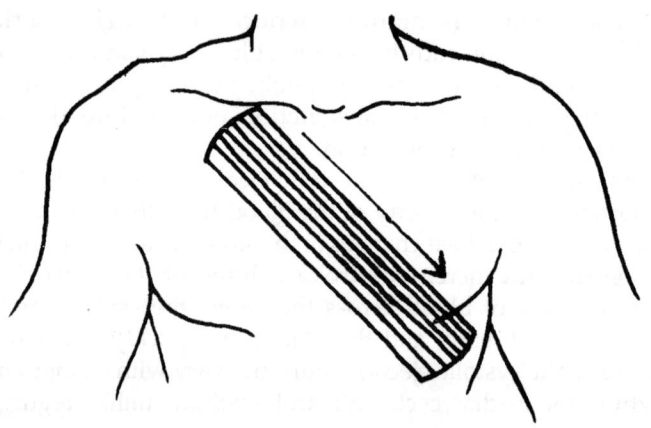

Fig. 39 Areas where aortic systolic murmur and clicks are best audible.

decreased intensity of the aortic valve closure sound.

The second heart sound is normal in aortic valve sclerosis and in hypertrophic obstructive cardiomyopathy. The systolic murmur in the latter condition is loudest along the left sternal border and radiates to the apex but may be poorly transmitted to the base or to the carotids. The murmur may increase in intensity when the patient changes from a squatting position to an upright position, and also during expiration. It decreases in intensity with an intense and a sustained grip (isometric exercise). An aortic ejection sound is not heard, but there is a loud left atrial gallop sound. The murmur of aortic stenosis may be accompanied by paradoxical splitting of the second heart sound and it implies the existence of hypertrophic obstructive cardiomyopathy rather than valvular stenosis.

In elderly persons a faint systolic murmur may be audible in the aortic area due to the stiffening and calcification of the aortic valves (aortic valve sclerosis). The murmur reaches its peak intensity early in systole and the second sound remains normal.

Flow murmurs: The flow murmurs of hyperkinetic circulatory states are not associated with a thrill. There is no ejection click and A_2 is diminished in its intensity. Innocent murmurs are always mid-systolic in timing and are caused by turbulent flow in the left (sometimes right) ventricular outflow tract. In severe aortic regurgitation there is an increase in the diastolic left ventricular blood volume leading to an increased left ventricular stroke volume. An increased amount of blood flows through the aortic valve during systole. It produces an ejection murmur, that may be faint or loud depending on the amount of stroke volume and velocity of ejection. The intensity of aortic component of the second sound may be faint. The systolic murmur of aortic stenosis is one of the loudest among the cardiac murmurs. There is a systolic thrill in the aortic area.

Pulmonary systolic murmur: Pulmonary systolic murmur is heard in pulmonary valve stenosis (congenital, rheumatic or carcinoid heart disease), absent pulmonary valve, pulmonary hypertension, dilatation of the pulmonary artery and increased blood flow through dilated main pulmonary artery as in secondum ASD and hyperkinetic circulatory states, or any condition that causes increased pulmonary flow such as anaemia, hyperthyroidism, pregnancy, anxiety or exercise and in straight back (narrow chest) syndrome due to compression of the heart. The murmur is diamond— or kite-shaped and is usually of low or medium frequency. It is localized to the second left intercostal space near the sternum, and it may radiate towards the neck. The murmur increases in its intensity on inspiration especially on standing. Inspiration increases the filling of the right ventricle, which leads to an increased flow across the pulmonary valve. The murmur may begin with a pulmonary ejection click. Ejection click if present, will decrease or disappear on inspiration. The pulmonary component of the second sound is decreased in its intensity. Severe pulmonary stenosis is accompanied by late peak of the murmur and very faint second sound.

Regurgitant Murmur

Regurgitant murmur is produced when there is flow between two chambers that have widely different pressures throughout systole such as LV and either the left atrium or the right ventricle. The pressure gradient occurs early in contraction and lasts until relaxation is almost complete. The late contraction of outflow tract is responsible for late peak of the crescendo. Regurgitant murmur is encountered when there is backward flow of the blood from the ventricles to the atrium through incompetent valves-mitral or tricuspid, or by the flow of blood through a ventricular septal defect, and under certain circumstances such as AP shunts.

The murmur is holo-(pan) systolic as blood flows over a constant intensity throughout the whole of the systole. Pansystolic murmurs are always organic murmurs. The murmur begins before aortic ejection and at the area of maximum intensity, it begins with S_1 and end after S_2

Mitral Regurgitation

A soft blowing, high-pitched pansystolic murmur is heard at the apex and it is conducted towards the axilla and the lower end of the left sternum. The radiation is great if the murmur is loud. The murmur varies little with respiration. It is frequently accompanied by a loud early diastolic filling sound (S_3). Very loud murmurs are accompanied by a thrill. The murmur may diminish in intensity during inspiration and during Valsalva manoeuvre. It may increase in intensity during isometric handgrip.

Mitral regurgitation represents a wide spectrum of disease. It can be acute or chronic. Acute mitral regurgitation occurs form rupture of chordae tendinae of the mitral valve cusps due to congenital attenuation or myxomatous degeneration or from a rupture of a papillary muscle or perforation or avulsion of a valve cusp or papillary muscle dysfunction which generally occurs as a result of acute myocardial infarction, infective endocarditis, or trauma or as a post-operative complication of cardiac surgery.

Chronic mitral regurgitation is due to rheumatic heart disease where the mitral valve leaflets are damaged and unable to coapt. Other causes of valve leaflet abnormalities include infective endocarditis, hypertrophic cardiomyopathy with outflow tract gradient, restrictive cardiomyopathy, Marfan's syndrome, prolapsed mitral valve syndrome, endocardial cushion defects or a single papillary muscle. Partial rupture of chordae tendinae or papillary muscle dysfunction due to ischaemia or fibrosis can result in chronic regurgitation also. Left ventricle dilatation also may cause regurgitation because of relative shortening of the papillary muscle preventing coaptation of the mitral valve leaflets. Calcification of mitral annulus may impair normal mitral ring systolic contraction and leaflet excursion and produce mild mitral regurgitation.

There is prolapse of markedly elongated chordae and billowing of mitral valve leaflets into the left atrium during left ventricular systole in mitral valve prolapse. It produces a high-high pitched chordal snap audible at the cardiac apex as an early systolic ejection click. It may or may not be followed by a systolic murmur. The murmur appears to increase in intensity during the late phase of systole as the leaflets become more redundant with marked contraction of the left ventricle. With the rupture of chordae tendinae or of the leaflets of mitral valve a loud high-pitched pansystolic murmur is audible at the cardiac apex. The murmur may radiate over a wide area to the second right intercostal space near the sternum, to the left of the cardiac apex, up and down the spine, and to the top of the head. There may be an atrial gallop.

Papillary muscle dysfunction and papillary muscle rupture due to myocardial infarction produce a high-pitched systolic murmur at the cardiac apex which may last throughout systole but usually tapers during late systole.

A cleft mitral valve associated with an ostium primum septal defect produces a pansystolic murmur at the cardiac apex and it radiates to the axilla. The dilatation of the mitral valve annulus in dilated left ventricle causes a loose and slightly untethered mitral valve. It produces a pansystolic murmur. It has a decrescendo configuration. It is often accompanied by atrial and ventricular gallop sounds. The murmur varies in its intensity according to the size of the left ventricle. It decreases in its intensity as the heart size decreases.

Tricuspid Regurgitation

The murmur simulating that of the murmur of the mitral regurgitation is heard over the tricuspid area (at the end of the sternum) in tricuspid regurgitation associated with pulmonary hypertension. It may be heard in the region of the cardiac apex when associated with marked right ventricular hypertrophy. It tends to get louder on inspiration due to an increased return of blood into the right ventricle, consequently a large stroke volume during systole. It is not conducted well into the axilla. The murmur may be accompanied by a right-sided gallop sound, a right ventricular gallop sound and a tricuspid valve diastolic rumble. Often the murmur of tricuspid regurgitation is due to the dilatation of the right ventricle, from pulmonary hypertension secondary to mitral valve disease or cor pulmonale, or a secondum ASD, rather than that of tricuspid valvular damage from infective endocarditis in drug addicts, rheumatic heart disease, carcinoid heart disease, Ebstein's anomaly of the tricuspid valve or right ventricular infarction.

Ventricular Septal Defect

A high-pitched pansystolic murmur is heard over the centre of the sternum or adjacent to the left side of the middle of the sternum at the level of the third and fourth left intercostal spaces. It is noted in congenital interventricular septal defect. Usually the defect is in the membranous septum. As it does not take part in the muscular contraction of the left ventricle the murmur is heard throughout the systole. The murmur decreases in its intensity near the end of systole if the defect is in muscular septum as the defect becomes small with the contraction of the left ventricle. It is frequently associated with a thrill. The murmur does not vary with respiration and it is not conducted to the axilla. Often there is a left ventricular gallop sound. Pulmonary valve closure sound increases in intensity with occurrence of pulmonary hypertension. There is decrease in shunt leading to a diminished intensity of the murmur (Eisenmenger's syndrome). The VSD as a result of myocardial infarction is associated with a murmur similar to that seen in congenital VSD. The murmur in the former condition may be better audible near the cardiac apex.

Late Systolic Murmur

Late systolic murmur is heard at the apex in mild mitral incompetence due to an unusual distortion of the mitral valve leaflet, chordae tendinae or papillary muscles (valves becoming incompetent in late systole). Similar murmur is heard in papillary muscle dysfunction or mitral valve prolapse. Dynamic outflow tract obstruction (hypertrophic cardiomyopathy) is associated with late systolic murmur and it gets accentuated on standing. These murmurs are separated from the first sound but extend up to the second sound.

Coarctation of the Aorta

There is an ejection murmur over the precordium. Often it is heard well in the left interscapular and infrascapular region. There is a slight delay in the appearance of a murmur and it occurs later than they systolic ejection murmur of aortic stenosis.

Diastolic Murmur

Diastolic murmur is always associated with cardiac disease. The murmur may be delayed (mid or late) diastolic arising from the mitral or tricuspid valves or early diastolic resulting from aortic valve regurgitation and rarely from pulmonary regurgitation.

Apical diastolic murmur: A diastolic filling murmur at the apex may arise due to a normal or deceased forward blood flow across a narrowed (stenotic) or distorted atrioventricular valve, or from an increased blood flow across normal atrioventricular valves. They occur during early ventricular period and are due to disproportion between valve orifice and flow rate. Occasionally it may be transmitted murmur from other sites.

1) With structural damage to the mitral valve:

a) *Mitral stenosis:* The narrowing of the orifice of the mitral valve due to the fusion of its cusps at the edges of the commisure results in four classical auscultatory signs. They are; opening snap mid-diastolic murmur, presystolic murmur, and loud first heart sound

The diastolic murmur begins just after a high-pitched opening snap (OS). There is a pause between the A_2 and the OS and no murmur is heard because of isovolumetric relaxation time. The diastolic murmur is low-pitched, and loud. After a very short crescendo, there is a decrescendo rumble that ends with a presystolic murmur. The diastolic rumble is like a growl and bark of a dog. It is localized to the apex or slightly inside the apex beat. Generally this murmur is constant in mitral stenosis. Frequently, it is associated with a diastolic thrill. The mid-diastolic murmur is produced by the flow of blood through the stenosed mitral valve from the left atrium than by gradient. The murmur is heard better by placing the bell of the stethoscope lightly over the cardiac apex (left ventricular impulse), and turning the patient to the left lateral position while lying down (Fig. 40). This manoeuvre brings the left ventricle into close contact with the chest wall and increases pressure gradient across mitral valve. Further it can be made prominent by increasing the blood flow across the valve (after exercise, and on coughing).

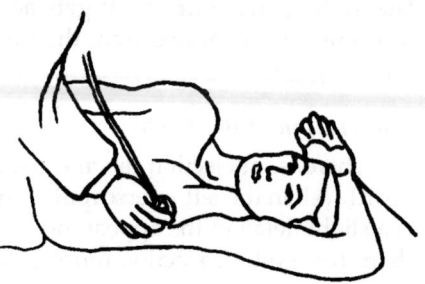

Fig. 40 Auscultation for presence of mitral diastolic murmur. Patient in left lateral position.

The duration of the murmur is a good guide regarding the severity of the stenosis. The longer the duration, the greater is the stenosis. The intensity of the murmur does not reflect the severity of valve obstruction. It must be noted that the opening snap and loud first heart sound are audible over the entire precordium and the diastolic rumble only at the cardiac apex.

A late crescendo presystolic murmur (atrial systolic ejection murmur) follows the mid-diastolic murmur and becomes continuous with an accentuated first sound.

It reflects the decrescendo gradient and flow across the stenotic valve from the left atrium to the left ventricle. Atrial contraction forces blood through the stenotic valve, and therefore occurs in sinus rhythm. The presystolic murmur disappears with the onset of the atrial fibrillation as there is no coordinated contraction of the atria. The mitral diastolic murmur is soft in mild mitral stenosis, obesity, emphysema, and low flow from severe pulmonary hypertension, tricuspid or aortic stenosis, a very dilated left atrium, cardiomyopathy, atrial fibrillation, a large right ventricle pushing the left ventricle posteriorly and a coincident ASD. The presystolic accentuation is not appreciable in the presence of mitral regurgitation and after successful mitral valvotomy. P_2 is loud when pulmonary hypertension is present.

Rheumatic valvular disease is the cause of mitral stenosis. Rare causes of mitral stenosis include left atrial myxoma, congenital mitral stenosis, a calcified bacterial vegetation and mitral ring constriction due to localized constrictive pericarditis.

b) *Carey-Coomb's murmur:* The inflammation of the mitral valve cusps (mitral valvulitis) in acute rheumatic fever or increased left atrial blood flow as a consequence of mitral regurgitation, causes a turbulence of blood flow through a distorted mitral valve and it results in a short diastolic murmur at the apex. It is soft and low-pitched and is not associated with any thrill. It is transient (Carey Coomb's murmur). It may be associated with a third heart sound, and not an opening snap as the obstruction to the valve is not significant,

c) *Calcification of mitral valve:* In elderly persons, there may be thickening and calcification of the mitral valve. It results in a blowing faint mid-diastolic murmur (Rytand's). The condition may present with syncopal attacks.

2) Without structural damage:

a) *Myoxoma of the left or right atrium:* The primary tumour of the heart arising from the lower atrial septum on the left or right atrium in middle age presents with a variable (postural) diastolic murmur at the apex. It is due to the obstruction to the flow of blood at the mitral or tricuspid orifice by the growth. The murmur changes in its intensity on alteration of the posture.

b) *Austin-Flint murmur:* In severe, chronic aortic incompetence, the regurgitating blood flow from the aortic root and the normal blood flow from the left atrium in the early part of the diastole cause ventricular filling. There is a functional partition separating the inflow and the outflow tracts of the left ventricle. The rapidly increasing left ventricular volume from increased ventricular filling makes the anterior leaflet of the mitral valve to partially close in mid-diastole and late diastole. Then the flow from the left atrium to the ventricle occurs through a narrowed orifice to result in a diastolic rumble. The murmur does not exhibit any presystolic accentuation. The murmur is not associated with a thrill or an opening snap. A third heart sound may be audible. The first heart sound is not loud. The murmur is named after Austin-Flint, a US physician.

In acute, severe aortic regurgitation, the left ventricular diastolic pressure may exceed left atrial pressure resulting in a mid-diastolic murmur due to 'diastolic mitral regurgitation'.

c) *Flow murmurs:* An increased velocity and volume of blood flow across a normal mitral valve, congenital heart diseases with a left-to-right shunt, for example VSD, PDA, hypertrophic cardiomyopathy with or without outflow obstruction, congenital complete AV block with a very slow ventricular rate, hyperkinetic circulatory states like severe anaemia, and thyrotoxicosis result in a short mid-diastolic rumble at the apex beginning after the S_3. There is no presystolic accentuation. No thrill is felt. A diastolic rumble may be heard in the lower edge of the sternum on either side due to an increased blood flow across a normal tricuspid valve (ASD). The murmur increases in its intensity on deep inspiration.

An increased blood flow across the mitral or tricuspid valve as in gross mitral regurgitation, or tricuspid regurgitation can result in a similar diastolic rumble. In mitral regurgitation the blood volume that traverses the mitral valve during ventricular systole is added to the normal amount of left atrial blood and an increased volume passes through the mitral valve during diastole.

3) *Transmitted murmurs:* The high pitched early diastolic murmur of aortic regurgitation, the diastolic murmur of PDA or tricuspid stenosis may be heard from their transmission at the apex.

Tricuspid Valve Stenosis

Tricuspid valve stenosis produces low-pitched murmur of a scratchy character and is audible near the lower end of the left sternum with the bell of the stethoscope. The diastolic rumbling of tricuspid stenosis is crescendo-decrescendo in character since the right atrial systole occurs earlier than the left. It increases blood flow through the tricuspid valve following reduction in intrathoracic pressure leading to a decreased right atrial and ventricular pressure. The intensity of the diastolic rumble is increased during inspiration and in right lateral decubitus position. It increases blood flow through the tricuspid valve following reduction in intrathoracic pressure leading to a decreased right atrial and ventricular pressure. It is associated with giant 'a' waves in the neck. The tricuspid opening snap occurs later than that of the opening snap of mitral stenosis. The increased blood flow into the right ventricle during ventricular diastole makes the large tricuspid valve leaflets to snap.

Rheumatic tricuspid stenosis never exists without mitral stenosis. In the absence of mitral stenosis, a presystolic murmur at the left parasternal area may be due to a right atrial myxoma, an ASD or carcinoid stiffening of the tricuspid valve.

Basal Diastolic Murmurs

1) *Aortic valve regurgitation:* At the end of ventricular systole the semilunar valves close. In aortic regurgitation, the cusps of the aortic valves fail to come in apposition, during the diastole, resulting in regurgitation of blood under aortic systolic pressure into the left ventricle, and is maximum at the beginning of the diastole.

The murmur begins with or shortly after the aortic component of the second sound (A_2) as the early (immediate) diastolic murmur. It may be of short duration or extend throughout the diastole. The severity of aortic regurgitation is correlated better with the duration of the diastolic murmur rather than with its intensity. It is high pitched, blowing in character and decrescendo (diminuendo) in its configuration as there is progressive diminution in the volume or rate of regurgitation during diastole. It is heard in the aortic area and conducted characteristically along the left sternal border and towards the cardiac apex. It is heard best in the left third or fourth intercostal spaces in the parasternal region. When the murmur is faint, often it is restricted to that region. The murmur may be heard loudly over the 2nd or 3rd interspace to the right of the sternum or in the 4th space when the condition is associated with dilatation of the aorta. The murmur can be mimicked by breathing out quickly with the mouth open or by whispering 'ah'. The intensity of the murmur gets diminished in the presence of increased diastolic pressure in left ventricle.

The intensity of aortic second sound is diminished in all conditions of aortic regurgitation associated with destruction of the aortic valve leaflets. The second sound is loud and ringing in aortic regurgitation of syphilitic origin. The murmur can be made prominent by asking the patient to sit up and lean forward and to hold the breath on full expiration (Fig. 41). It is best heard with the diaphragm of the stethoscope applied firmly against the chest wall. The murmur is accentuated by an acute elevation of the arterial pressure, such as occurs with handgrip exercise. The aortic regurgitation when not accompanied by other valvular lesions is considered very mild if the diastolic blood pressure is not below 70 mm Hg. In severe aortic regurgitation, the stroke output occurring through the aortic valve into the aorta during systole is doubled and it may give rise to an ejection sound and an ejection systolic murmur. It should not be mistaken for a concomitant aortic stenosis. The ejection sound is due to recoil of the aorta to a large ventricular stroke volume.

Aortic regurgitation is recognized in rheumatic, syphilitic, hypertensive, congenital (bicuspid aortic valve, fixed orifice subaortic stenosis) and arteriosclerotic (calcified aortic valve) processes. It can be heard in conditions associated with dilatation of the aortic ring as in aortic aneurysm, aortoannuloectasia, dissection of the aorta, myxomatous degeneration of the aortic valve, Marfan's syndrome, ankylosing spondylitis and may appear during subacute infective endocarditis

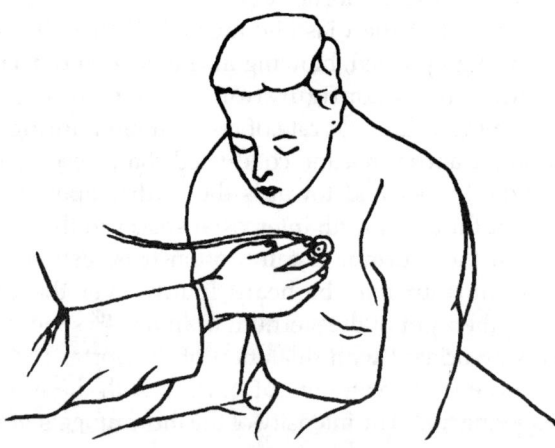

Fig. 41 Auscultation for presence of diastolic murmur of aortic regurgitation. Sitting and leaning forward, following forced expiration.

Causes of Aortic Regurgitation.

Rheumatic heart disease
Bicuspid/fenestrated aortic valve
Syphilis
Subacute infective endocarditis
Arteriosclerosis
Aortic aneurysm
Dissection of the aorta
Myxomatous degeneration of the aortic valve
Marfan's syndrome (dilatation of the aortic root)
Ehelers-Danlos syndrome
Paraprosthetic valve leaks
Idiopathic myxomatous degeneration of the aortic valve
Osteogenesis imperfecta (dilation of the aortic root)
Supravalvular aortic stenosis (fusion of a cusp with supravalvular membrane
    or adhesion of valve leaflets to the aortic wall)
Aortic arch syndrome (dilatation of the aortic ring)
Rupture of sinus of Valsalva
Ankylosing spondylitis
Giant cell arteritis
Aortic-annular ectasia
Trauma

The quality of the murmur will not be a guide to the aetiology except in the presence of a spinning top or a musical diastolic murmur, which usually denotes an evertion (subacute infective endocarditis, trauma) or retroversion and subsequent perforation of an aortic cusp or rupture of an aortic sinus of Valsalva. The rheumatic aortic regurgitation is usually accompanied with other valvular abnormalities and the murmur is better heard over the left parasternal area. The syphilitic aortic regurgitation is an isolated free regurgitation and has a tambour-like second sound and the murmur is better conducted in the right parasternal area.

The conduction of the diastolic murmur down the right sternal border points to the lesions, which cause dilatation of the root of the aorta, and rightward displacement of the ascending aorta such as aortic aneurysm, aortic dissection or aneurysm of sinus of Valsalva.

Severe aortic regurgitation may exhibit presence of four additional murmurs in addition to the high-pitched diastolic murmur. They are a systolic murmur in the aortic area due to large systolic stroke volume, a diastolic rumble at the apex, a mitral systolic murmur due to spreading of the base of the papillary muscle of the left ventricle and dilatation of mitral valve annulus and a systolic murmur of tricuspid regurgitation due to dilatation of the right ventricle and associated heart failure.

In dissection of the aorta, or aneurysm of the first part of the ascending aorta, or dilatation and rightward displacement of the aortic root, a high-pitched diastolic blowing murmur of aortic regurgitation is heard best along the right sternal border in the third interspace (Harvey sign).

Acute aortic regurgitation developing from aortic dissection, infective endocarditis or trauma is not associated with many of the peripheral manifestations (because of insufficiency to time to develop) of chronic aortic regurgitation. A 'to and fro' systolic murmur and a diastolic murmur are heard along left sternal border. The murmur is shorter in duration, and S_1 is soft or absent (due to premature mitral valve closure). A loud S_3 is heard.

3) Pulmonary valve regurgitation: The occurrence of pulmonary regurgitation is rare. It is due to dilatation of the pulmonary valve annulus secondary to long standing, very high pulmonary hypertension noted in mitral stenosis, left ventricular failure, chronic respiratory disease, congenital heart disease (VSD, PDA, ASD) with an Eisenmenger reaction, repeated pulmonary embolism or primary pulmonary hypertension. Rarely it may be noted in pulmonary valve stenosis due to a persistent opening at the centre of the valve.

The murmur of pulmonary valve regurgitation caused by pulmonary hypertension simulates the diastolic murmur of aortic regurgitation and is referred to as Graham Steell murmur, named after Graham Steell, an English physician. The early diastolic murmur is high-pitched with a decrescendo configuration. It is heard best in the second left intercostal space next to the sternum. If it is loud, it may be transmitted along the left border of the sternum. The murmur is not heard at the cardiac apex. The murmur begins immediately after loud P_2. P_2 is usually not heard in pulmonary valve stenosis (valvular type). It is associated with palpable impulse in the pulmonary area, and parasternal heave. It is not associated with the peripheral vascular signs as in aortic regurgitation. The Graham Steell murmur increases with inspiration when it is loud.

Very rarely, primary pulmonary regurgitation with normal pulmonary pressure (idiopathic dilatation of the pulmonary artery, pulmonary valvotomy. Congenital absence of pulmonary valve substance, loss of valve substance due to infective endocarditis may be noted. In such an instance, the murmur begins after slight delay following P_2. The murmur is short and then builds up quickly to a crescendo followed by a longer decrescendo character and increases with inspiration.

The diastolic murmur of congenital pulmonary regurgitation without pulmonary hypertension is low-to-medium pitched. The onset of the murmur is delayed because the regurgitant flow is less at the onset of pulmonary valve closure.

Continuous Murmurs

Continuous murmur is a murmur that is continuous throughout systole and diastole. There is a continuous flow of blood through an abnormal communication from a region of high pressure to a region of low pressure with a large pressure gradient between the two regions that persist through end of systole and the beginning of diastole. The flow of blood is in the same direction. The murmur begins in systole, peaks near S_2 and continues into all or part of diastole. Continuous murmurs are noted in thoracic aorta (persistent (patent) ductus arteriosus (PDA), collaterals of coarctation, mammary soufflé, an aorto-pulmonary septal defect (window), a rupture of a sinus of Valsalva into the pulmonary artery, right atrium, or ventricle, an internal mammary-to-pulmonary vein fistula) or cardia (a small ASD and mitral stenosis with high left atrial pressure, coronary artery to right heart fistula, surgically produced connections of the subclavian-pulmonary artery anastomosis, anomalous origin of the left coronary artery from the pulmonary artery, and cor atrium with all pulmonary veins forming a common chamber emptying into left atrium through a small opening).

In PDA, the murmur is continuous as there is a continuous aortic-pulmonary pressure gradient throughout systole and diastole. It is best heard in the second left interspace near the sternum. The next loudest site is the first left interspace. Often the murmur is referred to as a machinery (Gibson murmur, named after George Gibson, a Scottish physician) murmur and is accompanied by a thrill. A large PDA is accompanied by a paradoxically split S_2. Development of pulmonary hypertension allows disappearance of diastolic component of the murmur due to disappearance of the diastolic gradient. Pulmonary valve closure sound becomes loud.

Aortopulmonary window (septal defect) exhibits the maximum loudness of the murmur in the second left interspace and the site of next loudest site is third left interspace. However continuous murmur is uncommon as it is usually associated with severe pulmonary hypertension. In coarctation of the aorta, the systolic and diastolic gradient across a severe coarctation, and collateral intercostals vessel flow results in a continuous murmur audible over the posterior chest. In mild or moderate coarctation, only a systolic murmur is heard.

A dilated left or right coronary artery that communicates with the coronary veins, right atrium, right ventricle or pulmonary artery, and rupture of a sinus of Valsalva into right atrium or right ventricle are associated with continuous murmur in the parasternal region with diastolic accentuation of the murmur. The murmur in rupture of the sinus of Valsalva is louder and exhibits a musical quality.

In pulmonary arteriovenous fistula, there is a right-to-left shunt from the pulmonary artery to a pulmonary vein resulting in a continuous murmur over the lungs and it becomes louder on inspiration due to an increase in pressure gradient from the pulmonary artery-to-pulmonary veins. It is usually congenital and is associated with cyanosis, clubbing and telangiectasis in the skin or mucous membrane. In a small number of pregnant women a mammary soufflé is heard as a continuous arterial murmur along the left sternal border due to a large flow of blood into the superficial arteries of the breast during pregnancy and lactation.

The continuous murmur has to be differentiated from a to-and-fro murmur. The latter consists of the systolic murmur due to blood flowing in one direction and the diastolic murmur due to flow in opposite direction such as ejection murmur of aortic stenosis and aortic regurgitant murmur and the systolic murmur of ASD or mitral regurgitation, and an aortic regurgitant murmur. In the latter the forward and backward flow does not take place through the same orifice. It should be noted that the continuous murmur of PDA reaches a crescendo at about the time of the valve closure sound, and the to-and-fro murmur has, in fact, two components that can be differentiated. The systolic component fades and disappears before the onset of the semilunar valve closure sound.

The to-and-fro murmur (VSD with a defect in membranous part of interventricular septum and aortic valve regurgitation due to a poorly supported aortic valve) has, in fact, two components which can be differentiated. There is a pansystolic murmur which fades and disappears before the onset of the semilunar valve closure sound. It is followed by an early diastolic murmur.

Auscultation of Blood Vessels

Apart from the transmitted murmurs from the heart (Systolic murmurs of aortic stenosis and pulmonary stenosis), a murmur may arise in the arteries. The presence of the murmur (bruit) over a vessel has great diagnostic significance.

Systolic murmur: A systolic murmur is audible as a hissing systolic sound over an aneurismal sac affecting the innominate, carotid, and subclavian arteries, over the partially narrowed carotid artery in the neck and over the stenosed renal artery in the loins. The bell of the stethoscope is used to listen to the arterial bruit. A systolic murmur may be audible in the intercostal spaces in the presence of coarctation of the aorta. The murmur is caused by tortuous intercostal arteries. Even the murmur of aortic coarctation is heard in the interscapular region. An increased pulmonary blood flow noted in ASD may produce a systolic murmur over the lungs posteriorly. Obstruction of the iliac arteries may produce a systolic murmur in the right and left lower quadrants. Systolic bruit is audible over the bones (Paget's disease), thyroid (thyrotoxicosis), pregnant uterus (uterine soufflé) and lactating breast (mammary souffle).

A systolic murmur from an excessive forward flow is produced by applying chest piece on the femoral artery and gradually compressing the artery with the fingers proximal to the chest piece. A pistal shot sound (Traube's) coinciding with the first heart sound is audible loudly over brachial and femoral artery with the bell of the stethoscope, in aortic regurgitation and hyperkinetic circulatory states.

Diastolic murmur: In aortic regurgitation, a diastolic murmur is produced by gradually compressing the femoral artery with the fingers distal to the chest piece (Duroziez's sign, named after Paul Duroziez, a French physician). The diastolic murmur is due to backward flow of the blood as occurs normally in all large arteries.

Continuous murmur: A rough continuous murmur with a systolic accentuation is heard over the arteriovenous (AV) fistula. A continuous humming murmur is heard over the jugular veins from rapid blood flow and over dilated veins communicating portal with caval venous systems in cirrhosis of the liver. An AV malformation of the brain may produce a continuous murmur over the head.

EIGHT

NERVOUS SYSTEM

> *"God may forgive you your sins, but your nervous system won't"*
>
> Alfred Kovzybski (1879-1950)

Introduction

Nervous system is divided into the central and peripheral nervous system. The former consists of the brain and spinal cord encased in the cranium and the vertebral column respectively. The brain consists of forebrain (cerebral hemispheres, thalami, and hypothalamus), mid-brain and hind brain (pons, medulla oblongata and cerebellum). The emerging cranial nerves and the spinal nerves constitute the peripheral nervous system.

The diseases affecting the central nervous system result in a disorder of its function. A detailed neurologic examination is essential to determine the presence of neurologic abnormality. The clinical diagnosis in a neurologic case comprises four essentials: Physiologic diagnosis (right hemiplegia), anatomic diagnosis (left internal capsule), pathologic diagnosis (internal carotid artery occlusion), and aetiologic diagnosis (atherosclerosis). Based on the history and signs, and basic knowledge of neuroanatomy, the location (site) of the lesion in the nervous system and the nature of the lesion have to be determined.

It should be remembered that the neurologic examination may be normal even in patients with a serious neurologic disease such as seizures, a transient ischaemic attack (TIA) or chronic meningitis.

The clinical examination consists of examination of higher functions, cranial nerves, motor system, sensory system, cerebellum, peripheral nerves, neck, skull and spine. The examination has to be performed in an orderly manner to avoid errors and omissions.

Higher Functions

The intellectual state and mental functions of the patient are judged at the commencement of the physical examination. The ability to give a coherent and chronologic history, memory for recent or remote events, promptness to answer the questions gives an insight into his mental functions. Depending upon the educational background, upbringing and general knowledge of the surroundings, the questions may be framed to test the intelligence.

Mental status: The mini-mental status examination (MMSC) is used to assess cognitive function. It helps in making the diagnosis of moderate-to-severe dementia. It gives a true picture of the patient of current mental status of the patient.

The Mini-mental Status Examination.

Cognitive functions	points
Orientation	
Name season/date/day/month/year	5 (1 for each name)
Name hospital/floor/town/state/country	5 (1 for each name)
Registration	
Identify three objects by name and ask patient to repeat	3 (1 for each object)
Attention and calculation	
Serial 7s: subtract from 100 (e.g. 93-86-79-72-65)	5 (1 for each subtraction)
Recall	
Recall the three objects presented earlier	3 (1 for each object)
Language	
Name pencil and watch	2 (1 for each object)
Repeat 'no, ifs, ands, or buts'	1
Follow a 3-step command (e.g. 'take this paper, fold it in half, and place it on the table')	3 (1 for each command)
write 'close your eyes' and ask patient to obey written command	1
ask patient to write a sentence	1
ask patient to copy a design (e.g. intersecting pentagons)	1
Total	30

Level of consciousness: Level of consciousness refers to the patient's relative state of awareness of the self and the environment, and ranges from fully conscious to comatose.

The state of consciousness has to be noted. Consciousness refers to awareness of oneself and the surroundings in a state of wakefulness. The patient is in a fit mental state to give the history and relevant facts about oneself. The patient is alert about his surroundings and responds to stimuli. It is a function of the cerebellum and is affected by supratentorial lesions. Wakefulness is a function of hypothalamus and the reticular system.

The patient may be comatose (loss of consciousness) and it may be graded as light (semi-appropriate movements for the noxious stimuli) or deep (absence of any response except retention of primitive reflexes). The patient may be in a state of drowsiness (a state exhibiting excessive tendency to sleep, from which the patient can be roused to wakefulness, but tends to sink into sleep again if the stimulus is stopped), or stupor (a state wherein the patient shows response on vigorous stimuli but sinks as soon as the painful stimulus is withdrawn).

Altered consciousness is produced by the lesions affecting the brain stem, reticular formation, and the cerebral cortex. The important causes of coma and stupor are cerebrovascular accidents (cerebral haemorrhage, subarachnoid haemorrhage, brain stem haemorrhage or infarction, hypertensive encephalopathy), space occupying lesions (mass lesions above the tetorium cerebri, cerebral abscess, haematoma), head injury, infections (meningitis, encephalitis, cerebral malaria), metabolic disorders (hypoglycaemia, hyperglycaemia, hepatic failure, renal failure), endocrine disturbances (hypopituitarism, hypothyroidism, Addison's disease), hyperpyrexia, hypothermia, respiratory failure with hypercapnoea, epilepsy, narcotics and alcohol abuse.

Even when the patient is conscious, he may be in a state of confusion or delirium. Confusion is a state of altered consciousness in which the patient is bewildered and misinterprets the world around him. Delirium refers to a state of high arousal associated with confusion and often, visual hallucinations. Apathy is a state wherein the patient does not show any interest in the surroundings. However, he can talk and volunteer information.

Akinetic mutism is a variety of stupor wherein the patient cannot be aroused even with persistent painful stimuli even though eyes remain alert to moving objects. The condition results from damage to the reticular activating system. The "locked-in syndrome" is a state of unresponsiveness but wakefulness. The patient is not able to communicate or move. It is due to infarction of the brain stem.

Emotional state: The attention, interest in the surroundings, dress and personal cleanliness give an idea about the general appearance and behaviour pattern of the patient. The emotional state of the individual is assessed, by noting the presence of happiness, depression, apathy (absence of emotional response), anxiety or irritability. There may be laughter or tears in an incongruous manner. The individual may exhibit false perception mistaking something for what it is not (illusion), false beliefs (delusions) or false sensory impression (hallucinations).

Orientation: The orientation to time and surroundings is noted by asking about the time, day, place of examination and surroundings. The handedness has to be determined by asking the patient which hand he uses for routine work and skilled work. In right-handed individuals, the speech centre is situated in the left cerebral hemisphere. The muscular development is good on that side. Idiopathic epilepsy is common in left-handed individuals.

Speech

Speech is communication by language. The formation of speech is essentially a cortical function. It involves perception, formation and expression of thoughts. It is the outcome of visual and auditory stimuli, their comprehension and expression. The centres are situated in the left cerebral hemisphere in right-handed individuals. It is referred to as the dominant hemisphere. However, left hemisphere dominance is noted in left-handed individuals.

The speech centres are situated in the form of a quadrilateral, consisting of a visual area (calcarine sulcus of the occipital lobe), auditory area (superior temporal gyrus), Broca's (after Pierrre Paul Broca, a French anatomist and surgeon) area (3rd frontal convolution at the posterior portion of inferior frontal gyrus), writing centre (2nd frontal convolution) and their associated fibres in between. The visual and auditory impulses reach the visual and auditory areas in the occipital cortex and then they are carried through association fibres to different parts of the cerebral cortex. The efferent or motor centre is located in Broca's area. The muscles of articulation (larynx, palate, tongue and lips) are innervated by the cranial nerves arising from the bulbar region.

The defects of speech may arise from the lesion in the cortical centres (dysphasia or aphasia) or in the peripheral motor mechanisms (dysarthria). Speech defects may affect articulation, fluency, verbal comprehension, naming, repetition, reading and writing. The lesions, in front of the central sulcus affects articulation and fluency. Reading and writing are affected in lesions behind the central sulcus. They are referred to as anterior and posterior aphasic syndromes. Before examination of the patient the educational background, mother-tongue, level of consciousness, handedness, intelligence and hearing have to be assessed.

Speech defects fall into four main types:
1. Aphasia / dysphasia
2. Dysarthria
3. Aphonia
4. Mutism

1. Aphasia /dysphasia

Aphasia: Aphasia refers to a disturbance in the ability to use language. There is defective production and or comprehension of spoken and or written symbols. The individual loses his ability to express (motor) or comprehend (sensory). Expressive aphasia may be of spoken or written speech. Receptive aphasia may be auditory (word deafness) or visual (word blindness). The reception and interpretation of the speech is dependent on the integrity of vision and hearing. The centres concerned in the dominant hemisphere may be affected in injury, thrombosis, tumour, abscess or degeneration. It is rare to find an isolated variety of either motor or sensory aphasia. Generally it is of mixed type.

a) *Motor aphasia (Broca's or anterior aphasia):* There is an inability to speak or write (rarely). It is due to a lesion in the left frontal lobe that causes decreased fluency of speech with comprehension remaining relatively intact. Generally these defects are observed when the patient is allowed to talk on his own. All degrees of expressive aphasia may be met with. The patient may find an inability to speak or his speech may be limited to certain words. He may use wrong words or use words repeatedly or may construct incomplete sentences. He may use words or phrases inappropriately or coin a new word that does not exist (neologism). The patient may have difficulty in naming the objects presented to him (nominal aphasia). He finds it difficult to name familiar objects like a pen, book, matchbox, key, watch or pencil. It is caused by a left posterior temporal or inferior parietal lesion. To rectify the difficulty he may adapt a description, which is nearly, but not exactly, right (paraphasia) wherein for a pen he says that 'it is used for writing'. Then if a series of objects are enumerated before him, he readily agrees with the relevant word. There may be a difficulty or loss of ability to comprehend mathematical exercises (acalculia).

b) *Sensory aphasia (Wernicke's or posterior aphasia):* The sensory aphasia may be auditory where there is an inability to comprehend the words heard, or visual, where there is an inability to understand the written words in spite of the respective cranial nerves being intact. It is due to a left temporoparietal lesion.

In word deafness, though the patient hears the words, he is unable to grasp the meaning and they mean nothing to him. The individual is unable to carry out the simple commands like 'touch the nose with your finger', 'show the teeth', or 'open the mouth'. In word blindness (visual agnosia) there is an inability to understand written words. Vision is not affected. This is tested by asking literate patients, to perform written instructions.

As the motor speech centre, is influenced by the receptive centre, the expression is affected. To use a proper word the patient must be able to understand written or spoken words. The replies will be inappropriate if he is unable to understand. In dysgraphia, the patient is unable to write.

c) *Global (central) aphasia:* When both the receptor and expressive centres are affected it results in total aphasia. The patient loses the ability to understand. There is widespread damage to the areas concerned with speech. It is noted following a severe left hemisphere infarct.

Dysphasia: Dysphasia refers to a condition wherein the patient fails to put into properly constructed words or phrases to the thoughts he wishes to express. This happens in the lesion of the highest mechanism of speech located in the dominant cerebral hemisphere. The condition includes disturbances of writing (dysgraphia) and failure to comprehend the spoken word (receptive dysphasia) or the written word (dyslexia).

2. Dysarthria

Proper articulation requires proper coordination of the tongue, lips, palate, larynx and the muscles of respiration. It may be affected in lesions of the upper and lower motor neurons, muscles concerned with articulation, and influence of the extrapyramidal and cerebellar systems, to result in distortion of enunciation of the individual words and phrases. While taking the history, the clarity, fluency and rhythm of the speech have to be noted. Some of the common types of dysarthria are as follows:

Spastic dysarthria: Bilateral upper motor neuron disease such as motor neuron disease, pseudobulbar palsy and upper brain stem tumour, give an impression that the patient is trying to talk from the back of the throat. The speech is slurred.

Rigid dysarthria: The speech in Parkinsonism (named after James Parkinson, English physician) is monotonous with low volume, and words run into one another and sentences start and stop abruptly. The later words in long sentences may come out in a rush. There may be constant repetition of a particular word (palilalia) in severe cases.

Ataxic dysarthria: Absence of coordination of the muscles of speech results in an irregular, slurred speech. Sometimes the speech is too hard or too soft, and the words run into each other, or are spaced too far. The rhythm is jerky, sometimes explosive. Such staccato or scanning speech is encountered in chorea, cerebellar disease or tumours, and multiple sclerosis. In scanning, the speech is slow, and patient utters syllable by syllable.

Dysarthria due to lower motor neuron (LMN) lesions: Though speech is well maintained, individual words cause difficulty due to muscle weakness in facial palsy (labials), tongue paralysis (distorted speech) or palatal paralysis (nasal speech).

3. Aphonia

Aphonia refers to a condition wherein the patient while speaking, fails to produce any volume of sound or merely whispers. Diseases of the larynx (laryngitis) or vocal cords (bilateral adductor palsy) may result in the loss of voice even though the articulation is intact.

4. Mutism

Mutism is a psychological disorder wherein a conscious patient makes no attempt to speak or make sound. It may be encountered in lesions involving the anterior part of the walls of the 3rd ventricle and the posterior-medial surface of the frontal lobe bilaterally.

Memory

Memory is a higher mental faculty concerned with registration (ability to add new information to the existing memory stores), retention (ability to retain memory), recall (ability to remember an experience) or recognition (familiarity of person, event or object).

Memory loss (amnesia) can develop either suddenly or slowly. Defects of memory are either in the registration of recent images and ideas (antegrade) or the recall of past events (retrograde).

The recent memory is tested after noting special interests of the patient like sports, literature, films or current affairs. He may be asked about the literature, films or current affairs. He may be asked about the date, day of the week, or any event of major importance. He may even be asked to recall the names and numbers after five minutes of other conversation. The limbic system, including the mamillary bodies and hippocampus must be intact to register a new experience and recall recent events.

Antegrade amnesia is noted in gross dementia, following epileptic seizure, head injury, dysphasia, cerebrovascular disease, depression and in acute confusion states. The long-term memory is assessed, by asking details of remote events concerned with him and his family, and about important people or events. Loss of memory for recent events is more common than loss of memory for past events.

Confabulation refers to a defective memory being bridged by imaginary stories. It is encountered in toxic states (alcoholism, drug addiction) and head injury.

Cranial Nerves

There are 12 pairs of cranial nerves and they are classified into three categories depending on their function: 1) Sensory: Olfactory, optic and auditory; 2) Motor: Oculomotor, trochlear, abducent, spinal accessory and hypoglossal; and 3) Mixed: trigeminal, facial, glossopharyngeal and vagus. Amongst them, the olfactory and optic nerves are extensions of the central nervous tissue. Remaining nerves arise from the brainstem and innervate facial, cranial and cervical tissues. These nerves may be affected in the disease process in their intracranial and extracranial courses, and at their site of origin. The functions of these nerves are examined in detail.

Olfactory Nerve

The olfactory nerve fibres arise from the sensory cells in the olfactory epithelium located in the upper part of the nasal fossa and reach the olfactory bulb after passing through the cribriform plate of the ethmoid. It carries sensations of smell from the nasal mucosa to the olfactory bulb. The fibres forming the olfactory tract emerge from the olfactory bulb and reach the uncus of hippocampal gyrus (olfactory area) in the cerebral cortex.

The sense of smell is tested to determine presence of any impairment and to find out whether it is due to local nasal lesion or to a neurologic lesion. It is performed by using familiar aromatic substances, such as camphor, oil of lavender, oil of cloves, oil of peppermint, turpentine, eucalyptus, tooth paste, soap, fruit, or coffee. Each nostril is tested in turn by bringing the bottles containing these substances near it (Fig. 42). While testing one nostril, the other nostril is compressed by placing a finger over it. The patient has to close his mouth and is asked to identify the substances on sniffing. The test is repeated using the other nostril. After an interval to allow dispersal of the odour, the test is repeated with two further substances. Irritant substances such as ammonia or acetic acid are not used as they act by stimulating the sensory endings of the trigeminal nerve present in the nasal mucosa. This test is purely subjective and patient's word has to be taken.

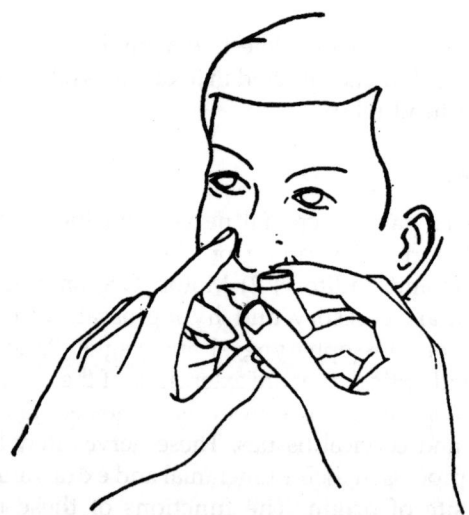

Fig. 42 Bottle with aromatic substance brought to each nostril.

Loss of Smell is called Anosmia. It may be lost in the Following Conditions.

Local nasal conditions
    coryza, sinusitis
    atrophic rhinitis
    nasal polyp
    heavy smoking
Neurologic conditions
    head injury
    fracture of the anterior cranial fossa
    atrophy of olfactory bulb
    olfactory groove meningioma, inferior frontal glioma
    basal meningitis
    Parkinson's disease
Kallmann's syndrome (agenesis of olfactory bulb, hypogondotropic
    hypogonadism)
Hysteria

Anosmia is considered significant if it is unilateral. Anatomical location of olfactory nerve, makes it liable to be damaged by tumours especially subfrontal meningioma or by head injuries especially that involving anterior cranial fossa. Often the patient confuses anosmia with loss of taste, as flavour depend upon the sense of smell not the sense of taste. The loss of smell may be a feature of hysteria. The sense of smell is diminished in nasal obstruction.

Parosmia refers to a perversion of smell where offensive substances appear to have a pleasant odour and *vice-versa*, and it may be noted in incomplete recovery following head injuries, aura in epilepsy, lesions in the uncus and pyriform cortex, schizophrenic or depressive states, and hysterical conversion syndromes. Hallucination of smell may occur as an aura in temporal lobe epilepsy.

Optic Nerve

The optic nerve, concerned with vision is a sensory nerve and is considered as a forward extension of a part of the brain. It carries visual impulses from the retina to the optic chiasma and in the optic tract to the lateral geniculate body. In addition, it acts as an afferent pathway for the papillary reflex by the fibres traveling to the superior colliculus of the mid brain.

The fibres originating in the retina pass behind as the optic nerve and enter the cranial cavity through the optic foramen. The nerves of both sides meet at the optic chiasma lying in close contact with the pituitary gland. Here the fibres from the medial (nasal) half of each retina representing the temporal fields decussate. The outer (temporal) half, representing the nasal field continues to remain on the same side. The fibres from the macular region lie centrally.

The optic tracts that result from this partial decussation contain fibres from the temporal half of the same side and nasal half of the retina of the opposite side. They pass posteriorly to terminate in the lateral geniculate body. Some fibres carrying the afferent pathway for pupillary reflex pass forward to reach the tectum of the midbrain. The optic radiation arising from the lateral geniculate body passes through the posterior limb of the internal capsule on either side to reach the visual (calcrine) cortex in the occipital lobe (Fig. 43). The visual field projected to each optic tract, optic radiation and cortex is referred to as homonymous (different).

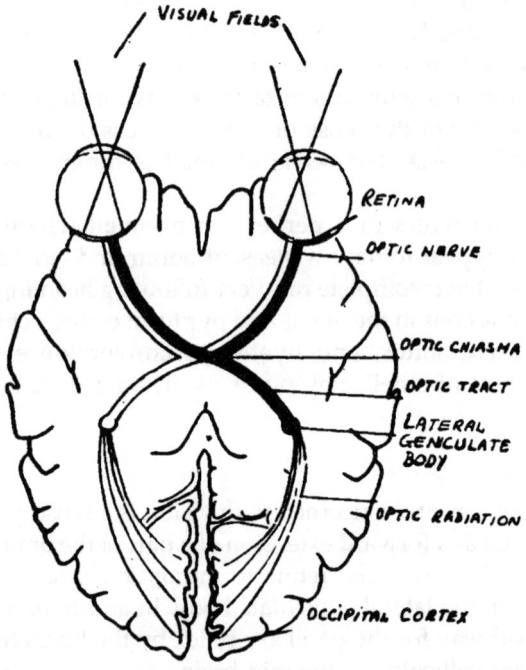

Fig. 43 Visual pathways.

The examination of the optic nerve includes the following functions: 1) acuity of vision, 2) field of vision, 3) colour vision, and 4) funduscopic examination.

1) Acuity of vision: The acuity of vision (distant) is tested by asking the patient to read the letters of a Snellen's chart (named after Hermann Snellen, a Dutch ophthalmologist, who devised the chart) at a distance of six metres. The construction of the letters is such that the top letter is visible to the normal eye at 60 meters; the seventh (penultimate) line can be read at a distance of six metres.

Each eye is tested separately while the other is covered. The individual stands at a distance of six metres from the chart and reads the letters that decrease in size progressively. The individual having normal vision is able to read all letters and the acuity is described as 6/6 vision. The visual acuity is 6/60, if he is able to read only the top letter of the chart. The visual acuity (S, from German, Sehscharfe, means acuity) is expressed as a fraction (d/D), the numerator indicates the distance at which the patient is standing from the chart (d), and the denominator indicates the distance at which a normal person is able to read the same (D).

The near vision is tested, by using Jaegar type cards (named after Edward Jaeger, an Austrian oculist). The card must be held 30 cm from the patient's eye and a similar test is then carried out. The different types are labeled according to their size, and average acuity lies between J.1 and J.4. Near vision is tested by asking the patient to read small newspaper print.

In the wards, the vision is often determined by finger counting. This method is used generally for individuals who are unable to read the letters from any distance or who are illiterate. The patient is asked to count the number of fingers shown to him at varying distances by the examiner. Each eye is tested separately. To determine the presence of diplopia, the fingers are to be counted with both eyes open. If the acuity of vision is markedly diminished the patient is asked to identify motions of the hand in front of his eyes or to distinguish light from darkness (perception of light). The visual acuity is decreased (amblyopia) in diseases of the eye (refractory errors, cataract, corneal opacity). Inspection of the eye reveals the presence of some of these abnormalities.

In those having refractory errors, the acuity of vision is tested with glasses on. The type of lens is determined by looking at an object through it. The object is watched while moving the lens from side-to-side. The lens is said to be concave if the object moves in the same direction and convex if it moves in the opposite direction to the lens. The individuals with short sight (myopia) use concave lenses, and convex lenses are used by individuals with long sight (hypermetropia). Optic nerve lesions are associated with unilateral visual loss. The loss is total when there is complete lesion of the nerve. The blind eye exhibits loss of papillary reflex (direct and consensual) when it is illuminated.

2) *Field of vision:* Determination of visual fields help in locating a lesion in the visual pathways. It is determined by the confrontation method wherein the examiner compares the patient's visual field with that of his, using the movement of the finger. It is tested in one eye while the other is covered. The examiner sits in front of the patient at a distance of approximately 0.6 to 1.0 m. If the right eye is to be tested, the patient is asked to cover the left eye with the palm and the examiner covers his right eye. Both of them look into each other's eye without moving them. The examiner extends the arm and then brings the forefinger wriggling gradually inwards from the various directions-medial, lateral, above and below-on the periphery. The patient is instructed to tell when he recognizes the wriggling of the finger. Then the test is repeated on the other eye. It is always necessary to move from blind areas to areas of vision, as it is easier to detect appearance than disappearance of objects. The examiner compares the field of vision of the patient with that of his provided his own field of vision is normal.

As a screening test, it is sufficient to test both visual fields simultaneously (binocular vision) without closing the eyes while the patient has fixed the gaze with both eyes of the examiner. The moving fingers of both hands are to be brought to the lateral portion of the visual fields. Instead of the examiner's fingers, a large white pin may be used to give more accuracy. This test helps in recognition of the phenomenon of visual inattention, seen in parietal lobe disorders. Though the fields tested in each eye separately are normal, only one object is recognized when both are moved simultaneously.

For those who show defects, the field of vision can be charted using a perimeter.

The field of vision may undergo concentric contraction (tunnel vision) all round the periphery (papilloedema, retinitis pigmentosa) or may show an area of blindness (scotoma) in the central field as in diseases of the choroids, or retina near the macula (retrobulbar neuritis). The macular fibres concerned with central vision show a great vulnerability. The defects of the field of vision are of various types depending on the site of lesion in the visual pathways. Hemianopia is blindness in one-half of the visual field (temporal or nasal). Homonymous hemianopia is a condition of hemianopia in both eyes, on the same half from a lesion any where from the optic tract to the optic cortex (tumour or aneurysm). The lesion in the occipital cortex (unilateral posterior cerebellar artery infarct) results in homonymous hemianopia. The macula is spared in such a lesion as it has blood supply from the middle cerebral artery. There can be involvement of one acqueduct (quadran-tanopia). Temporal lobe lesions (tumour, infarction) may involve the lower portions of the optic radiation and produce upper quadrantianopic defect in opposite visual field and parietal lobe lesions may produce lower quadrantianopic defect.

Bitemportal (heteronymous) hemianopia occurs in lesions at the level of the optic chiasma (pituitary tumours, vascular aneurysms, secondary neoplasm, trauma) interrupting the impulses from the nasal halves of both retina thus resulting in loss of vision from the temporal side. Binasal hemianopia exhibits loss of vision from the nasal half of each field. The field defect may be symmetrical (congruous) or asymmetrical (incongruous). Involvement of the occipital lobe causes contralateral homonymous hemianopia sparing central vision.

3) Colour vision: This is tested, by reading the Ishihara colour plates. At the bedside, the patient is asked to identify the different colours of the objects shown to him. Familiar objects like a *saree*, tie, pen, book, blanket, bed-sheet are used to identify the colour. Colour blindness (red-green blindness) may be congenital. The colour sensitivity is essentially confined to the central (macula) field corresponding to the central part of the retina, which is rich in cone cells.

4) Funduscopic examination: The examination of the fundus using an ophthalmoscope gives an opportunity to view the retina, optic disc, macula and blood vessels. A good view of the fundus is obtained if the pupil is dilated and the field still. The right eye is examined by the right eye of the examiner. Then the examiner has to walk around the bed to examine the left eye with the left eye.

The vessels are to be followed to their point of convergence, the disc. Its colour, the clarity of its edges and the optic cup (depression in the centre) are to be viewed; then the vessels that leave and enter the disc are to be seen. The veins are wider and darker than the arteries. Arteries are lighter and narrower than veins. Often they exhibit a central reflecting line ('silver wire' appearance).

The optic disc appears as a round disc with clear-cut margins and the retinal vessels appear radiating from it in all directions. The disc may become pale with clear-cut margins (optic atrophy) or swollen with indistinct margins (papilloedema). In primary optic atrophy, the whole disc is white standing like a full moon against a dark red sky. In consecutive optic atrophy, developing long time after severe papilloedema the disc is pale and the edges blur out into the immediately surrounding retina. Lesions of the papillomacular bundle (multiple sclerosis) is associated with temporal pallor (strikingly pale disc on the temporal half).

Papilloedema is due to raised intracranial pressure. It begins as blurring of the nasal edge of the disc. Then it extends to the upper and lower margins and ultimately the temporal edges. The optic cup becomes less evident. The disc margins merge with the retina exhibiting a uniform colour. The veins become swollen and engorged. A tumour in the posterior inferior frontal region causes optic atrophy on one side by compression of the optic nerve and papilloedema on the other by causing obstruction to the venous return or by raised intracranial tumour (Foster-Kennedy syndrome, described by Robert Foster Kennedy, an American neurologist).

The arterial crossings of veins, haemorrhages and exudates are to be looked. Haemorrhages may appear as small streaks near the vessels. They can be long and linear or flame shaped. Exudates appear fluffy like cotton-wool patch. When the patient looks directly at the light, the vessel-free macula is visualized.

Oculomotor, Trochlear and Abducent Nerves

The external ocular muscles are innervated by oculomotor, trochlear and abducent nerves (III, IV and VI cranial nerves). As their action is closely related in controlling the ocular movements, these nerves are examined together. These nerves control all the external ocular muscles and the elevators of the eyelids. Autonomic fibres in these nerves and the trigeminal nerve regulate pupillary muscles.

Oculomotor Nerve

Oculomotor nerve supplies the medial, superior and inferior recti, inferior oblique, levator palpabrae superioris, iris and sphincter pupillae muscles. The nerve takes its origin from a series of nuclei in the mid brain. The nuclei in the front supply parasympathetic innervation to the ciliary muscles and iris (Edinger-Westphal nucleus) and the nuclei behind are concerned with innervation to the extraocular muscles.

Trochlear Nerve

Trochlear nerve supplies the superior oblique muscle. It arises from the mid brain caudal to the nucleus of oculomotor nerve concerned with nerve supply to the external ocular muscles. The nerve fibres of trochlear nerve decussate unlike other cranial nerves, before it emerges near the roof of the fourth ventricle between the superior cerebellar and posterior cerebellar arteries.

Abducent Nerve

Abducent nerve innervates the lateral rectus muscle and it takes its origin from the abducent nerve nucleus situated in the floor of the fourth ventricle at the level of the pons and emerges between the medulla and pons. This is the only cranial nerve that has a very long intracranial course, making it vulnerable to the effects of pressure.

All these nerves pass through the cavernous sinus and the superior orbital fissure before reaching the eyeball.

Ocular Movements

The eyeball can move horizontally (adduction) and outwards (abduction), vertically upwards (elevation) and downwards (depression) and diagonally at any intermediate angle. It can make rotary movements either moving towards the nose (internal rotation) or away from the nose (external rotation) as a reflex compensation. The participant muscles are grouped into three pairs depending on their movements. Medial and lateral recti are concerned with adduction and abduction (in horizontal plane) respectively. Superior and inferior recti are concerned with elevation and depression respectively when the eye is in abduction. Inferior oblique and superior oblique act as elevators and depressors respectively when the eye is in adduction.

Cardinal movements of the eye are concerned with the horizontal and vertical movements of the eye from the mid position of the gaze. Gaze movements are to be tested when the eye is elevated or depressed. The muscles work in unison symmetrically so that the visual axes meet at the point towards which eyes are looking horizontally or vertically. This is called conjugate movement of the eyes and it is the result of integrated action of the oculomotor, trochlear and abducent nerves in the brain stem. Normally the eyes move 50° laterally, 50° medially; 30° upwards and 50° downwards.

While making the examination of these three nerves together the following are noted while the patient looks at a clear and definite point:

1) ocular movements and conjugate deviation of the eyes
2) ptosis
3) squint
4) diplopia
5) nystagmus, and
6) pupils

1) Oculomotor movements: The ocular movements are tested, by fixing the head of the patient stationary while his eyes follow the movement of the tip of the finger of the examiner. The finger is moved slowly in the horizontal and vertical planes. The eyeball can move horizontally inwards (adduction) and outwards (abduction); vertically upwards (elevation) and downwards (depression) and diagonally at any intermediate angle. It can make rotary movements either moving towards the nose (internal rotation) or away from the nose (external rotation) as a reflex compensation. The participant muscles are grouped into three pairs depending on their movements. Medial and lateral recti are concerned with adduction and abduction (in a horizontal plane) respectively.

Superior and inferior recti are concerned with elevation and depression respectively when the eye is in abduction. Inferior oblique and superior oblique act as elevators and depressors respectively when the eye is in adduction. Cardinal movements of the eye are concerned with the horizontal and vertical movements of the eye from the mid-position of the gaze. Gaze movements are to be tested when the eye is elevated or depressed. The muscles work in unison symmetrically so that the visual axes meet at the point towards which eyes are looking horizontally or vertically. This is called conjugate movement of the eyes and it is the result of integrated action of the oculomotor, trochlear and abducent nerves in the brain stem. Normally the eyes move 50° laterally, 50° medially, 30° upwards and 50° downwards,

The eyes remain synchronized if the brain stem is intact when the head is turned from side-to-side (conjugate gaze). The eyes turn in opposite direction from the way the head is turned as in a toy doll's eyes in injury to the brain stem (doll's eyes reflex, oculocephalic reflex). The test is not advised in a patient with injury to the neck.

In the involvement of the oculomotor, trochlear and abducent nerves, the lesions may be supranuclear (upper motor neuron), nuclear or infranuclear (lower motor neuron). There is paralysis of conjugate movements of the eyes in supranuclear lesions and it does not affect the muscles. The eyes are turned in one direction persistently. In the irritative phase of the lesion (cerebral haemorrhage), the eyes are turned away from the side of the lesion. The nuclear lesions are recognized by the presence of paralysis of ocular muscles ipsilaterally and hemiplegia contralaterally. In the infranuclear lesions there is paralysis of the individual eye muscles or groups of muscles.

The lesion affecting the oculomotor nerve will greatly restrict eye movements. There will be ptosis of the lid. The eye turns down and out and the pupil is dilated. Paralysis of superior oblique muscle is indicated by an inability to depress the eye in adduction. When lateral rectus muscle is paralysed, abduction of the eye is not possible.

Conjugate deviation and ocular movements: There may be a tendency to look to one or the other side (sidewards, upwards, or downwards) in conjugate deviation. To test the ocular movements, the examiner has to fix the head of the patient with one hand, and then the forefinger of the other hand has to be brought to the midline 30 cm in front of the patient's eyes. The finger has to be moved to right and left horizontally upwards and downwards in the midline, and vertically when the eyes are deviated to one side. The patient is asked to follow the finger with his eyes without moving the head to test the ocular muscles, to note the presence of inability of the movement of the eyes in any one direction (conjugate deviation).

2) Ptosis: Ptosis refers to the drooping of the upper eyelid. It may be congenital or acquired. A congenital ptosis may be unilateral and is due to the absence of muscle. Acquired ptosis is unilateral in situations of paralysis of oculomotor nerve and of the cervical sympathetic nerve. It is bilateral in situations of myopathy, tabes dorsalis and myasthenia gravis.

Ptosis occurs from the paralysis of the levator palpabrae superioris in oculomotor nerve palsy and from weakness of tarsal (unstriated) muscles in cervical sympathetic paralysis. Ptosis, in the latter situation is slight and the lid can still be raised by the contraction of levator and frontalis muscles. The degree of ptosis, is assessed by eliminating the action of frontalis muscles. This is done by pushing the muscle downwards thus bringing the eyebrows to the same level and then asking the patient to look upwards thus allowing the levator to rise.

In oculomotor paralysis, ptosis may be associated with dilated and fixed pupils. The involvement of all muscles supplied by oculomotor nerve suggests the lesion to be in the nerve in its peripheral course. Nuclear lesion may involve a single muscle. In cervical sympathetic paralysis (Horner's syndrome, named after a Swiss Ophthalmologist, Johann Horner), ptosis is associated with miosis (papillary constriction). There may be enophthalmos and absence of sweating on the corresponding half of the face and neck. The ciliospinal reflex is abolished. The pupil does not dilate on 'shading the eye'.

The lesion of the sympathetic pathway is on the same side. The lesion may be central (cerebral infarction, pontine glioma, lateral medullary syndrome) associated with loss of sweating on the entire half of the head, arm, and upper trunk or in the neck proximal to the superior cervical ganglion associated with loss of sweating on the face (cervical cord lesion such as syringomyelia, cord tumour) or distal to superior cervical ganglion without loss of sweating (lesions of thoracic root or of sympathetic chain in the neck).

In myopathy, often there is head retraction as the ptosis is fixed. There is involvement of other extraocular muscles giving rise to ophthalmoplegia. The ptosis is due to muscular weakness in myasthenia gravis and it can be made to appear by fixing the eyes in an upward gaze. In tabes, ptosis is due to hypotonia and loss of power in the levator muscles and it is often compensated, by wrinkling of the forehead. The pupils are often small, irregular and unequal with loss of light reflex. Local conditions of the eyes (conjunctivitis, blepheritis and trachoma) can lead to ptosis.

3) *Squint:* Normally the eyes do not move independently. The muscles controlling the movement of the eyeballs move in an organized way so that visual axes remain in the same relationship throughout. The image of an object falls on the corresponding part of the retina when the eyes are looking at it. This is dependent on the conjugate action of the ocular muscles. The central nervous mechanism keeps the eyes in unison based on the sensory input from each eye and motor output from the third, fourth and sixth cranial nerve nuclei coordinated in the midbrain, facilitating the conjugate action of the ocular muscles. In a squint (strabismus), the visual axes fail to meet at the point of fixation and they are not parallel in both eyes. There is a deviation of the eyes, and it is most common in horizontal axis.

Squint may develop from either sensory or motor deficiencies. There are two types of squint: concomitant (non-parlaytic) and paralytic. In the concomitant type there is interruption of the sensory input from one eye. It results in an imbalance in the action of opposing muscles. The squint is present at rest in all directions of gaze and it is not associated with diplopia (double vision) as the images from the squinting eye, is suppressed by the brain. There is no limitation of the movement of the eye, in which one eye either turns in or less often turns out. This is the common form of squint found in children. The cause may be familial. It may be due to refractive errors and rarely from congenital cataract or ocular tumour.

Squint is recognized by 'cover test' performed slowly in each eye separately. The squinting eye can be recognized by seeing that it takes up fixation on a distant object and later on a near object when the straight eye is covered. It is referred as a convergent squint if the eye moves outwards and if it moves towards it is referred to as a divergent squint.

Paralytic squint occurs most frequently in adults. It is due to weakness of one or more extraocular muscles. There is failure of movement of the eye towards the side of action of the paralysed muscle (primary deviation). The unaffected eye will exhibit deviation more than the primary deviation of the affected eye (secondary deviation). The squint may or may not be obvious at rest but becomes noticeable when the patient attempts to move the eye in the direction of the action of the paralysed muscle. Diplopia occurs in such positions of the eyes that depend upon the contraction of the paralysed muscle. The deviation of the images is greatest when the gaze is in the direction of the defective movement. The images fall on different parts of the retina as the visual axes are not parallel.

Double vision forms the outstanding symptom of a paralytic squint. The causes may be neurogenic (interruption of the nerve pathways), muscular (thyroid disorders, and myasthenia gravis or mechanical (tumour within the orbit). Mano-ocular diplopia may occur from corneal or lens opacities. There is diplopia even when one eye is closed.

4) *Double vision:* Diplopia is appreciated by the patient due to ocular muscle weakness, even before it is evident to the examiner. There is a failure of light rays to fall on exactly corresponding parts of the two retinae, resulting in failure of binocular fusion in the visual cortex and the person perceives two separate images.

In these situations, the individual can see distinctly the image falling upon the macula of the healthy eye (true image). The image falls upon the retina outside the macula in the affected eye and it appears indistinct and blurred (false image). The false image is projected into that part of the field of vision in which the paralysed muscle should move the eye if it were normal. The patient turns his head in the direction of action of the paralysed muscle (head tilt) to overcome the diplopia. The patient complains of diplopia when looking downwards and medially in abducent nerve paralysis and when looking laterally in trochlear nerve paralysis. There is maximal separation of images when the eyes are moved in the direction towards which the paralysed muscle would normally move the eye.

Mono-ocular diplopia is seen in lens opacities and astigmatism. In those situations in which both eyes are functional and if one deviates, there is occurrence of binocular diplopia.

5) *Nystagmus:* There is a balance of tone between opposing ocular muscles and any disturbance of this balance results in a drift of the eyes in one or other directions. If this drift is corrected, by a quick movement back to the original position and frequent repetition of this cycle results in nystagmus.

Nystagmus refers to a disturbance of ocular movements characterized by involuntary, often rhythmic oscillations of the eyes and are independent of their normal movements. The axis of the movement may be horizontal, vertical or rotary. The oscillations may be pendular or jerky, and the amplitude fine or coarse.

Pendular nystagmus: In pendular nystagmus the eyes move

with equal velocity and amplitude in both directions on either side of the midline but at a variable speed. It is noted in blindness (cataract, central scotoma), congenital conditions such as albinism, total colour blindness, or absence of iris and in weakness of ocular muscles concerned with the maintenance of posture of conjugate movements as noted in myasthenia gravis, acute polyneuritis or botulism. It is also noted in high infantile myopia, opacities of the media and macular abnormalities.

Jerky nystagmus: Jerky nystagmus (slow-quick) consists of quick movement in one direction and slow movement in the opposite direction. The quicker jerk indicates the direction of the nystagmus. It is seen in lesions of vestibular apparatus (Meniere's disease, named after Prosper Meniere, a French physician) or labyrinthine disorders. In the former, the quick phase is away from the lesion and in the latter, towards the lesion. Nystagmus (central pathways-medial longitudinal fasciculus-concerned with ocular movements) from the medullary and pontine lesions, is more prominent in one direction. The quick phase is towards the lesion. It may be horizontal or rotatory. In cerebellar lesion, nystagmus is marked on looking to the side of the lesion. Nystagmus may be pendular or jerky in the lesions near the fourth ventricle.

Horizontal nystagmus: Horizontal nystagmus is the commonest form and it is seen in the peripheral (ear, vestibular nerve) or central (brain stem/cerebellum) lesions and the condition may be congenital or acquired.

Vertical nystagmus: Vertical nystagmus is noted in acquired brain diseases or intoxication (codeine, barbiturates, alcohol or dilantin). The peripheral lesions are commonly associated with fine amplitude except in severe vertigo. Coarse amplitude indicates a central lesion.

While testing for nystagmus, the effect of the eye position (gaze centre, to right or to left) and the effect of head position is noted. The patient is asked to look straight (gaze centre position) in front of him and the eyes are looked at whether or not they remain steady. In blindness or congenital nystagmus, there will be pendular movements in gaze centre position. Then the examiner should bring his finger in front of the eyes of the patient and ask him to follow it. The finger is moved quickly to the extreme right and then to the left and then upwards and downwards from the central gaze. The eyelids, must be held up by the other hand. Normally the eyeballs move freely.

Nystagmus is graded into 3 grades: Grade 1: Nystagmus with fast component to left, looking toward left; Grade 2: Nystagmus with fast component to left, looking straight ahead; and Grade 3: Nystagmus with fast component to the left, looking toward right.

In the presence of nystagmus, the eyeballs show oscillations. The rate, rhythm and amplitude of the oscillations in each direction are to be noted. The oscillations may be in a constant horizontal direction in differing directions of horizontal gaze (peripheral lesion), or the oscillations may be to right, or to the left on gaze left (central lesion). In vertical nystagmus the oscillations may be upwards (sometimes in phenytoin intoxication or in lesions of the medulla, pons, or cerebellum), or downwards (lower medullary) or medullocervical lesions as in Arnold-Chiari malformation, named after Julius Arnold, a German pathologist and Hans Chiari, an Austrian pathologist).

A paroxysmal and rotary nystagmus may accompany benign positional vertigo or in posterior fossa tumours, when the head position is changed rapidly (erect to head hanging position to right or to left).

Not all nystagmus are pathologic. An end point nystagmus is horizontal and is commonly found in many normal persons. The oscillations occur to the right on far gaze right and to the left on far gaze left. Often a few irregular jerky movements of the eyes are noted in full lateral deviation of the eyes in normal individuals. However they are not persistant and regular like nystagmus.

Optokinetic nystagmus can be demonstrated while the eyes follow a passing scenery (railway nystagmus) due to excessive gaze deviation and in badly lit mines requiring the miners to move the eyes continuously to avoid fatigue (Miner's nystagmus). The movements are pendular.

6) Pupils: Normally the pupils are central, regular, equal and reactive to light and accommodation. The pupils are examined to note their size, shape, position, equality and mobility (reaction to light and accommodation). Normally the size is 2-6 mm and it is dependent on the balance of contraction of the sphincter pupillae and dilator pupillae innervated by the oculomotor and cervical sympathetic nerves respectively. Pupils are small in early infancy, old age, during sleep and in bright light; and large in poor light, and myopia.

The shape may be distorted instead of being round as in iritis, following iredectomy or corneal perforations. It may be placed eccentrically. The pupils may be unequal (anisocoria) due to miosis (constriction) or mydriasis (dilatation) of one of the pupils. The pupil exhibiting less mobility is usually the abnormal one. A unilateral dilatation of the pupil occurs in increased intracranial tension and may appear as an early sign of oculomotor nerve involvement.

Miosis occurs from sympathetic paralysis unilaterally. Bilateral constriction is seen in tabes and the size may become pin-point in pontine lesions or poisoning (opium, morphine, diazinon). Mydriasis occurs from oculomotor nerve palsy, sympathetic over activity, glaucoma, adhesions following iritis, effects of atropine and d-amphetamine.

Light Reflex

The reaction to light is dependent on reflex consisting of the afferent fibres in the optic nerve, oculomotor nerve nuclei and the efferent fibres in the oculomotor nerve. The efferent fibres reach the papillary sphincter through the ciliary ganglion. The light reflex is tested in two parts: direct and indirect.

Direct light reflex: When the patient is looking straight with one eye while the other is closed, a bright beam of light suddenly from a torch is shone from the side of the pupil. Normally there is rapid constriction of the pupil. Then it dilates a little and after undergoing a few slight oscillations, settles down to a smaller size.

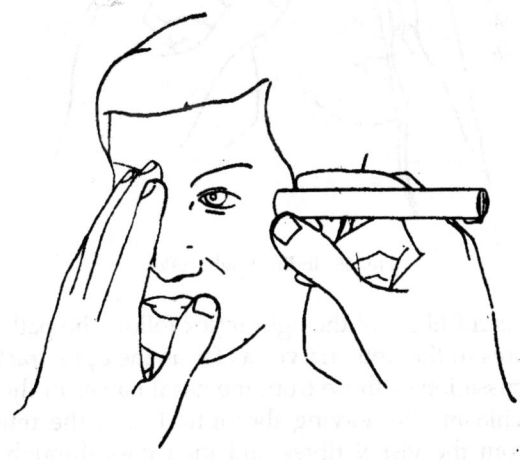

Fig. 44 Direct light reflex.

The pupil will rapidly dilate to its previous diameter after switching of the light. The test is repeated on the other side and the results compared (Fig. 44).

Indirect light reflex (consensual or swinging light test): Both eyes are kept open and the examiner places his hand vertically between the eyes to prevent the light falling on the opposite side eye when the bright light is shown in one eye. There is contraction of both pupils indicating a consensual papillary reaction. The opposite pupil not exposed to the light contracts as quickly as the pupil on which the light is shone. If light is shone immediately into such an eye, the pupil may show slight dilatation and oscillate in the originally illuminated eye, indicating that consensually mediated light reaction of the second eye is more active than its direct reaction. This phenomenon is due to the decussation of some of the fibres in the optic nerves at the optic chiasm and the impulses from one eye are conveyed to brainstem oculomotor nuclei concerned with papillary constriction bilaterally (Fig. 45).

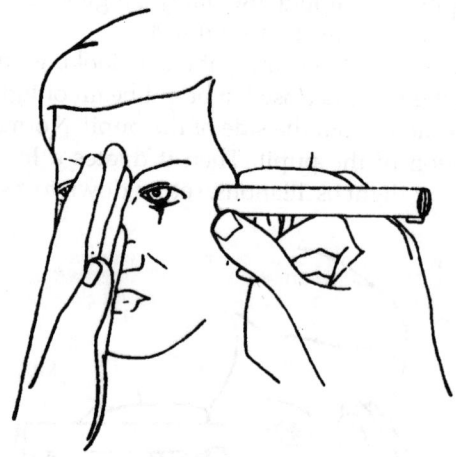

Fig. 45 Indirect light reflex.

The afferent fibres of the light reflex follow the path of visual afferent fibres to the optic nerves as far as the optic tracts, with a similar decussation of those from the nasal halves of the retina at the optic chiasm. On leaving the optic tracts, the reflex fibres separate from the visual fibres and then pass through superior colliculus, on to the pretectal region and synapse in the oculomotor nuclei. The efferent path of the reflex runs from the oculomotor nuclei (Edinger-Westphal nucleus) through the iridoconstrictor fibres. They enter the oculomotor nerve and terminate in the ciliary ganglion, from which postganglionic fibres arise and reach the circular muscles of the iris through the short ciliary nerves (Fig. 46).

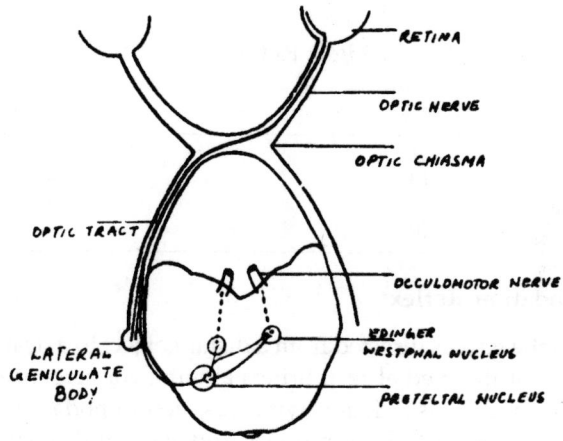

Fig. 46 Pathways for light reflex.

Both the optic tracts must be connected with the oculomotor nuclei on either side, since a beam of light falling upon either half of either retina evokes a contraction of both pupils (consensual). The light reflex is lost in any condition that interferes with the reflex pathway at some point. The lesion may be in the afferent (the retina, optic nerve or chiasm) or efferent (parasympathetic supply from the midbrain running with the third nerve) loop. It is lost in oculomotor palsy, cerebral haemorrhage, optic atrophy with blindness and tabes dorsalis. Brain stem injury is associated with dilated pupils. The prognosis is grave when they do not react to light. The injury is reversible if there is reaction to light. A unilaterally dilated pupil that remains active to light may be the earliest sign of increasing intracranial tension. Light reflex may be lost in meningitis.

Lesions of ipsilateral optic nerve lead to absence of direct and consensual light reflex as no stimulus can be received (retrobulbar neuritis, compression or ischaemic lesions of the optic nerve) and lesions in ipsilateral oculomotor nerve cause loss of direct light reflex, but there is retention of consensual light reflex. It becomes reversed in contralateral oculomotor nerve lesion. There is absence of consensual light reflex but the direct reflex is preserved. The direct and consensual light reflexes are retained in contralateral optic nerve lesions. Thus when the lesion is unilateral, both pupils will react when the normal side is stimulated.

Light Reflex.

Lesion	Nerve	Direct	Consensual
Ipsilateral	II	−	−
Ipsilateral	III	−	+
Contralateral	II	+	+
Contralateral	III	+	−

Accommodation Reflex

When the gaze is directed from a distant object to a near object, contraction of the medial recti brings about a convergence of the ocular axes and in association with this, accommodation occurs by contraction of the ciliary muscles and the pupils contract. In eliciting this, the patient is asked to look at a distant object about 22 cm in front of the bridge of the nose. This position prevents lowering of the lids that obscures the normal papillary constriction. Then he is asked to look quickly at the examiner's finger brought towards the bridge of the nose within 5 cm of the eyes. The reflex activity of convergence of the eyes, accommodation and miosis are closely related.

The reaction of accommodation will be lost in any lesion of iridoconstrictor fibres, along with the light reflex. But the selective impairment of light reflex with preservation of the accommodation indicates a midbrain lesion (neurosyphilis, encephalitis, diabetes). Accommodation is only rarely lost in brain stem lesions.

Accommodation and associated iridoconstriction can occur in the absence of vision as in the lesions of the optic nerve. It is demonstrable in a blind individual by asking him to look at the end of his nose. The lesion of the oculomotor nerve may abolish the reaction to light, but not accommodation. Hence the reflex pathway of accommodation reaction is a complex one. The afferent pathway probably is mediated through the proprioceptive impulses resulting from the contraction of both medial recti (convergence) and the efferent impulses arise from the unpaired median nuclei of the oculomotor nerve in the midbrain (n. Perlia), and thereafter the fibres bypass the ciliary ganglion and terminate in the ciliary muscle.

Argyll Robertson pupil: The pupils are small, irregular, unequal and eccentric. The irides are light coloured. There is absence of constriction of either pupils under the influence of light but on accommodating the eyes to a near object, both pupils contract. The abnormality is bilateral but it may be more obvious in one eye. The papillary abnormality was described by Douglas Moray Cooper Lamb Argyll Robertson, a Scottish physician. Miosis is not an invariable feature and there is poor response to mydriatics like atropine, physostigmine and methacholine. The condition is the result of a lesion in the periaqueductal grey matter at the level of superior colliculi interrupting decussating pathways from the oculomotor complex to the Edinger-Westphal nucleus (named after Ludwig Edinger, and Carl Westphal, German neurologists) whose rostral portion contains the reflex to light whereas the caudal portion regulates accommodation. The lesion appears to be localized in the area immediately rostral to Edinger-Westphal nucleus. The abnormality is seen classically in neurosyphilis (tabes, general paresis of insane) and occasionally in non-leutic conditions such as diabetes mellitus (pseudotabes), multiple sclerosis, tumours and haemorrhage in the midbrain, sarcoidosis, Wernicke's encephalopathy, Charcot-Marie-Tooth syndrome (named after Jean Martin Charcot, and Pierre Marie, French physicians, and Howard Tooth, English physician), Dejerine-Sottas hypertrophic neuritis (named after Joseph Dejerine, and Jules Sottas, French neurologists), Herpes zoster, lymphocytic meningoradiculitis and von Economo's encephalitis). Thus the sign is specific to an anatomic lesion, and not to a disease.

Adie-Holmes (myotonic) pupil: A rare abnormality of pupil, named after William Adie, a British neurologist and G.M. Holmes, an Australian neurologist in England, characterized by abnormality of absent direct and consensual constriction of pupil under the influence of light, and accommodation is sluggish. The papillary abnormality is unilateral and is of mid-size. Mydriatics cause good dilatation. The cause appears to be due to denervation in the ciliary ganglion. There may be absent tendon reflexes on the side of papillary abnormality. The condition is seen in young women and it has no pathologic significance.

Hippus: There can be alternate dilatation and constriction of the pupils either in response to light or spontaneously. It has no clinical significance and it may be noted prominently in bulbar neuritis.

Ciliospinal reflex: Normally there is dilatation of the pupils when the skin of the neck is pinched. It is due to reflex excitation of the pupil dilating fibres in the cervical sympathetic nerve. This reflex is abolished in cervical sympathetic paralysis. Sometimes, it is lost in medullary, cervical and upper thoracic cord lesions.

Types of Paralysis

In the involvement of the oculomotor, trochlear and abducent nerves, the lesions may be supranuclear, nuclear or infranuclear. In supranuclear paralysis the muscles are not affected. There is paralysis of conjugate movement of the eyes. The eyes are turned in one direction persistently. In the irritative phase of the lesion (cerebral haemorrhage) the eyes are turned away from the side of the lesion.

The nuclear palsies are recognized by the presence of palsy of ocular muscles in isolation ipsilaterally and hemiplegia contralaterally. In the infranuclear paralysis, the ocular muscles are paralysed either singly or in groups.

Oculomotor palsy: The eye is deviated downwards and outwards. There will be ptosis, pupils are dilated and fixed. There is an inability to move the eyeball inwards and upwards. There will be an overaction of frontalis to raise the eyelids. The paralysis is not complete in many cases thus demonstrating a few of the above-mentioned features. Diplopia is not apparent as there is closure of the eye by the drooped upper eyelid. Isolated third nerve palsy may occur in upper midbrain vascular accidents, and demyelinating conditions.

Trochlear nerve paralysis: The eye is deviated inwards. There is difficulty to move the eyeball downwards and outwards. Diplopia is evident when attempting to look down and away from the affected side. To prevent it, the patient may tilt the head on to the paralysed side so that the eye is elevated above the plane of the normal eye. The squint is rarely evident. The isolated paralysis of trochlear nerve is uncommon. It may occur in lesions of the cerebral peduncles, and in head injury. Generally it is associated with oculomotor palsy.

Abducent nerve paralysis: The sixth cranial nerve has a long intracranial course and it can be involved in many conditions at or near the base of the skull. In abducent nerve paralysis, the eye is deviated inwards. There is an inability to move the eye outwards beyond the midline. On looking in that direction, diplopia is evident. The isolated palsy has a limited localizing value as it occurs in any condition resulting in raised intracranial tension (false localizing sign). The nerve may be damaged in the brain stem (multiple sclerosis), in raised intracranial pressure (from compression against the tip of the petrous temporal bone) or in tumour infiltration. An isolated sixth nerve palsy may be noted in diabetes mellitus. Paralysis of both lateral recti gives rise to deviation of both eyes medially (convergence).

Trigeminal Nerve

The trigeminal nerve is a mixed cranial nerve containing sensory and motor fibres. It carries somatic sensations from the face, anterior part of the scalp, eyes, and oral cavity. The sensory part has three divisions-ophthalmic, maxillary and mandibular. The motor part is present in the mandibular division and it innervates the muscles of mastication (ptery-goids, masseter, temporalis, tensor tympani and tensor palati). The ophthalmic division carries sensations from the upper eyelid and its medial part of the conjunctiva, nose up to the tip, forehead and anterior part of the scalp. The maxillary branch carries sensations from the cheek, upper lip, lower eyelid and its conjunctiva, side of the nose, mucous membrane of the nose, upper teeth, roof of

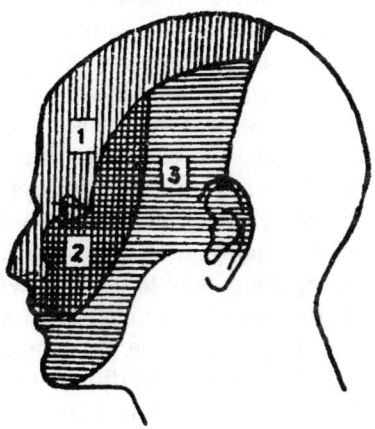

Fig. 47 Divisions of the trigeminal nerve over the face: (1) ophthalmic; (2) maxillary; and (3) mandibular.

the mouth, soft palate, upper part of the pharynx and the tonsils. Mandibular division carries sensations from the lower part of the face, the lower lip, ear, tongue and the lower teeth (Fig. 47). Skin on the scalp region supplied by the trigeminal nerve meets that by the second cervical segment just posterior to vertex. Upper cervical segments also supply the skin on the angle of the jaw.

The sensations carried through the sensory divisions reach, the Gasserian ganglion in the petrous portion of the temporal bone. The sensory root originating from the ganglia terminates in the brain stem (ascending fibres transmitting touch and postural sensibility into a large nucleus in the pons, which cross and ascend to the thalamus; thermal and pain sensibility in the descending or bulbospinal tract extending up to the second cervical segment of the spinal cord before ascending in medial laminiscus and cross midline and ascend in the quintothalamic tract). The fibres of the ophthalmic division reach the lowest level.

The trigeminal nerve has a long sensory nucleus extending from the pons to the upper cervical portion of the spinal cord, and a small motor nucleus lying medial to the main sensory nucleus in the pons near the floor of the fourth ventricle.

The examination of the trigeminal nerve includes the tests for sensory and motor functions.

1) Sensory function: Sensation is tested as elsewhere in the body by the use of cotton wool and a pin over each area of the face and the buccal mucosa supplied by the three sensory divisions of the fifth nerve on each side of the face. The sensation of touch, pain and temperature are tested over three different areas of the face on either side corresponding to the three sensory divisions: ophthalmic (forehead and upper part of the side of the nose), maxillary (cheek and upper lip) and mandibular (chin and anterior part of the tongue). The sensations inside the mouth is tested by asking the patient to drink water from a tumbler. The patient feels the tumbler to be broken in situations of involvement of the nerve.

The pattern of sensory impairment depends on the site of the lesion. Lesions of the different divisions peripheral to the ganglion or in their sensory nucleus result in loss of cutaneous sensibility in their territory. A total loss of sensation in the skin and mucous membrane of the face and nasopharynx occurs in the lesions affecting the Gasserian ganglion and the sensory root or extensive lesion anterior to the ganglia where the motor root is usually involved (tumours on the base of the skull, neurofibroma of the trigeminal nerve, meningitis and basal injuries). The lesion near the thalamus may result in the loss of sensation on one side of the body including the face.

The conditions like acoustic neuroma, herpes zoster, carotid aneurysm, and tumours in the orbital fossa may cause a loss of sensation over different parts of the opposite face. There may be a loss of touch sensation of the face on the same side alone in pontine lesion, affecting the sensory nucleus from vascular disease, pontine tumour, brain stem displacement by large tumour. In syringobulbia, there will be loss of pain and temperature sensation with retention of touch sensation, due to a lesion of descending root. Such an abnormality may be noted in foramen magnum tumour or anomalies and bulbar vascular accidents. In thrombosis of posterior inferior cerebellar artery, there will be ipsilateral loss of pain and temperature on the face and loss of sensations over the contralateral part of the body. In trigeminal neuralgia, there is spontaneous spasmodic pain over one-half of the face without any objective sensory loss. There can be loss of facial sensations as a part of total hemianaesthesia and it indicates a lesion high in the brain stem or in the region of opposite thalamus.

2) Motor function: Before testing the power of the muscles of mastication, the presence of any wasting around the zygoma (wasting of temporalis and masseter) or deviation of the jaw on opening of the mouth towards the paralysed side due to the action of normal muscles (pterygoid weakness) are to be noted.

i) *Temporalis and masseter:* The patient is asked to clench his teeth or jaw in an edentolous situation. The temporalis and masseter muscles are palpated in the region of the temple and cheek respectively. Normally they become prominent and are felt firmly contracted on each side.

ii) *Pterygoids:* The patient is asked to move the lower jaw from side to side against resistance to test the pterygoids. The patient fails to move the jaw to the opposite side in conditions of weakness of pterygoids. The normal jaw tends to deviate towards the weak muscle.

A lower motor neuron or a muscle lesion causes hollowing of the temple and flattening of the angle of the jaw. There is wasting of temporalis and masseter muscles. The conditon may occur due to nuclear lesion (motor neuron disease-bilateral) or a peripheral nerve lesion or compression of motor root (unilateral) or muscular dystrophy. Unilateral weakness of the muscles supplied by trigeminal nerve indicates disease of proximal mandibular division or a lesion of the ipsilateral pons if associated with sixth and seventh cranial nerve abnormalities or contralateral hemiplegia. Unilateral weakness of these muscles is not a feature with lesion of cerebral hemisphere as each muscle receives bilateral cortical innervation.

The maxillary division is rarely involved alone. Unusually it can happen in local trauma. It is affected in the cavernous sinus. Basal tumour involving the mandibular division affects both sensory and motor roots.

Corneal reflex: The patient is asked to look upwards as far as possible. An elongated wisp of clean cotton is brought from the side and the lateral edge of the cornea is touched gently. Care should be taken not to wipe the cornea with cotton. The central part of the cornea should never be touched (Fig. 48). The procedure is repeated on the other side. There will be blinking in both eyes, whichever side is tested. The procedure is explained to the patient before hand. Sometimes, the reflex is tested by blowing a puff of air into each cornea in turn while shielding the other. The ophthalmic branch of the trigeminal nerve and the facial nerve, form the afferent and efferent pathways of the reflex respectively. The centre is in the pons.

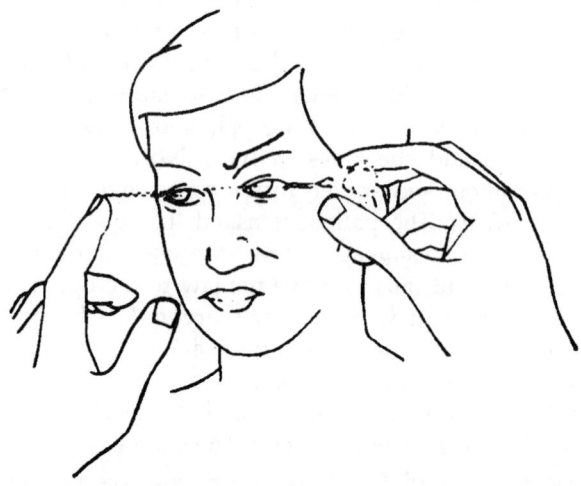

Fig. 48 Corneal reflex.

The reflex is lost in a lesion either of the fifth or the seventh nerve. When there is involvement of the ophthalmic division of the trigeminal nerve there will not be any blinking on either side when the affected side is tested; however there will be a normal response when the normal side is tested (consensual response). Such an abnormality is noted in tumours and aneurysms near cavernous sinus and orbital fissure. In facial palsy and in cerebello-pontine angle tumours, there will be no response on the affected side, irrespective of the test being carried out on the affected or healthy side. There will be blinking in the normal eye when the affected side is touched, provided the ophthalmic division is intact. The reflex is lost bilaterally in comatose patients. Absent corneal reflex with unilateral sensorineural hearing loss implies cerebello-pontine angle tumour (acoustic neuroma of 2 cm or more).

Loss of Corneal Reflex.

Lesion (side)	direct	consensual
Fifth nerve		
affected	loss	loss
healthy	present	present
Seventh nerve		
affected	loss	present
healthy	present	loss

Conjunctival reflex: Conjunctival reflex is dependent on the integrity of the trigeminal (afferent) and the facial (efferent) nerves. It is elicited by touching the conjunctiva with a wisp of cotton. It results in the closure of the eyelids. It has the same significance as corneal reflex, but gives added information as to the integrity of the upper cervical sensory neurons. The cornea has only pain fibres. Conjunctiva when touched evokes the feeling of touch only. The impulses from conjunctiva are carried down up to the second cervical segments, before ascending and joining the pain fibres from the cornea.

Facial Nerve

The facial nerve is almost entirely a motor nerve (Fig. 49). The motor fibres take their origin from the nucleus situated in the lower part of the pons lateral to that of the abducent nerve. On leaving the nucleus, the fibres encircle the abducent nucleus and emerge at ponto-medullary junction. At the cerebellopontine angle, the nerve lies medial to the auditory nerve and enters the internal auditory meatus with it, and reaches the geniculate ganglion.

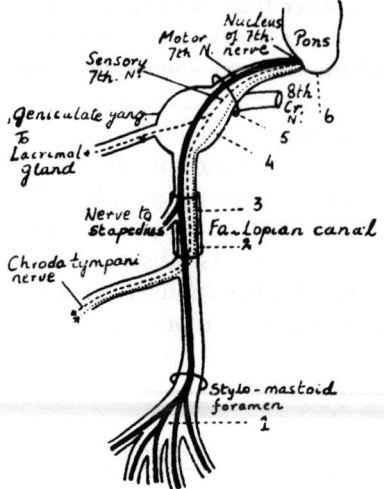

Fig. 49. Facial nerve—its course and lesions :
(1) Outside the stylomastoid foramen;
(2-3) Fallopian canal
(4) Geniculate ganglion;
(5) Internal auditory meatus; and
(6) Lower border of the pons.

During its course through the temporal bone the greater superficial petrosal nerve leaves the facial nerve carrying the secretomotor fibres to the lacrimal gland. The facial nerve pursues its course in the facial canal. The canal is related closely to the middle ear. It gives off a branch to the stapedius muscle. The taste sensations from the anterior two-thirds of the tongue is carried by the lingual nerve and the taste fibres leave to join the chorda tympani nerve, which joins the facial nerve beyond the branch to the stapedius and reach the geniculate ganglion. Secretory fibres to the salivary glands reach through the chorda tympani. The axons from the ganglia pass along the facial nerve (nervus intermedius) and reach the medulla oblongata wherein they terminate in the tractus solitarius.

The facial nerve leaves the facial canal through the stylomastoid foramen and passes through the parotid gland wherein it divides into many branches. The branches supply the muscles of the scalp and of facial expression and facial movement except the levator palpabrae superioris (supplied by oculomotor nerve). The facial nerve also supplies platysma, and stapedius.

Effect of paralysis: On inspection, the paralysed side of the face is expressionless and it exhibits smoothened furrows of the forehead, less pronounced nasolabial fold, a drooped corner of the mouth and a widened palpebral fissure.

The functions of the facial nerve are tested under the following heads: motor, sensory (taste) and emotional.

1) Motor: The patient is asked to perform the following movements which are compared on both sides.

a) Raise the eyebrows to wrinkle the forehead (frontal belly of occipitofrontalis). The furrows on the forehead are smoothened out in facial palsy.

b) Close the eyes as tightly as possible (orbicularis oculi). In facial palsy the affected eye remains open with a wide palpebral fissure and when the patient tries to close the eye, the eyeball rolls upwards and outwards under the upper eyelid which has failed to descend (Bell's phenomenon, described by Charles Bell, a Scottish physiologist in London). The eye can be opened easily while the patient attempts to keep it closed.

c) Blow the cheeks by inflating the mouth with air (Buccinator). During expiration the involved side puffs out. Air escapes easily when the cheek is tapped with the finger. The tone of buccinator muscle is lost in facial paralysis.

d) Whistle by pursing the lips (orbicularis oris). The patient fails to do it in facial palsy.

e) Show the upper teeth (levator anguli oris). The angle of the mouth is dragged towards the unaffected side by the unopposed action of the nerve on the opposite healthy side.

f) Depress the lower lip downwards and outwards (platysma)

2) *Taste:* The patient is asked to protrude the tongue. The tip is held gently by the examiner with a piece of gauze. The surface is dried with a gauze. There are four basic tastes (sweet-sugar, sour-lime, salt and bitter-quinine). These solutions are used for the purpose of testing. The cotton swab is dipped in the solution and is applied on either side of the tongue separately. The various test substances are enumerated before the patient. When the patient finds it coinciding with the perceived taste, he must nod his head. Then the mouth is rinsed and the other substances applied. The taste sensation of the posterior one-third of the tongue (carried by glossopharyngeal nerve) should be tested in the same sitting. The quinine test has to be done at the end, as its effect lasts for a longer time.

3) *Emotional expression-smile or cry:* Emotional facial weakness is present when there is deviation of the mouth on smiling, which disappears on voluntary movement. This is noted in deep-seated lesions of the opposite thalamus or its connections with the frontal

lobe. The spontaneous movements (smiling) are preserved in the upper motor neuron lesions.

Facial Palsy

Facial palsy is classified into three types: Supranuclear, nuclear or infranuclear, depending on the location of the lesion, above the facial nucleus, at the nucleus or below the nucleus respectively. The palsy may be unilateral or bilateral.

Supranuclear (upper motor neuron) palsy: Upper motor neuron (UMN) facial palsy is associated with deviation of the mouth and deepening of the nasolabial fold. There will be normal wrinkling over the forehead. To some extent the function of orbicularis oculi is preserved. In an infranuclear facial palsy, one-half of the face is completely paralysed. This difference is due to the fact that the facial nucleus receives the fibres controlling the muscles of the upper face (occipito-frontalis and orbicularis oculi) from the corticobulbar tracts of either side (bilateral innervation of the muscles of the upper part of the face), unlike the fibres controlling the lower half of the face (Fig. 50). The lesion in UMN palsy is present at some point between the opposite cortex and the facial nucleus in the pons.

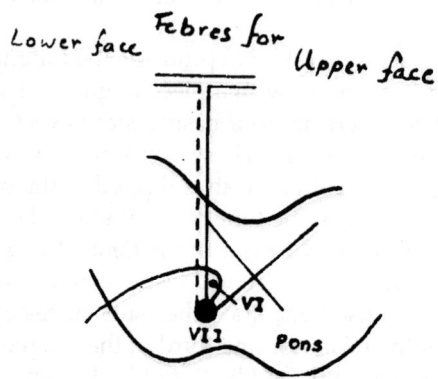

Fig. 50 Fibres for the facial nucleus.

Supranuclear facial palsy is associated with hemiplegia on the same side. Rarely the supranuclear facial palsy may affect the fibres concerned with emotional movement (mimic paralysis). The taste sensation remains unaffected.

In a comatose patient, the facial weakness is recognized by the drooping of the angle of the mouth. The paralysed cheek puffs out greatly with each expiration.

Nuclear facial palsy: The involvement of the facial nucleus is associated with paralysis of the abducent nerve with loss of lateral rotation of the eye on the side of the facial palsy. There is an associated contralateral hemiplegia. The condition may arise from pontine tumours, vascular lesions and demyelination. Facial nucleus may be involved in motor neuron disease (bilateral) and poliomyelitis.

Infranuclear facial palsy: The affection of the facial nerve beyond its nucleus, in the peripheral course, results in facial palsy on the same side. There is paralysis of one-half of the face resulting in an expressionless facies on the side, smoothened out furrows of the forehead, wide palpebral fissure, less pronounced nasolabial fold and drooped angle of the mouth. Saliva may be seen dribbling from the mouth and tears flow over the lower lid. The nerve can be affected at various levels. Depending on the location, the facial palsy is associated with any of the following features:

1) The lesion at the level of the stylomastoid foramen and beyond results in the commonest type of facial palsy of lower motor neuron type without any other associated neurologic deficit (Bell's palsy).

2) Involvement of the nerve in the facial canal just above its junction with the chorda tympani nerve results in the loss of taste (ageusia) on the anterior two-thirds of the tongue on the affected side.

3) Involvement of the nerve in the facial canal above the branch to the stapedius muscle— in addition to the loss of taste, the sounds are heard with unusual loudness on the affected side (hyperacusis) as the dampening influence on the stapes is affected by the paralysis of the stapedius muscle.

4) Involvement of the nerve above the geniculate ganglion is associated with facial paralysis and absence of lacrimal secretion.

The manifestations noted in (2), (3) and (4) are due to the lesions within the petrous temporal bone and the causes include trauma, infections of the middle ear, herpes zoster (Ramsay Hunt's syndrome) and tumours (glioma).

5) Involvement of the nerve in the internal auditory meatus or in the cerebello-pontine angle is associated with the eighth nerve paralysis with nerve deafness. The fifth and sixth nerves are also affected.

The nuclear or infranuclear facial palsy can lead to atrophy of the facial muscles, and atrophy is not produced by supranuclear lesions. Aberrant regeneration of facial nerve fibres during partial recovery from Bell's palsy may produce spasmodic movements of facial muscles. Apart from Bell's palsy, lower motor neuron facial palsy may be encountered in tumours of pons or of cerebellopontine angle, chronic middle ear infection resulting in osteomyelitis of the petrous temporal bone, parotid tumours and herpes zoster affecting the geniculate ganglia (associated with herpetic eruptions in the pinna of the ear), sarcoidosis, and facioscapulo-humeral muscular dystrophy.

Partial facial palsy: Peripheral lesions such as parotid tumour may cause weakness of the lower face due to partial facial nerve lesion.

Localisation of Facial Palsy.

Features	Supranuclear	Nuclear	Infranuclear
Hemiplegia	ipsilateral	contralateral	no
Involvement of sixth cranial nerve	no	yes	no
Facial paralysis	lower face	one half of face	one half of face
Taste	unaffected	unaffected	yes (chordatympani)
Hyperacusis	no	no	yes (stapaedius)
Facial reflexes (light tapping of the facial muscles around the mouth)	increased	normal	normal/decreased
muscular atrophy	no	yes	yes

Bilateral Facial Palsy

1) Bilateral LMN facial palsy: Bilateral LMN facial palsy is encountered in infective polyneuritis, leprosy, heredo-familial muscular dystrophies, basal meningitis, myotonica dystrophia and myasthenia gravis.

2) Bilateral UMN facial palsy: Bilateral UMN facial palsy is seen in cerebrovascular accidents. multiple sclerosis and motor neuron disease.

Auditory Nerve

The eighth cranial nerve has two divisions: cochlear and vestibular. The former is concerned with hearing and the latter with equilibrium. Their dysfunction manifests in altered hearing (deafness, tinnitus) and loss of equilibrium (vertigo) respectively. Distubances of the vestibular functions are dramatic in their development.

The auditory fibres arising from the cochlear ganglion terminate in the dorsal and ventral nuclei situated in the pons. The vestibular fibres arising from vestibular ganglion terminate in a group of nuclei in the pons and medulla. The secondary auditory tracts after partial decussation end in the inferior colliculi and the medial geniculate bodies. The fibres arising from them pass through an internal capsule to the cortical centre for hearing in the first and second temporosphenoid convolutions. The sounds received in one ear predominantly reach the opposite cerebral hemisphere. However in unilateral cerebral or brain stem lesions, unilateral deafness does not occur due to partial decussation of secondary auditory tracts. The vestibular fibres are connected with the cerebellum.

1) Acuity of hearing: Generally the power of hearing is tested by means of a watch. While the patient is looking straight, or has closed his eyes, the examiner standing behind, has to bring the watch near the ear. Each ear is tested separately. One ear is closed, by placing a finger in the patient's external auditory meatus, when the other ear is tested for the audibility. The distance at which the patient is able to hear the sound of the tick is noted and compared with the other ear. The presence of wax must be excluded before concluding about loss or impaired hearing. The patient's ability to hear with each ear, can also be tested by rubbing a finger or by whispered voice.

If there is any impairment of hearing, it is necessary to find out whether it is due to the disease of the auditory nerve (nerve or perception deafness) or of the middle ear (middle ear or conduction deafness). Perception deafness can occur at cochlear (Meniere's disease, advanced otosclerosis, drug-induced deafness, internal auditory occlusion, prolonged exposure to loud noise), nerve trunk (oldage, trauma, post-inflammatory conditions, meningitis, cerebellopontine angle tumours) or at brain stem (severe pontine vascular lesions, severe demyelinating lesions) levels. Conduction deafness is encountered in all diseases of external meatus, middle ear and Eustachian tubes.

   a) Rinne's test: Acuity of hearing is tested by the use of a tuning fork. Normally the sound is conducted through the air to the drum and bony ossicles. This normal method of hearing is twice as effective as conduction through the bone. The base of a vibrating tuning fork (512 Hertz per second) is placed on the mastoid process on one side while the other ear is closed. When the patient stops hearing the sound the tines of the fork are to be brought near the ear and it is noted whether the patient still hears the sound (Rinne's test Fig. 51). The vibrations will still be heard normally.

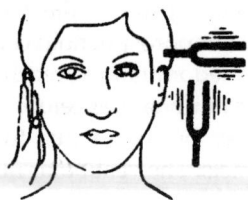

Fig. 51 Rinne's test.

In diseases of the middle ear or obstruction to the outer ear, the conduction through the air is decreased, hence the vibrations are not heard. In complete loss of hearing due to nerve deafness, though air conduction is better than the bone conduction, the patient is unable to hear the sounds. However in situations of partial loss of hearing or perception deafness, the patient can still hear the sounds when the vibrating tuning fork is brought near the ear.

In a normal ear, the air conduction is better than bone conduction and is referred to as Rinne positive. In nerve deafness though both air and bone conduction are diminished, the normal relationship is still maintained. Rinne negative implies that the bone conduction is better than air conduction. It is a middle ear deafness.

b) *Weber's test:* Normally the sounds are heard to an equal degree in both ears when a vibrating tuning fork is placed on the middle of the forehead or mandible. The sounds are heard better on the affected side in conduction deafness. In nerve deafness the sounds are better heard on the healthy side only (Fig. 52). The test was described by Friedrich Weber, a German otologist.

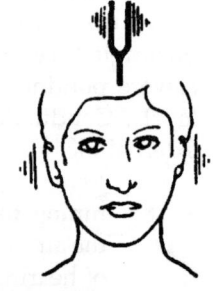

Fig. 52 Weber's test.

The test helps in lateralisation of the lesions wherein the sound is better heard by the affected ear in conduction deafness and by the normal ear in perception deafness.

2) *Vestibular function:* In disorders of vestibular function, the objects surrounding the individual appear to move round him or there is a feeling of a subjective sensation of rotation. The resulting manifestations—described as giddiness or dizziness—are noted in labyrinthitis, motion sickness, Meniere's disease, effect of drugs (salicylates, streptomycin) and vascular insufficiency in the brain stem. The involvement of the nerve results in an alteration in the current of the endolymph within the semicircular canals. Rotational test and calorie test are employed in recognizing the abnormality.

a) Rotational test: While the patient sitting on a rotating stool with his head well supported and fixed in a head rest, the horizontal and vertical canals are tested.

Horizontal canals are tested by flexing the head 30°, so that the eye/external auditory meatus plane is horizontal. Vertical canals are tested, by flexing the head to 120°. The stool is rotated ten times in 20 seconds. When rotation is stopped, for example right, the endolymph continues to flow in that direction, resulting in nystagmus with its slow phase to the right. It is always in the direction of the current. Since the test stimulates the labyrinths on both sides, the calorie test is preferred.

b) Calorie test: When the patient lies supine with head flexed 30°, the horizontal canals lie in the vertical plane with the ampulla at the highest point. In such a position warming or cooling the endolymph produces current upwards or downwards respectively. This movement produces nystagmus by stimulating the ampullae of the canal. This phenomenon is absent in affections of the vestibular nerve.

Warm water is poured into the right external ear through the external auditory meatus when the patient is lying supine with head flexed 30°. The irrigation is carried with about 250 ml of water at 40°C and later at 44°C. The current flows upwards in the right horizontal canal towards the ampulla. It displaces endolymph in an arc curving forward towards the left. The patient fixes his eyes on to a given point immediately above his head and after completion of irrigation, the time is measured in seconds during which nystagmus on forward gaze persists. The slow phase of nystagmus appears towards the left. This phase is always in the direction of the flow. The quick phase is to the right. Irrigation of the right ear with warm water produces nystagmus to the right;

with cold water to the left. In a similar fashion the irrigation of the left ear with warm water results in nystagmus to the left; and with cold water to the right.

Glossopharyngeal and Vagus Nerves

The glossopharyngeal and vagus nerves are mixed cranial nerves, and they take their origin in an elongated nucleus in the floor of the fourth ventricle and emerge by several roots along the lateral aspect of the medulla and leave the base of the skull through the jugular foramen along the accessory nerve. As the area of innervation and action of these nerve overlap, they are examined together.

The glossopharyngeal nerve innervates certain muscles concerned in swallowing such as the stylopharyngeus muscle and middle constrictor of the pharynx. The motor function overlaps with the vagus nerve. The ninth nerve conveys sensations from the upper part of the pharynx and taste as well as somatic sensations from the posterior-third of the tongue.

The vagus nerve has a wide distribution and it carries sensations from the pharynx, larynx, oesophagus, heart, respiratory passages and abdominal viscera. It forms an important part of the autonomic nervous system. The motor fibres innervate the voluntary muscles of the soft palate, pharynx, larynx and the upper oesophagus.

These nerves are tested as follows:

1) The taste sensation of the posterior third of the tongue is tested in a way similar to that done while testing the anterior third of the tongue. The procedure is difficult. Loss of taste sensation may be noted in a lesion of the trunk of the glossopharyngeal nerve.

2) Pharyngeal ('gag') reflex: The afferent and efferent pathways of gag reflex is by the ninth and tenth nerves respectively. Each side of the back of the pharynx is tickled using a sterile swab stick. Normally there will be a reflex contraction of the pharynx, elevation of the palate, retraction of the tongue and cough. In unilateral paralysis, the pharyngeal reflex is absent and the posterior pharyngeal wall moves to the normal side like a curtain. The reflex may be absent in normal individuals also. Pharyngeal weakness results in accumulation of mucus in the throat.

3) Movement of the soft palate: The position and symmetry of the palate and uvula at rest and with phonation has to be observed.

The patient is asked to open the mouth and say 'Ah'. During phonation both sides of the soft palate arch upwards. The uvula remains in the midline. In unilateral lesion of the vagus, the soft palate remains flat and immobile on the affected side. The median raphe and uvula will be pulled towards the healthy side. In bilateral paralysis, the whole palate does not exhibit any movement.

4) In bilateral involvement of these nerves there is difficulty in swallowing, especially of fluids. The patient may notice regurgitation of the fluid through the nose. This is due to defective elevation of the soft palate during swallowing. There is a nasal quality to the voice due to improper closure of the nasopharynx. These manifestations are assessed, by asking the patient to drink water, and by asking him pronounce words such as big, hug, or tub. Hoarseness of the voice is noted if there is paralysis of the recurrent layrngeal nerve, a branch of the vagus. The nerve supplies all muscles of the larynx except the cricothyroid.

The left recurrent laryngeal nerve is more commonly affected than the right. It may be affected from mediastinal tumours, aneurysm of the aorta, and injury to the neck. Bilateral lesions of recurrent laryngeal nerve leads to respiratory obstruction.

Isolated paralysis of any of these nerves is rare. Generally they are seen together. Unilateral paralysis of these nerves may be encountered in bulbar palsy (poliomyelitis, diphtheria, encephalitis, and botulism), syringomyelia, infective polyneuritis, posterior fossa tumours, tumours at the jugular foramen, aneurysms and posterior inferior cerebellar syndromes. Bilateral upper motor neuron paralysis is seen in pseudobulbar palsy and amyotrophic lateral sclerosis. Bilateral lower motor neuron paralysis is seen in progressive bulbar paralysis.

Accessory Nerve

The eleventh cranial nerve is pure motor in function and it has two roots: cranial and spinal, arising from a nucleus in the floor of the fourth ventricle along the glossopharyngeal and the vagus nerves and the upper cervical portion of the spinal cord respectively. The former emerging from the lateral aspect of the medulla joins the vagus nerve contributing to the innervation of the larynx and pharynx, hence it is considered part of vagus nerve. The spinal accessory emerging from the lateral side of the cord supplies the upper part of the trapezii and sternomastoid muscles influencing the posture and movements of the head and shoulder girdles.

The accessory nerve is tested to detect wasting and weakness-unilateral or bilateral—of sternomastoid and trapezius muscles and to determine if the lesion is located in the nucleus, nerve trunk or its branches or local muscle disease. Atrophy indicates that the lesion is either in the nucleus or the peripheral nerve.

The upper part of the trapezius, is tested by placing the hands over the shoulder from behind while the patient is sitting symmetrically upright (Fig. 53). The patient is asked to raise his shoulders towards his ears, while they are pressed downwards by the examiner. Shrugging of the shoulder is weak in weakness of trapezius muscle. It may be noted that part of the muscle is supplied by cranial nerves. In the paralysis of the muscle, there is drooping of the shoulder with displacement of the scapula downwards and laterally. These changes are accentuated when the arm is abducted against resistance. There is rotation of the scapula directing its superior angle further from the spine than the inferior angle. The vertebral border of the scapula stands out like winged scapula as in serratus anterior palsy (see page 266). The head is bent forwards due to the weakness of the muscle.

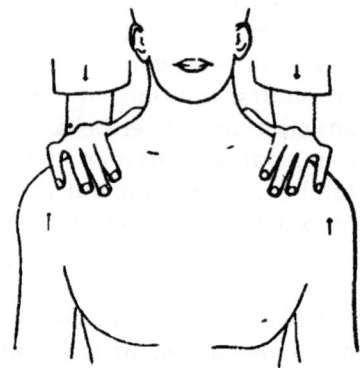

Fig. 53 Testing upper part of the trapezius.

The sternomastoid is tested by placing the hand on right side of the cheek and asking the patient to turn it against resistance (Fig. 54). The belly of the left sternomastoid stands out prominently on movement of the cheek to the right. The procedure is repeated on the other side. It demonstrates the power of the opposite sternomastoid. In paralysis of the sternomastoid muscle, the chin deviates to the affected side. There is weakness of rotation of the chin towards the opposite side. Both sternomastoids can be tested simultaneously by asking the patient to depress the chin against resistance. Normally both sternomastoids stand out together. Paralysis of the muscle results in drooping of the head backwards.

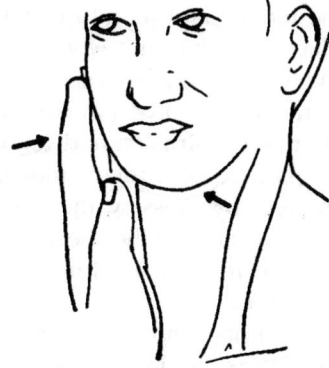

Fig. 54 Testing sternomastoid.

The Accessory Nerve can be Affected Unilaterally or Bilaterally.

Unilateral lesion
  Trauma in the neck or base of skull
  Poliomyelitis
  Syringomyelia
  Tumours at jugular foramen
  Bony anomalies at base of skull
Bilateral lesion
  Motor neuron disease
  Spinal muscular atrophy
  Poliomyelitis
  Polyneuropathy

Paralysis of the sternomastoid is characteristic in dystrophia myotonica.

Hypoglossal Nerve

The hypoglossal nerve is a motor cranial nerve, and it arises from a nucleus situated in the lower part of the floor of the fourth ventricle, close to the midline in the medulla. It leaves the skull through the anterior condylar foramen. It supplies extrinsic and intrinsic muscles of the tongue and the depressors of the hyoid bone, thus controlling all movements of the tongue and some movements of the hyoid bone and larynx during and after deglutition. As the nerve contains only motor fibres, the tests carried out on the nerve are truly objective.

Before testing the strength of the tongue, its size, shape, surface and position are to be observed by asking the patient to protrude the tongue and then to move it from side-to-side. It is normally placed in the centre when protruded. Involuntary movements of the tongue may be noted in Parkinsonism (rapid protrusion and retraction), chorea (an up and down flapping movement with alternate protrusion and retraction) and intake of phenothiazine drugs (irregular rotary movements). It is possible to assess the strength by pressing the tongue with a finger when the patient protrudes it into the cheek on either side. Fasciculations are to be looked at with the tongue within the mouth and not when extended.

In upper motor neuron type of paralysis, the normal-looking tongue is deviated towards the paralysed side due to the unopposed contraction of the genioglossus muscle. Commonly it is associated with hemiplegia on that side. It does not occur as an isolated phenomenon. The asymmetry of the mouth noticed after facial palsy may give an erroneous impression of deviation of the tongue onto one side. The relation of the median raphe with the central incisor teeth will help in the detection of it. In a very short frenum, the tongue is held back and it curves downwards.

In bilateral upper motor neuron type of paralysis, there is difficulty or inability to protrude the tongue beyond the lips. The tongue lies immobile on the floor of the mouth. Its size appears small and feels firm in consistency. Its surface does not show any folds. There are no fasciculations. It is associated with gross dysarthria and even dysphagia. It is noted in cerebral atherosclerosis, pseudobulbar palsy, motor neuron disease, tumours of the brain stem and multiple sclerosis.

In the lower motor neuron type of paralysis, the tongue may exhibit unilateral wasting and wrinkling. It feels soft and flabby, which can be judged by holding the tongue in between the finger and the thumb with a gauze piece. The longitudinal folds are prominent on the paralysed side. The median raphe and tip are curved round towards its affected (wasted) side. This is due to its unopposed, pushing action of the normal genioglossus. The speech is little affected. The tongue deviates towards the weaker side on protrusion. There may be fasciculations. In bilateral involvement of the hypoglossal nerve (progressive bulbar palsy) the tongue is wasted, and shrunken and it may demonstrate generalized fasciculations. Fasciculations are marked in lesions such as motor neuron disease. Protrusion of the tongue becomes difficult and it lies on the floor of the mouth. The tip of the median raphe remains central. The jaw jerk will be exaggerated. There is dysarthria. The condition is associated with paralysis of the lips due to the close connection of hypoglossal nucleus with the nucleus of facial nerve controlling the orbicularis oris.

Bulbar palsy: The term bulbar palsy refers to lower motor neuron type of weakness of the muscles supplied by lower (ninth to twelfth) cranial nerves having nuclei in the medulla (bulb). The condition arises from the lesions of the lower cranial nerves or their nuclei or from neuromuscular diseases. The common examples are lesions of brain stem (infarction, syringobulbia, motor neuron disease and poliomyelitis), tumours in the jugular foramen or neck or nasopharynx, or polyneuropathy.

Pseudobulbar palsy: Pseudobulbar palsy refers to bilateral upper motor neuron type of lesions of the lower cranial nerves. It is associated with weakness and poor movement of the tongue and of the pharyngeal muscles. The tongue is small due to spasticity. There are no fasciculations. There is dysarthria. The gag reflex and palatal reflexes are preserved. The jaw jerk is exaggerated. There is emotional lability. The condition is noted in motor neuron diseases (both upper and lower motor neuron lesions), late stage of multiple sclerosis and cerebrovascular disease with multiple infarcts, double hemiplegia of vascular origin and brain stem tumours.

Motor System

The voluntary motor activity is dependent on the integrity of the various parts of the nervous system. The initiation of the voluntary movements takes place at the motor cortex (anterior aspect of the central sulcus, and adjacent parts of the precentral gyrus) and the impulses are carried along the pyramidal tract (corticospinal tract, the upper motor neuron). The pyramidal tract passes through the internal capsule (posterior one-third of the anterior limb, genu and the anterior two-thirds of the posterior limb), midbrain, pons and medulla. At the junction of the medulla and spinal cord, the fibres of the pyramidal tract undergo partial decussation and descend down to terminate in the internuncial neurons in the grey matter of the spinal cord, which in turn synapse with the anterior horn cells. During the course in the brain stem, the pyramidal tract gives fibres to the motor nuclei of the cranial nerves. A second relay of fibres originate from the motor nuclei of the brain stem as cranial nerves, and from the anterior horn cells of the spinal cord as peripheral nerves (lower motor neurons) and terminate in the muscles. The extrapyramidal system consists of the basal ganglia, the subthalamic nuclei, the substantia nigra and other structures present in the brain stem concerned with movement and posture. The cerebellum receives afferent fibres from the spinal cord, vestibular system, basal ganglia and cerebral cortex and modulates movements. The integrity of the sensory system is necessary for the reflex movements.

Motor abnormality presents with two basic patterns as the upper and the lower motor neuron lesions. Upper motor neuron (UMN) lesion causes weakness of the muscles that is incomplete except in the acute stages, or in the presence of an extensive destructive lesion. It affects particular movements rather than particular muscles. It is markedly seen in the abductors and extensors of the upper limb, and the flexors of the lower limb. There is increased tone of the muscles and exaggerated reflexes.

Lower motor neuron lesion affects muscles having that segmental supply. After some time there is marked wasting of the muscles and loss of tendon reflexes in the affected muscles are involved. A lesion either of the anterior horn or anterior root affects the muscles supplied by specific segment and the muscles may show fasciculations. A lesion at the periphery of the nerve affects all muscles supplied by the nerve.

The Functions of the Motor System are examined under the Following Separate Headings.

Nutrition (bulk, size) of the muscles,
tone of the muscles,
power (strength) of the muscles,
coordination of movements,
involuntary movements,
reflexes, and
gait.

Nutrition of the Muscles

The nutrition of the muscles is affected in various disorders of the neuromuscular system. Wasting (atrophy) of the muscles is detected by making a comparison with the other muscles in the same or other limbs. When the wasting is asymmetrical on either side, it is detected without difficulty by inspection and palpation.

The wasted (atrophic) muscles appear soft, small and flabby. When fibrosis supervenes, the wasted muscles become inelastic and hard (muscular dystrophy or polymyositis). They later become shortened to cause contractures. Then there is difficulty to stretch the muscles passively to a normal degree.

The existence of wasting, can be assessed by taking the measurement of the circumference of the two limbs kept in identical positions at a fixed level from a bony point. Generally the measurement of circumference of the limbs is taken at clearly defined places such as 10 cm above or below olecranon; 18 cm above patella; 10 cm below tibial tuberosity. The symmetrical wasting has to be carefully evaluated. The presence of other systemic diseases must be looked for, to determine the cause of generalized wasting (cachexia) seen in patients with malignancy, thyrotoxicosis, diabetes mellitus, tuberculosis, malnutrition and malabsorption syndrome. Generalised wasting is also encountered in advanced neurologic diseases, especially myopathies and motor neuron disease.

Localised muscle wasting may be seen following injury or disease of the joint. The power is retained in such muscles. Wasting is seen in the interossei muscles when the metacarpophalangeal joints are showing evidence of arthritis. Similar wasting is seen in the thenar muscles when there is arthritis of the first metacarpophalangeal joint, and in the extensor muscles proximal to the knee, shoulder and hip when these joints are affected in arthritis.

There may be evidence of hypertrophy of certain groups of muscles. This hypertrophy of muscles is noted in athletes, and in individuals engaged in heavy manual work. In pseudo-hypertrophy, the muscles (calf muscles, glutei, infraspinatus and deltoid) are globular and give a tense rubbery feeling due to deposition of fat (pseudohypertrophy of Duchenne and Becker muscular dystrophy). However, the muscles are weak in spite of their size indicating that 'all that glitters is not gold'. There may be more diffuse hypertrophy of muscles in myotonia congenita, including thighs and shoulder girdles.

The wasting of the muscles may be noted in primary diseases of the muscles (myopathy) or diseases involving the anterior horn cells (motor neuron disease, poliomyelitis, syringomyelia) or nerves (peripheral neuropathy). Wasting of the muscles is thus a characteristic feature of the lower motor neuron lesions. Though wasting of the muscles is not a feature of the upper motor neuron lesions, disuse atrophy of muscles is noted in muscles that have not been used for a prolonged period. The extrapyramidal disorders do not exhibit wasting of the muscles.

The distribution of the wasting seen during the early stages of the neuromuscular disease is characteristic: myopathy (proximal muscles), peroneal muscular dystrophy (distal segments of the limbs with transverse demarcation in between normal and wasted portions of the muscles), motor neuron disease (distal muscles), diabetes mellitus (extensor digitorum brevis), and cauda equina lesions (glutei). In advanced stages of the neuromuscular diseases the individual becomes crippled and the wasting is seen over widespread regions.

The wasting of the small muscles of the hand involving the segmental nerve supply-C_8 and T_1, is caused by the lesions at different levels:

1) Anterior horn cells: motor neuron disease, poliomyelitis, syringomyelia, cervical cord tumours

2) Anterior roots: cervical spondylosis, pachymeningitis, cervical tumours

3) Brachial plexus: injuries, cervical ribs, bronchogenic carcinoma (apical segment of the upper lobe)

4) Peripheral nerves: (i) Ulnar nerve-injury, leprosy (wasting of the small muscles except opponens pollicis and abductor pollicis brevis (ii) Median nerve-injuries, carpal tunnel syndrome (wasting of the thenar muscles), myotonic dystrophy.

5) Others: rheumatoid arthritis, peroneal muscular atrophy, distal muscle dystrophy of Wellander.

Proximal muscle wasting is noted in myopathies (symmetrical) and spinal muscular atrophy. In muscular dystrophy there is a selective pattern of individual muscle involvement (Facio-scapulohumeral dystrophy, limb-girdle syndrome, X-linked muscular dystrophies of Duchenne and Becker).

Isolated peripheral wasting of muscles of leg is less common. It occurs as a part of extensive cauda equina lesion and as a part of a polyneuropathy. It will follow poliomyelitis and peripheral nerve trauma (lateral popliteal nerve). Peripheral wasting in all four limbs is rare. It is seen in peroneal muscular atrophy and rarely in chronic polyneuropathies.

Muscle Tone

Tone is the constant degree of tension in the skeletal muscles at rest. It enables the joints to maintain the posture. It is of the nature of a stretch reflex, and is dependent on the spinal reflex arc. Further, the tone is regulated, by pyramidal and extra-pyramidal tracts. The movements are coordinated under the influence of the cerebellum and its related tracts.

The tone of the muscles is assessed by estimation of the degree of resistance offered to a passive movement of the extremity through its full range of motion. The full range of flexion and extension movements is carried out passively by the examiner at the shoulder, elbow, wrist, hip, knee and ankle joints.

In the upper limbs, tone is assessed by rapid pronation and supination of the forearm and flexion and extension at the wrist. In the lower limbs, while the patient is supine, the hands are to be placed behind the knees and rapidly raised. With normal tone, the ankle is dragged along the bed for a variable distance before rising. An increased tone results in an immediate lift of the heel off the surface. The muscles are felt during the movement. The patient has to be encouraged to relax during the examination. Normally there is a slight degree of resistance. It may be increased (hypertonia) or decreased (hypotonia). In stuporose or comatose patients, the arm or leg can be raised and allowed to fall back on the bed. On the side of paralysis, it falls without any check as if it does not belong to him. Muscular contracture is characterized by shortening of the muscle and the range of motion is decreased.

Hypotonia: The muscles feel soft and flabby. The condition is called flaccidity. As there is little or no resistance, the range of movement at the joint is increased. There is looseness of the extremities on shaking. There is difficulty to maintain the position of the limb. The condition is seen in lesions of lower motor neuron (poliomyelitis), in lesions of afferent sensory pathways (tabes dorsalis), in lesions of motor side of reflex arc (neuropathies), in lesions of peripheral nerves (polyneuropathy, peripheral nerve injuries), in cerebellar disorders, in disorders of myoneural junctions (myasthenia gravis), in muscle disorders (myopathies, spinal muscular atrophies), states of neurological shock (severe cord lesion, profound hemiplegia), and in chorea.

The tone may be decreased during sleep and under the effect of sedatives. Flaccidity is accompanied by sluggish tendon reflexes, except in myasthenia gravis. An acute lesion of corticospinal tract produces flaccidity, however the tone increases within a few days due to a loss of the inhibiting effect of the corticospinal pathway and an increase in spinal reflex activity.

Hypertonia: The increase in muscle tone may be present in two forms-spasticity and rigidity due to the lesions of pyramydal and extrapyramidal tracts respectively.

Spasticity: Though there is an increased tone in all muscle groups, the tone is more in one group of muscles (agonist, e.g. the quadriceps) than in the other (antagonist, e.g. the hamstrings). The resistance is felt greatly at the beginning of passive flexion and it gives way suddenly on continued pressure (clasp-knife type lengthening reaction). It is most easily demonstrated at the elbow and knee. The muscles feel firm. Spasticity is an important sign of the upper motor neuron lesion. The spasticity is more marked in the flexors of the upper limb (antegravity muscles) than the extensors of the lower limb.

Rigidity: There is an increase in tone and resistance in all groups of muscles-both agonists and antagonists—to an equal degree on the affected side. This is an important sign of disease of the basal ganglia and is called extrapyramidal rigidity. The resistance may be felt to the same degree throughout the range of passive movement (plastic or lead pipe rigidity), or may be less uniform diminishing in jerky steps due to the contraction of agonists and antagonists alternatively and is greatly increased when there is superimposition of tremors (cog-wheel rigidity). Patients with catatonic states and frontal lobe disease may exhibit a similar plastic type of rigidity. There is a persistent abnormal posture (dystonia). There is a progressive increase in resistance during all phases of passive movements (paratonic rigidity). In hysterical rigidity, the resistance to passive movements is proportional to the amount of force applied. There is an increasing resistance occurring in a jerky manner.

Paratonia: There can be fluctuating changes in resistance as in the lesions of the frontal lobe pathways. Such an abnormality may be encountered in normal difficulty in relaxing.

Myotonia: Myotonia refers to a state of muscle contraction that continues beyond the period of time needed for a particular movement to be made. It is encountered in the muscles of the face and hands. The condition is seen in myotonic dystrophy and myotonia congenita. The patient is asked to show his teeth and then to 'let go'. There is a delay in relaxation. To test the hand muscles the patient is asked to grip the fingers and then suddenly relax his hold. It will result in flexion of the wrist, adduction and opposition of the thumb and incomplete extension of the fingers. Ultimately the patient has to drag his hand away.

Muscle Power (Strength)

Major groups of muscles such as flexors and extensors of the neck; the adductors, abductors, and rotators of the shoulder; the flexors and extensors of the elbow, wrist and fingers; the hand grip; the abdominal muscles; the extensors of the spine; the flexors and extensors of hip and knee; the dorsiflexors and plantar flexors of the feet; and the flexors and extensors of the toes, especially the great toe are tested for their power.

Upper limb weakness is screened by testing 'pronator drift'. The patient is asked to hold both arms fully extended and parallel to the ground with eyes closed. This position should be maintained at least for 10 seconds. Any flexion at the elbow or fingers or pronation of the forearm, especially if asymmetric, is considered a sign of potential weakness.

If the examination reveals weakness, tests are to be carried out for individual muscles responsible for the defective movement. The limb has to be placed in a correct position. Then the power is tested by the following manoeuvres carried out by the patient against resistance offered by the examiner. The patient should exert maximal effort for the particular muscle or muscle group being tested.

Grading of weakness: The power is graded on an index of 0 to 5 from total paralysis (0) to normal power (5) against gravity and resistance respectively.

0	total paralysis (no movement)
1	presence of a slight flicker of the contraction of muscle without any associated movement at a joint
2	a normal range of power when the opposing force of gravity is removed by appropriate position
3	a normal range of power against gravity but not against resistance
4–	movement against a mild degree of resistance
4	a normal range of power against moderate resistance
4+	movement against strong resistance
5	normal or full power

Unilateral or bilateral weakness of the upper limb extensors and lower limb flexors, referred to as pyramidal weakness suggests lesions of the pyramidal tract. Bilateral proximal weakness suggests myopathy and bilateral distal weakness suggests peripheral neuropathy.

Testing of the muscles: The power of the muscles is tested by the following manoeuvres carried out by the patient against resistance offered by the examiner.

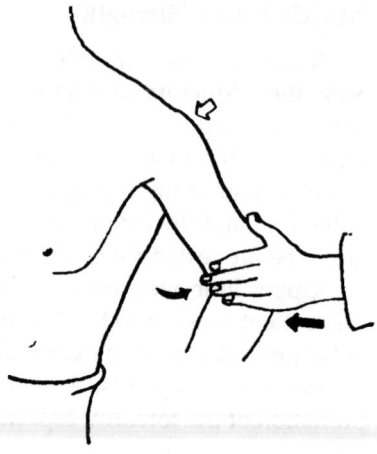

Fig. 55 Testing deltoid.

The alphabets C (cervical), T (thoracic), L (lumbar), and S (sacral) refer to spinal segments. The number of appropriate segments is given as a subscript.

Upper limb: Muscles of the shoulder girdle and scapula-Supraspinatus (C_5): Abduct the arm from the side to 30° while the scapula is fixed.

Deltoid (C_5): Abduct the arm held at 30° further to right angle (Fig. 55).

Infraspinatus (C_5): Push the arm backwards when the elbow is held by the side and fixed at right angle.

Serratus anterior ($C_{5, 6}$): Push against the wall with the hands while the upper limb is lifted forwards. The vertebral border of the scapula stands projecting in the paralysis of the muscle (winged scapula. Fig. 56).

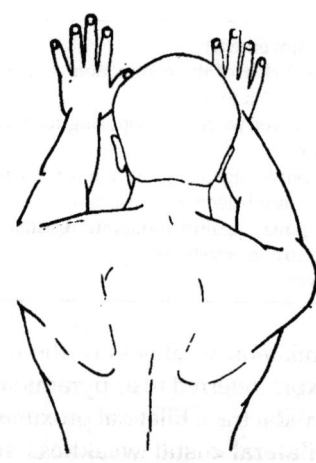

Fig. 56 winged scapula.

Pectoralis major ($C_{5, 6}$): Bring the hands together when the arm is raised to 60° (sternal) and 90° (clavicular) Fig. 57).

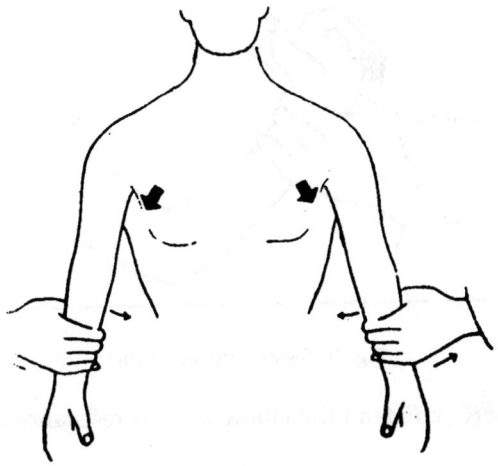

Fig. 57 Testing pectoralis major.

Latissimus dorsi (C_6): Adduct the arm while it is abducted above 90° to the side.

Lower part of the trapezius (C_4): Approximate the shoulder blades.

Rhomboides (C_5): Try to force the elbow backwards while the hand is placed on hip.

Muscles of the elbow joint Biceps (C_5): Flex the elbow while the forearm is kept supinated (Fig. 58).

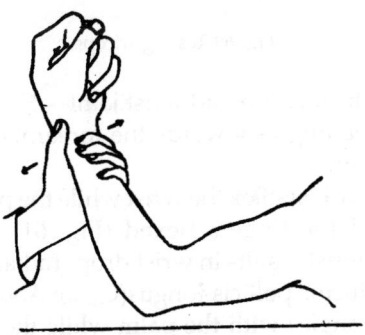

Fig. 58 Testing biceps.

Brachioradialis ($C_{5, 6}$): Flex the elbow while the forearm is kept midway between pronation and supination (Fig. 59).

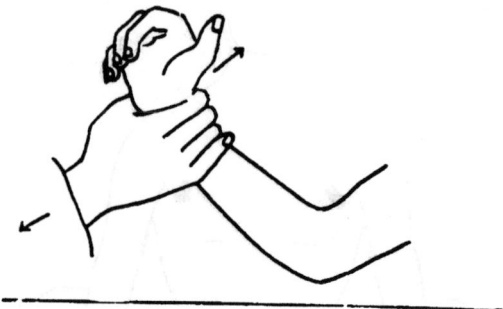

Fig. 59 Testing brachioradialis.

Triceps (C_7): Extend the elbow against resistance (Fig. 60).

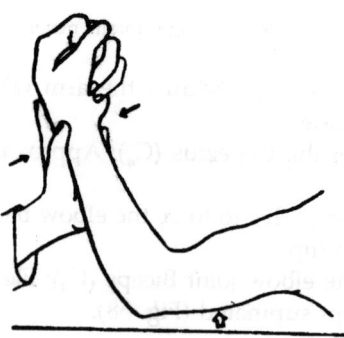

Fig. 60 Testing triceps.

Muscles of the forearm and wrist joint— Flexors (C_7): Flex the wrist to bring the fingers towards the forearm while the palm is kept facing upwards.

Extensors (C_7): Dorsiflex the wrist while the palm is kept facing downwards and the fingers flexed (Fig. 61). Paralysis of the extensors of the wrist results in wrist drop (radial nerve paralysis).

Thumb-Abductor pollicis longus($C_{6, 7}$): Abduct the thumb to bring it at right angles with the palm while the metacarpal bone of the thumb is fixed.

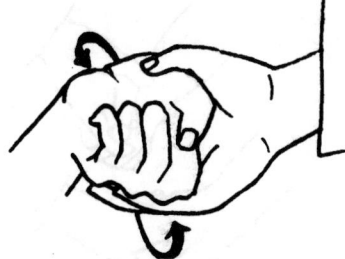

Fig. 61 Testing extensors of the wrist.

Abductor pollicis brevis (median nerve, $C_{6, 7}$): Abduct the thumb in a plane at right angles to the palmar aspect of the index finger. In paralysis, the thumb lies on a level with the fingers giving 'ape-hand' deformity.

Opponens pollicis ($C_{6, 7}$): Touch the tip of the little finger with the point of the thumb.

Adductor pollicis ($C_{6, 7}$): Hold a piece of paper tightly between the thumb and palmar aspect of the forefingers (Fig. 62).

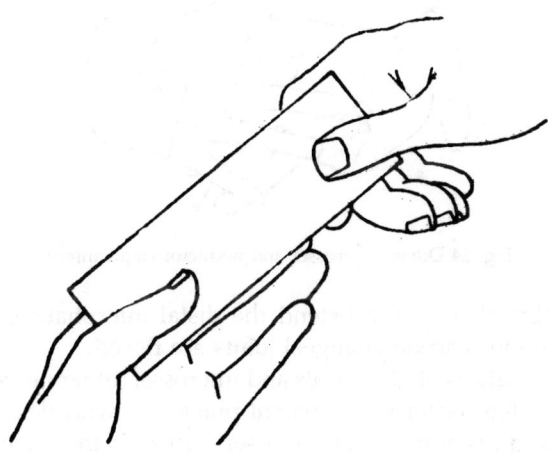

Fig. 62 Testing adductor polices.

Fingers-Flexors: Squeeze the examiner's index and middle fingers with the hand, thus enabling him to assess the grip (Fig. 63).

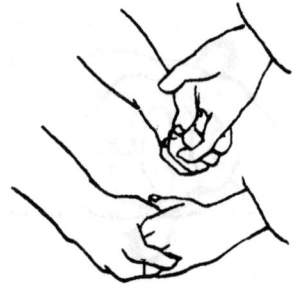

Fig. 63 Squeeze by finger flexors.

Extensors: Extend the proximal and distal phalanges
First dorsal interosseus (ulnar): Abduct the index finger.

Interossei (C_8, T_1): Abduct the index, ring and little fingers away from the midline (dorsal interossei and abductor digiti minimi (Fig. 64), and adduct the above fingers towards the midline (Palmar interossei).

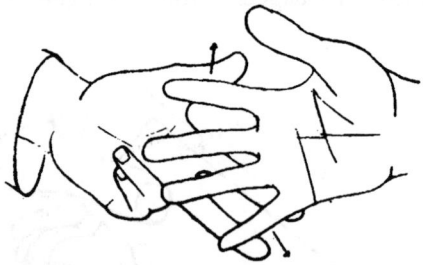

Fig. 64 Dorsal interossei and abductor digiti minimi.

Lumbricals (C_8, T_1): Extend the distal interphalangeal joints while the metacarpophalangeal joints are flexed.

The paralysis of lumbricals and interossei (ulnar nerve) results in hyperextension of the proximal phalanges with flexion of the middle and distal phalanges and separation of the fingers (claw-hand) as the power is retained in the long flexors and extensors of the fingers.

Lower part of the trapezius (C_4): Approximate the shoulder blades

Trunk-Extensors (Erector spinae) of the spine: Raise the head from the pillow by extending the neck and back while lying in a prone position with hands clasped over the back.

Abdominals (T_5-_{11}): Raise the head while lying in a supine position. In the paralysis of the muscles, the patient finds it difficult to get up from the bed without the aide of his arms. The umbilicus gets displaced to the sound side in paralysis of a portion of the anterior abdominal wall when the head is raised from the pillow against resistance. In paralysis of the lower abdominal muscles, the umbilicus moves upwards and in paralysis of the upper abdominal muscles the umbilicus is pulled downwards (Beevor's sign, named after Charles Beevor, a British neurologist).

In organic spastic paralysis of a leg the affected limb rises first when the patient lying on his back with extended legs tries to get up without using his hands (Babinski's rising-up sign, after Joseph Babinski, a French neurologist). This does not happen in hysterical paralysis.

Lower limb: Thigh-Flexors (Iliopsoas, L_3): Raise the extended leg from the bed while in supine position.

Adductors (L_3): Adduct the limb to the midline when it is kept abducted.

Abductors (Gluteus medius and minimus, L_4): Abduct the legs from the midline (Fig. 65)

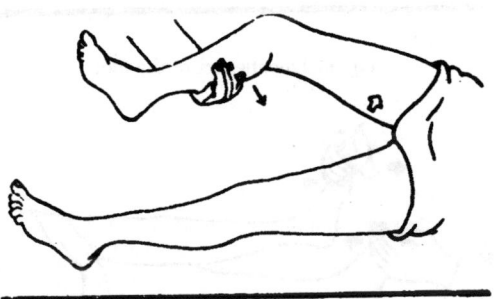

Fig. 65 Testing Gluteus medius.

Rotators (L_4): Rotate the thigh so as to move the foot medially and laterally when the lower limb is kept extended.

Extensors (Gluteus maximus, $L_{4, 5}$): Push down the foot of the extended knee that is lifted off the bed.

Knee-Flexors (hamstrings, L_5): Flex the knee of the raised leg from the bed.

Extensors (Quadriceps femoris, L_4): Extend the bent knee (Fig. 66).

Foot-Dorsiflexors (Tibialis anterior, L_5, S_1) and Plantar flexors (Gastrocnemius, L_5, S_1): Elevate (dorsiflexion—Fig. 67) and depress (plantar flexion—Fig. 68) the foot respectively.

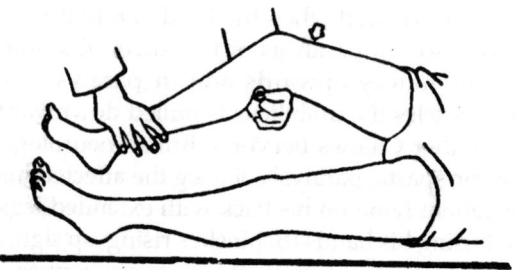

Fig. 66 Testing Quadriceps femoris.

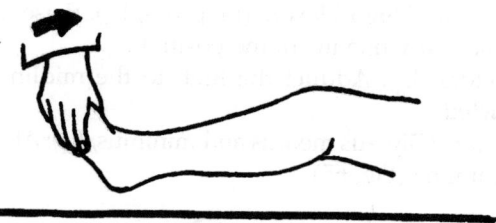

Fig. 67 Dorsiflexors of the foot.

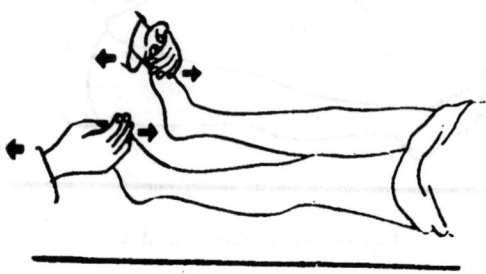

Fig. 68 Plantar flexors of the foot.

Eversion and inversion (Peronei and tibialis posterior, L_5, S_1): Turn the plantar flexed foot outwards and inwards.

Intrinsic muscles of the foot (L_5, S_1): Weakness or paralysis of the interossei results in a 'claw foot' deformity.

Patterns of weakness: The term paralysis is applied if no contraction is elicited in a muscle or a group of muscles, and paresis refers to existence of a feeble power of contraction. Paralysis of one side of the body especially of the arm and leg is called hemiplegia. It may involve one side of the face also (facio-brachial-crural hemiplegia). An upper motor neuron lesion above the decussation causes paralysis (hemiplegia) or weakness (hemiparesis) of the contralateral limb. The lesion below decussation causes the paralysis on the same side as the lesion. Paralysis of muscles supplied by the motor cranial nerves on one side and paralysis of the upper and lower limbs of the opposite side of the body are referred to as crossed paralysis (brain stem disorders). The term paraplegia is used to describe paralysis of both legs. Paralysis of one limb is called monoplegia and it may involve an arm (brachial) or a leg (crural). The term quadriplegia (diplegia) is applied to the paralysis of all four limbs. The term paresis is applied when there is weakness in a limb or other parts of the body.

Motor Weakness.

Type of paralysis	location of paralysis	site of lesion	type of lesion
Hemiplegia	paralysis of one side of body	corticospinal tract	UMN
Crossed paralysis	weakness of ipsilateral cranial muscles and contralateral hemiparesis	brain stem	UMN
Paraplegia	paralysis of both legs	spinal cord	UMN
Monoplegia	paralysis of one limb	nerve root or plexus	LMN
Quadriplegia	paralysis of all four limbs	cervical cord	UMN

In an acute severe lesion at the internal capsule (infarct) there is complete weakness in the limbs (pyramidal lesion, spastic hemiplegia). In partial lesion the weakness appears selective. The limbs are affected more than the trunk. The finger movements of the hands are affected more than the trunk. The finger movements of the hands are affected much more than the grosser movements of the shoulder. The extensors are stronger than flexors in the lower limb and the flexors are stronger than extensors in the upper limb. Hence there is weakness in the lower limb in the abductors and flexors of the hip, flexors of knee, dorsiflexors of the foot and toes, in the upper limb in the abductors and extensors of the shoulder, extensors of the elbow and in dorsiflexors of the wrist.

Sometimes the detection of hemiplegia in a comatose patient offers difficulty. However in recent paralysis of the limb there is hypotonia of the muscles. The arm raised from the side, if allowed to drop, falls like a log of wood as if it does not belong to the individual. The face appears asymmetrical and the angle of the mouth appears widely open on the paralysed side, and the affected cheek is seen moving outwards and inwards with respiration. The reflexes may be absent on both sides, but the plantar response is extensor on the paralysed side.

In lower motor neuron lesion paralysis, there is involvement of individual muscles or group of muscles controlled by particular segments of the cord. Upper motor neuron lesion paralysis affects movements rather than muscles.

Coordination of Movements

Coordination is the ability to perform skilled movements in the upper and lower limbs. Coordinate movements require efficient, smooth, adequate movement of a group of muscles together with an appropriate smooth relaxation of antagonist group of muscles and knowledge of the position of the moving part before, during and at the end of each movement, and the knowledge of the position of the point to which the part has to be moved. The muscles are also under the influence of cerebellar, extrapyramidal and vestibular systems. The deficiency in any one of the systems results in incoordination (ataxia).

All procedures to assess the coordination have to be carried out with the eyes open first, and later with the eyes closed. This enables one to assess the integrity of the sensory path in the posterior column and cerebellar tracts. In the sensory ataxia, the incoordination is corrected partially by vision.

Coordination is tested, by asking the patient to walk along a straight line if he is able to walk. The patient becomes unsteady and deviates to one side or the other, if there is incoordination.

Upper limbs: Finger-to-nose test: The patient is asked to stretch out his arm and then to bring the tip of the index finger to touch the tip of his nose. The finger has to be held on the nose to a count of 5 (Fig. 69). The procedure is to be done with the index finger of each hand in turn. Each time the test is repeated with the eyes closed. The smoothness of the movement and the accuracy of placing and the steadiness with which the finger is held on the nose are to be noted.

In conditions associated with intention tremor (cerebellar

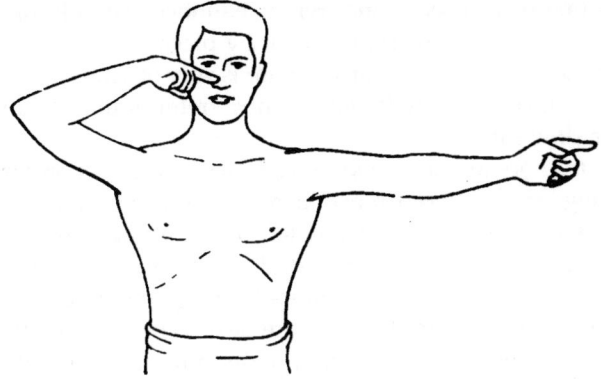

Fig. 69 Finger-to-nose test.

disease) there will be oscillations of the finger from side to side as it approaches the nose. In place of normal smooth movement there is a tendency to overshoot the object. There will be oscillations of the finger in various directions when it approaches the nose in the posterior column lesions impairing the position sense of the limb and this is made prominent by closure of the eyes.

Lower limbs: Heel-to-knee test: The heel has to be kept on the opposite knee and then it should be drawn along the shin towards the ankle. The procedure is done on either side. In cerebellar disease, the heel overshoots the knee sideways and exhibits oscillations from side to side while it is moved down the leg. In sensory ataxia, the heel is lifted too high and falls off several times during the downward course.

Abnormal Movements

The presence of involuntary muscular contractions has to be noted. They are of several varieties. They may be localized or widespread.

Tremors

Tremors are involuntary, rhythmic to and fro oscillatory movements from alternate contractions of opposing (agonist and antagonist) groups of muscles. Unlike chorea, tremors of athetosis, tics, and myoclonus are regular and are absent during sleep. The frequency and amplitude of tremors are variable; the movement may be fine or coarse. A fine tremor is noticeable only on close inspection, and it can be brought out by placing a piece of paper on the patient's fingers. A coarse tremor is very obvious, producing a movement of a few millimetres only. Tremors may occur at a rapid or slow rate.

The tremors are classified as rest (static) and action tremors depending on their occurrence at rest, or on voluntary activity respectively. Static tremors are noted in a limb at complete rest. The action tremors are subdivided as intention tremors and postural tremors. Hysterical tremors form a separate entity.

Static tremors: Static tremors are seen classically in Parkinsonism. The tremors are rapid, and rhythmically alternating in the flexor and extensor muscles in an involved limb. They may even appear as rotary movements between the index finger and the thumb (pill-rolling tremor). The tremors are marked at rest, and are suppressed briefly during voluntary activity like buttoning the coat. The tremor is absent in total relaxation, or in sleep and often immediately after walking. The tremors are increased by emotion. The tremors are more prominent in the distal than in the proximal muscles; in the arm than in the leg. Often they are unilateral. The lips and the tongue show tremors frequently.

Postural tremors: Fine tremors at a fast rate are noted when a limb is held in an antigravity posture. They are usually most evident in the hands. Tremors appear when the patient is asked to outstretch the arms to the front and keep the hands extended. The tremors can be felt by touching the fingers lightly or by placing a thin piece of cardboard on the outstretched hand. They are noted in situations of catecholamine excess, such as anxiety states, thyrotoxicosis, hypoglycaemia, and in alcoholism, and excess smoking (toxic tremors). They are also noted after ingestion of drugs such as caffeine, salbutamol, theophylline, amphetamines, tricyclic antidepressants, levodopa, lithium, sodium valproate, and steroids, and in mercury poisoning.

Tremor due to nervousness is very common. It is rapid, varying from fine to coarse, affecting mainly the fingers. It is noticed at rest and increased by any voluntary movements. Anxiety states are associated with tremors similar to that seen in nervousness, but are more marked, coarser and more persistent and are greatly influenced by emotions. It is accompanied by dilated pupils, tachycardia and cold, clammy sweating extremities. Thyrotoxicosis is associated with a fine, rapid tremor and is present constantly and is greatly influenced by emotion. It is accompanied by sweating and tachycardia, but the extremities are very warm.

A variable postural tremor, often coarse is noted in chronic alcoholism. Tremor may affect the whole limb and trunk. Though it is not greatly influenced by emotion or voluntary movement, it may be sufficiently severe to interfere with fine movement. Drugs taken in excess over a prolonged period of time may give rise to a tremor that resembles alcoholic tremor.

Essential tremor may occur as coarse, postural tremor and is noted in the upper extremities, head and neck. It may be hereditary, spasmodic, or may occur in association with other neurologic disorders. It may be noted in early adult life or in late life (senile tremors). Generally the tremors are noted with muscle contraction, and may occur at rest and severe. They are exaggerated by emotional and physical stress. There may be rhythmic oscillations of the head (titubation).

Hepatic precoma, respiratory and renal failure may be associated with tremors. They are demonstrated as follows: The examiner holding the forearm in its middle asks the patient to extend the hand, and rapid flexion and extension are noted at the wrist and metacarpophalangeal joints. As the movements simulate the beating of the wings of a bird, they are referred to as wing-flapping tremors. The 'liver-flap' is often a warning of impending hepatic coma.

Intention tremors: In brain stem or cerebellar diseases, the tremors are noted in a limb with a goal directed action. This appears to be due to loss of the modulating effect of the cerebellum on voluntary movement. They are noted when the patient is asked to perform the finger-to-nose test. The tremors appear when the finger approaches the tip of the nose. There is past-pointing accompanied by slowness and incoordination of rapid alternating movements.

Hysterical tremors: The tremors are variable and are not constant. It presents a bizarre picture involving a limb or the whole body.

Fasciculations

Fasciculations are irregular, flickering involuntary contractions of a bundle of muscle fibres. They are variable as twitchings of the muscle. They are irregular and inconstant with a variable intensity. They may be fine or coarse. Fasciculations have to be observed carefully over the body under good light. They are most easily seen in the larger muscles (deltoid or calves). The muscles must be completely relaxed. If the fasciculations are not obvious, they can be evoked by percussing or flicking the muscles. They occur during the active degeneration ('death cry') of the anterior horn cells and of the motor nuclei of the brain stem, or irritation of the anterior roots. They are seen over widespread regions in motor neuron disease where they are associated with progressive wasting of the muscle groups.

Fasciculations may also be seen in syringomyelia, cervical spondylosis, peroneal muscular atrophy and in the muscles recovering from poliomyelitis. The spontaneous contraction of the individual muscle fibres is called fibrillation and it is too fine a movement to be seen. Due to nicotinic effect, widespread fasciculations may be noted in organophosphorous insecticide (diazinon) poisoning and on administration of neostigmine. Benign fasciculations may be noted by the patient, commonly in arms and calves unaccompanied by other signs. Benign fasciculations may be noted objectively in some nervous individuals during convalescence or after exh ustion.

Epilepsy

During an epileptic attack, the muscular spasm demonstrates tonic and clonic phases. The term convulsions is applied when the muscle spasms are clonic and widespread. The movements may be generalized or confined to a limb and are characterized by their stereotyped repetitions. If an attack is observed, the following features should be noted— distribution, site of commencement and spread, tonic or clonic spasm, the presence of froth in the mouth and the behaviour of the patient after the fit.

Athetosis

Athetosis are slow, writhing stereotyped movements of the limbs due to degeneration of the basal ganglion. The movements increase on voluntary effort and disappear during sleep. They are more pronounced in distal than in proximal muscles, best seen at wrists, fingers and ankles. The fingers writhe, the wrists flex, the forearm and arm rotate inwards, abduct and then rotate outwards in abduction and foot is inverted.

Chorea (Dance)

Involuntary, irregular, non-repetitive, and purposeless movements of a group of muscles may occur in a disorderly fashion in the face, limbs and or sometimes all over the body. These movements are referred to as choreiform movements (rheumatic chorea, Huntington's chorea, senile chorea). They begin abruptly and end suddenly as jerky movements without being sustained. They are aggravated by excitement and voluntary effort and disappear during sleep. The face exhibits twitching and grimacing movements. The tongue is protruded and retracted rapidly (jaw in the box tongue). There is an inability to hold the protruded tongue steadily. The limbs are often flung forwards. There is respiratory irregularity. There is flexion at the elbow and wrist and the fingers are hyperextended at the metacarpophalangeal joints. The patient is unable to maintain the arm steadily when it is raised above the head. The condition is called hemichorea if the movements are restricted to one side of the body. The occurrence of choreiform movements during pregnancy is called chorea gravidarum.

Choreo-Athetosis

Choreo-athetosis is a combination of chorea and athetosis, and either may predominate. The movements are more apparent on voluntary effort. The condition commonly accompanies syndromes causing mental retardation.

Dystonia

Dystonia refers to a movement caused by a prolonged muscular contraction when a part of the body is thrown into spasm. It may be generalized (idiopathic dystonia muscularum deformans, after metoclopromide intake, after encephalitis lethargica) or focal (spasmodic torticollis, Writer's cramps). In dystonia, an abnormally maintained flexed posture is noted , which often is associated with continuous, plastic rigidity. It is encountered in Parkinson's disease and after recovery from hemiplegia.

Spasm

A spasm is an involuntary contraction of the muscles occurring in an exaggerated form (tetanus, hydrophobia, strychnine poisoning). The contractions may occur continuously (tonic) or interrupted by relaxations (clonic).

In tetany, the spasm of the muscles occurs periodically and is commonly noted in the distal parts of the limb bilaterally. The thumb is adducted and the fingers are brought together closely. There is plantar flexion with hollowing of the soles of the feet. Trousseau's sign and Chvostek's sign are used to bring forth the features of tetany in between the attacks.

Trousseau's sign is elicited by compression of nerves in upper limb by sphygmomanometer cuff inflated above diastolic pressure for four minutes. There will be contraction of wrist and finger flexors going into *main d'accoucheur* position. Chvostek's sign is elicited by percussing the facial nerve or its branches. It evokes marked twitching and retraction of the corner of the mouth. Chvostek's sign may be seen apart from tetany, in muscular irritability during regeneration of a damaged facial nerve.

Oculogyric Crisis (Conjugate Ocular Spasm)

Spasmodic conjugate ocular deviation upwards with an inability to look downwards may be noted as a sequelae to encephalitis or sometime following administration of phenothiazine drugs.

Myokimia

Myokimia is the most common involuntary movement of the muscles. It can present in 2 forms. There can be a fine very rapid ripping of the muscle fibres. They persist in the same group of fibres such as orbicularis oculi for minutes at a time. Myokimia can be recognized by the patient and examiner. A much coarser contraction of bundles of muscle fibres may be noted in the outer aspect of the thigh or arm, and also due to fatigue.

Myoclonus

Sudden, shock-like contraction or asymmetrical jerks of a single muscle or a group of muscles of the limb or of the whole body is referred to as myoclonus (encephalopathies, myoclonic epilepsy). Often it occurs in response to an outside stimuli (sudden loud noise). Nocturnal myoclonus is noted on falling asleep. Hiccough (myoclonic spasm of the diaphragm) is another classical example.

Torsion Dystonias

Slow rhythmic involuntary movements of the limb ar vertebral column result in rotation (torsion). In torticollis (wi neck) the head is rotated and abducted due to the contraction the muscles of the neck.

Tics (Habit Spasm)

Repeated, purposive movements of a part of the body withoi change in character or site of occurrence like frequent blinking the eyes, nodding of the head, smacking of the lips, movement the shoulder and facial grimace occur as part of normal motc gestures.

Cramps

Cramps refer to spontaneous contractions of part or whole c a muscle (e.g. calf muscle). It may occur in normal persons, or a a feature of chronic progressive neurogenic muscle weakness motor neuron disease, or as a manifestation of hyponatraemia, o hypomagnesaemia.

Reflexes

The reflex is an involuntary motor response to a stimulus. The reflex is dependent on the integrity of sensory receptor, an afferen pathway in the peripheral or cranial nerve centre in the spina cord, brain stem or midbrain, an efferent path in the peripheral oi cranial nerve and an effector in the muscle. An inhibitory influence is exerted by the upper motor neurons on the reflex response.

The elicitation of the reflexes is an important part of neurologic examination. The presence or the absence of a reflex response has to be noted. The reflexes are classified into three types: superficial (skin), deep (tendon) and organic (visceral). For routine clinical purposes, the superficial and deep reflexes are elicited.

Superficial Reflexes

These reflexes are elicited by stimulating an area of the skin (scratching) or mucous membrane (touching). The reflexes are corneal, conjunctival, palatal, ciliospinal, abdominal, cremasteric and the plantar response.

Palatal reflexes (the ninth and the tenth cranial nerves): On touching the posterior wall of the pharynx, there is a reflex contraction and an elevation of the soft palate and uvula are noted. Any damage to the reflex function is associated with a loss of the reflex.

Abdominal reflexes (T_{5-12}): Abdominal reflexes are elicited by scratching the abdominal wall with a key, or with a blunt point, or with a wooden end of a cotton-tipped swab, while the patient is recumbent and relaxed, and the abdomen is uncovered. Pin should not be used. The stimulus is applied obliquely from the outer aspect towards the midline in the place of the dermotome on either side of the epigastric (T_{5-7}), supraumbilical (R_{7-9}), umbilical (T_{9-11}) and infraumbilical

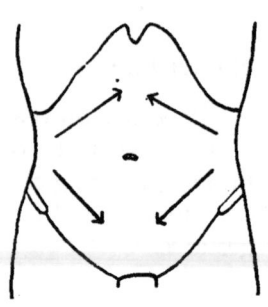

Fig. 70 Abdominal reflexes-sites of stimuli.

(T_{11-12}) regions and the movement of the umbilicus is observed (Fig. 70). The stimulus is applied firmly but lightly across four quadrants of the abdomen.

In a positive response, the abdominal muscles show contraction, and the *linea alba* and the umbilicus are drawn towards the area stimulated. The response to the stimulus is generally brisk in upper part of the abdomen. It is difficult to elicit the reflex in people having a flabby or fatty abdomen and in anxious patients, in elderly persons and in multiparous women. In infants the response is not elicited as the pyramidal fibres are not myelinated. The reflex gets fatigued easily and may disappear after repeated stimuli. Sensory loss may abolish the reflex. The reflex is lost in acute abdominal conditions and in abdominal distension. The reflex is lost early in upper motor neuron lesions. The reflex is lost on the affected side in hemiplegia and its reappearance has a good prognostic significance. Abdominal reflex is bilaterally lost in multiple sclerosis. The segmental level is determined in the lesions of the spinal cord as the reflex is absent below that level. The reflex has great significance when there is preservation of the upper (spinal cord level T_9) but not lower (T_{12}) abdominal reflex. It indicates a spinal lesion below T_9 or a breach of the appropriate reflex arc (herpes zoster, surgical operation destroying the peripheral nerve or the muscle).

The reflex has two pathways: (i) a local arc ending in a short spinal pathway; and ii) the fibres ascending in the pyramidal tract. Any lesion in the course of a pyramidal tract will damage the reflex fibres and result in the loss of reflexes. However, in lesions affecting the motor neurons selectively, such as motor neuron disease, and cerebral diplegia, the abdominal reflex is retained. Disseminated sclerosis is associated with loss of abdominal reflexes bilaterally early.

Cremasteric reflex ($L_{1,2}$): It is elicited by stroking the inner side of the upper thigh in male patients with a blunt point in a downward and inward direction while the patient is lying down or standing up. The testicle is drawn upwards due to the contraction of cremaster muscle. It is not elicited in pyramidal tract lesion and in conditions associated with hydrocoele, orchitis and in elderly men. Impaired sensation over the skin of the thigh or scrotal operations which have damaged the peripheral nerves or muscle, affect the reflex arc and the response is absent. The reflex is not to be confused with *dortos* reflex in which the scrotum contracts due to cold.

Bulbocavernous reflex: There is contraction of bulbocavernosus muscle when the dorsum of glans penis is pinched. The $S_{3/4}$ segments are concerned with the reflex.

Ciliospinal reflex: The pupil normally dilates when the skin of the neck is pinched. It is due to a reflex excitation of the pupil-dilating fibres in the cervical sympathetic. It is abolished in the lesions in the sympathetic trunk and pathway in the spinal cord. The loss of this reflex is useful to assess the depth of coma and to diagnose 'brain death'.

Released reflexes: It is possible to elicit certain reflexes released from the control of higher centres in patients, with diffuse degenerative disorders especially dementia, organic confusional states, and in old age. Normally these reflexes are present in infants (primitive reflex) but disappear in childhood, during normal development of nervous system. They can reappear when the inhibiting influence of central nervous system is removed, hence called released reflexes,

Sucking reflex: A sucking movement of the lips and deviation of the mouth in the direction of the stimulus is noted on lightly touching the corner of the mouth. The head turns towards the source of the stimulus. It is seen in diffuse cerebral atrophy and in stupor from diffuse encephalitis or traumatic lesions. It is normally seen in infants.

Pouting or snout reflex: Pouting of the lips from puckering of orbicularis oris occurs when the region above the upper lip is gently tapped. It may be noted in bilateral pyramidal tract lesions above upper brain stem, and in chronic dementia. Large doses of phenothiazine therapy may cause appearance of pouting reflex.

Grasp reflex: There may be grasping of the examiner's finger when the finger is drawn across the patient's palm between the thumb and the index finger. There is flexion of the fingers with adduction of the thumb and grasping of the examiner's hand. The reflex may be noted on one side in the lesions affecting the contralateral frontal lobe (tumour and vascular accidents). The reflex may be bilateral in diffuse cortical atrophy. Such a reflex is normally present in infancy.

Palmomental reflex: There can be contraction of the mentalis (chin) muscle drawing the lower lip upwards ipsilateral to a scratch stimulus applied diagonally to the palm of the thenar eminence of the palm from above downwards. The reflex is noted bilaterally in dementia, Parkinsonism and in frontal lobe lesion.

Glabellar reflex: Persistent blinking occurs by contraction of orbicularis oculi when the centre of the forehead above the level of the nose (glabella prominence), is tapped with a finger about two times per second. However, it stops quickly even if the tapping is continued in normal individuals (Fig. 71). In senile dementia, and in Parkinsonism, the blinking continues to occur rhythmically while the tapping is done. The reflex arc has trigeminal nerve as afferent and facial nerve as efferent.

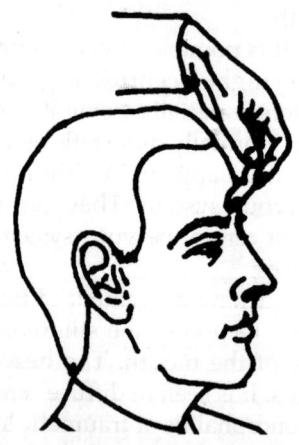

Fig. 71 Eliciting the glabellar reflex.

Plantar response (L$_5$, S$_s$): The plantar reflex is the most important reflex in the body. Normally when the outer side of the sole of the foot is stroked firmly, it results in flexion of the great toe at the metacarpophalangeal joint and the flexion and adduction of the outer toes. The ankle gets dorsiflexed and inverted. While eliciting the response, the knee is slightly flexed, and the thigh externally rotated. The leg is kept straight with the examiner's left hand over the ankle to prevent flexion of the leg and its withdrawal. To achieve proper relaxation, the patient may be asked to take a deep breath or his attention drawn elsewhere.

The outer side of the sole is stroked firmly with the blunt point such as the end of the percussion hammer, or a key, by moving it forward slowly from the heel end towards the base of the little toe, and then curved medially across the metatarsus towards the ball of the big toe (Fig. 72). The stimulus must be firm but not painful, and it should be performed slowly. A pin should not be used. Normally, there will be a flexor response by the time the stimulus has reached the middle of the outer aspect of the foot. The big toe is flexed at the metacarpophalangeal joint and the other toes are flexed and come together. There should be adequate relaxation to elicit the response.

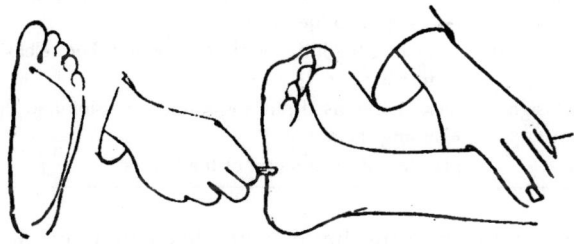

Fig. 72 Extensor plantar response.

Instead of a flexor response if an extensor response is elicited, it is referred to as the extensor plantar response, or as the upgoing great toe, or as a positive Babinski's sign, named after Joseph Babinski, French physician, who gave the first description of the phenomenon in 26 lines. There will be an extension (upgoing) of the big toe at the metatarsophalangeal joint due to the contraction of the extensor hallucis longus and usually the interphalangeal joint as well. It is accompanied by the extension and spread of the other toes like a fan and are dorsiflexed. This sign has a great diagnostic significance. It indicates disease involving the corticospinal tract above S_1 level of spinal cord. When the lesion is gross, the extensor plantar response is associated with dorsiflexion of the foot and flexion of the knee and hip joints (triple flexion). In such an instance, one can feel the contraction of the responsible muscles. When the big toe is fixed due to osteoarthritis, flexion seen in the hip or knee may be an important sign. Occasionally a crossed response, in the form of an extensor plantar response on the stimulated side and a plantar flexion of the opposite side, may be noted in cases of paraplegia in extension.

An extension of the big toe with slight dorsiflexion of the foot can be elicited in the following ways (Fig. 73). These tests have the same significance as the Babinski sign, but each is less reliable.

Sign	Method
Oppenheim's sign	pressing with the thumb and the index finger along the medial side of the anterior border of the tibia
Chaddock's sign	scratching / stroking the lateral part of the dorsum of the foot below the lateral malleolus
Gorden's sign	squeezing the calf muscles
Shaffer's sign	squeezing the Achilles tendon
Gonda's reflex	pressing one of the smaller toes downwards and then releasing it suddenly
Stranksy's method	abducting the little toe rigorously and then releasing it suddenly
Rossolimo's sign	flicking the distal phalanges into extension and then releasing them
Bing sign	pricking of the dorsum of the big toe

Some of these signs have been described by Hermann Oppenheimer, a German neurologist, Charles Chaddock, an American neurologist, Alfred Gordon, an American neurologist, Max Shaffer, a German neurologist, and Gregori Rossolimo, a Russian neurologist.

On recovery the area which is sensitive becomes smaller until only the outer side of the sole is receptive. Sometimes, the stimulus may elicit only dorsiflexion of the big toe without any fanning of the toes, or fanning of the toes without dorsiflexion of the big toe, and it is referred to as an equivocal plantar response. It is noted in early pyramidal disease, or in its minimal involvement.

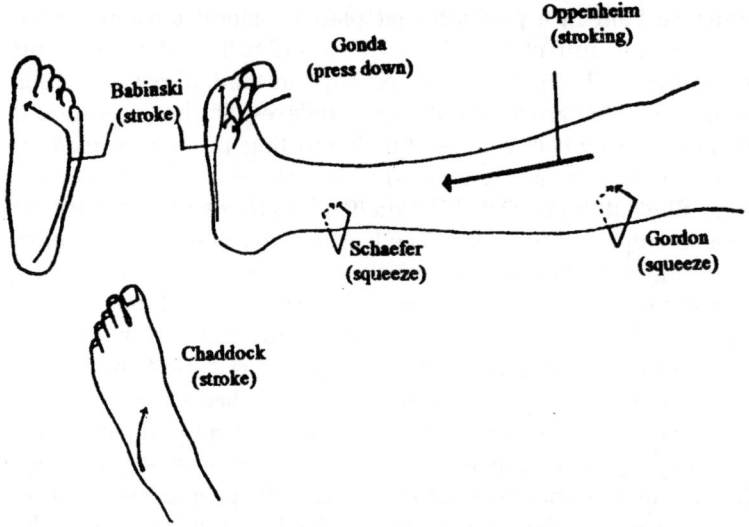

Fig. 73 Different methods to elicit extensor plantar response.

The plantar response may not be elicited if the patient is not relaxed, or has a thick sole, cold feet, a severe degree of loss of sensation interfering with the sensory arc of the reflex (peripheral neuropathy), or total loss with paralysis of the muscles failing to demonstrate any movement, or cauda equina syndrome (interruption of reflex arc passing through the first sacral segment). A bilateral extensor plantar response is noted in deep sleep, in infancy, following an epileptic seizure and in comatose conditions. An extensor plantar response does not necessarily mean a structural lesion of the pyramidal tract.

Deep Reflexes

Deep reflexes are referred to as muscle, or monosynaptic stretch reflexes. A single sharp tap on the tendon of a slightly stretched muscle, results in a brief contraction of the muscle. Stretch receptors in the muscle send impulses via afferent fibres in the peripheral nerves and dorsal roots to the anterior horn cells. These cells are excited and send efferent impulses via anterior roots and motor nerves to the same muscles leading to a brief contraction of muscle.

The soft rubber hammer is used to give an adequate stimulus. While eliciting the reflex the patient must be relaxed. The part must be held in a position that places a slight tension on the appropriate muscle (midway between full contraction and relaxation). The limbs are to be kept in similar position thus enabling a comparison of the elicited reflexes. The hammer should be held loosely between the thumb and fingers, so as to make it swing freely in an arc. It is raised by an extension of the wrist, and then allowed to fall and strike the tendon. In instances where the reflexes appear absent or reduced, excitability of the anterior horn cells, and sensitivity of the muscle spindle may be reinforced by asking the patient to clench his teeth (for upper limb reflexes), or to interlock the flexed fingers of both hands and pull them apart (for lower limb reflexes) while the tapping is done (Jendrassik's manoeuvre, after Erno Jendrassic who described in 1885).

Generally, the reflexes increase excitability of the anterior horn cells in the spinal segment, and the sensitivity of sensory endings in the muscle spindle to stretch. The reflex helps in demonstrating the integrity of the afferent and efferent pathways, and of the excitability of the anterior horn cells in the spinal segment of the stretched muscle. The reflex may be diminished or lost with interruption of sensory fibres, motor fibres and anterior horn cells. When the reflex is released or destroyed from the influence of suprasegmental fibres (pyramidal tract) there is hyperreflexia.

The reflexes are elicited with the patient lying on a bed comfortably. The deep reflexes are the jaw jerk, biceps, brachioradialis, triceps, the knee (quadriceps), and the ankle (gastrocnemius and soleus) jerks. For each reflex tested, the two sides should be tested sequentially. It is important to determine the smallest stimulus required to elicit a reflex rather than the maximum response.

Jaw jerk: To elicit the reflex, a finger is placed firmly on the chin, and the patient is asked to open the mouth slightly. Then the finger is tapped in a downward direction with the hammer suddenly. Normally there is no response. An upward jerk closing the jaw occurs in the upper motor neuron lesions above the level of the pons as in pseudobulbar palsy, amyotropic lateral sclerosis and disseminated multiple sclerosis (Fig. 74). The trigeminal nerve acts as the afferent and the efferent of the reflex, and the centre is in the pons.

Deep reflexes in the upper limb: While eliciting the reflexes, the elbow of the patient is flexed slightly and the forearm is drawn across in a semiprone position allowing the wrist to rest on the

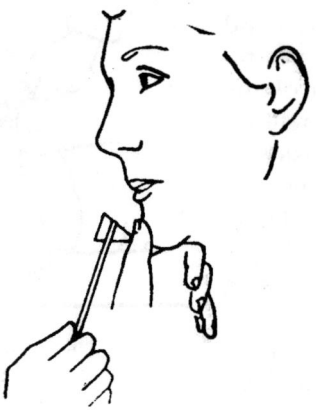

Fig. 74 Jaw jerk.

lower part of the abdomen. The reflexes biceps, brachioradialis and triceps depend on cervical segments of the cord $C_{5,6}$; $C_{5,6}$ and $C_{6,7}$ respectively.

Biceps jerk ($C_{5,6}$ musculo-cutaneous nerve): The elbow is flexed to a right angle and the forearm is slightly pronated. The biceps jerk is elicited by striking the left thumb or the index finger of the examiner placed over the biceps tendon, with the percussion hammer. It results in the contraction of biceps muscle causing flexion of the elbow (Fig. 75). The reflex is considered inverted if there is contraction of the triceps without flexion of the elbow.

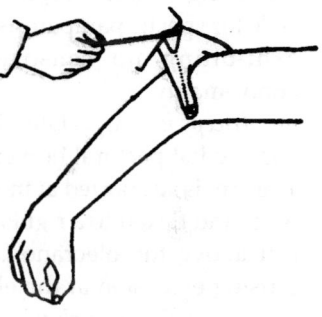

Fig. 75 Biceps jerk.

Brachioradialis (Radial, supinator) *jerk* ($C_{5,6}$ radial nerve): The elbow is flexed to a right angle and the forearm is placed midway between pronation and supination. There is contraction of the brachioradialis causing flexion at the elbow and partial supination of the forearm, when the styloid process of the radius is struck with the percussion hammer. There may be a slight flexion of the fingers (Fig. 76). There may be a slight flexion of the fingers. The reflex is considered inverted when there is a brisk flexion of the fingers without flexion of the elbow and supination of the forearm.

An inversion of the biceps and radial reflexes indicates a cord lesion at the level of C_{4-5} causing a lower motor neuron lesion at C_{5-6} segments. If the same lesion is compressing the spinal cord involving the pyramidal tract, reflexes innervated by lower segments of the cord (triceps) are exaggerated (cervical disc disease, syringomyelia, cervical trauma and cervical tumour). This is very important in localizing lesions responsible for spastic paraparesis exhi-biting no sensory abnor-mality.

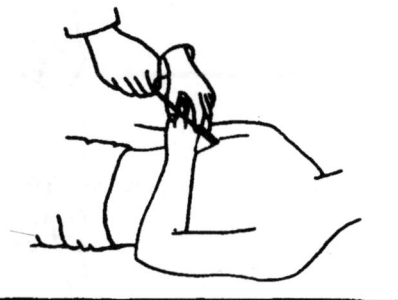

Fig. 76 Supinator jerk.

Triceps jerk ($C_{6,7}$) lateral and medial pectoral nerve: The arm is supported at the

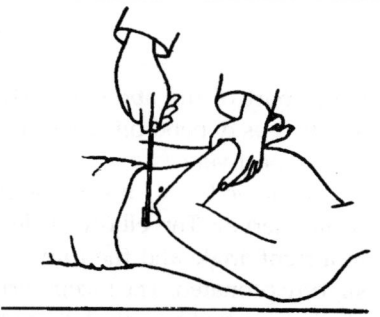

Fig. 77 Triceps jerk.

wrist and flexed to a right angle. Then the triceps tendon is tapped just above the olecranon. There is a contraction of the triceps causing extension at the elbow (Fig. 77).

Finger flexion jerk ($C_{7,8}$ median nerve): A brisk flexion of the fingers is noted in theupper motor neuron lesion when the examiner's fingers placed in contact with the palmar aspect of the tips of slightly flexed fingers of the patient, are tapped.

Hoffmann's sign: The tendon reflex activity, named after Johann Hoffmann, a German neurologist, in the hand is tested, by flexing and abruptly releasing the distal phalanx of the middle finger held between the fingers. In situations of the upper motor neuron lesion, in the upper limb there is flexion and adduction of the thumb and the index finger. Its presence on one side has significance and it can be an early sign of unilateral pyramidal tract lesion. It indicates an increased tendon reflex activity in the finger flexors.

Wartenberg's sign: When a patient has supinated his hand, slightly flexing the fingers, the examiner pronates his hand and links his similarly flexed fingers with that of the patient. Then, both have to flex their fingers further against each other's resistance. Normally there is extension of the thumb. In pyramidal tract lesions the thumb adducts and flexes strongly. Its presence on one side indicates an early stage of pyramidal lesion. The reflex is named after Robert Wartenberg, an American neurologist.

Deep Reflexes in the Lower Limbs

Knee (patellar or quadriceps) *jerk* ($L_{2,3,4}$ Femoral nerve): While the patient is recumbent, both the knees are semiflexed together, and are supported with one hand. The patient is encouraged to relax. The patellar tendon is tapped midway between its origin and insertion with the hammer. The contraction of the quadriceps causes extension of the knee joint (Fig. 78). The leg is momentarily shot forward in presence of sufficiently great contraction. The reflex can also be elicited with the patient sitting. The patient should either cross one leg over the other and allow the upper leg to hang loosely, or allow both legs to dangle freely over the edge of the cot. Then the patellar tendon is tapped with the hammer.

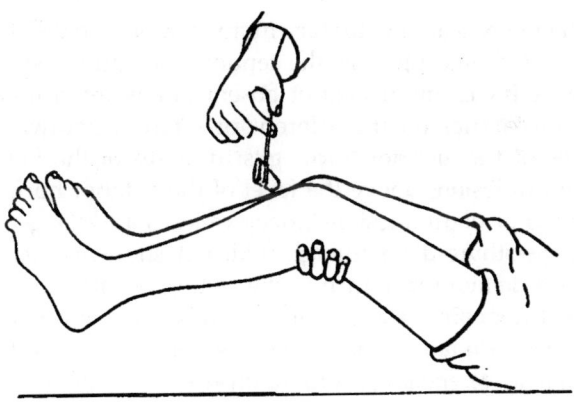

Fig. 78 Knee jerk.

The reflex is considered inverted if the attempt to elicit knee jerk causes a paradoxical knee flexion. This occurs due to denervation of L_{2-4} leading to paralysis of quadriceps and conduction of the blow to hamstrings innervated by $L_5 S_1$ segments.

In chorea, the knee jerk appears sustained, and the raised leg hovers for a short while, and then falls to the resting position. The knee jerk becomes pendular in cerebellar disorder on the same side of the lesion.

Ankle (Achilles) jerk ($S_{1,2}$ medial popliteal nerve): The leg is flexed slightly at the knee and rotated externally while the patient is supine. With one hand the foot is slightly dorsiflexed, so as to stretch the tendon of calcaneus (Achilles tendon) and then it is tapped with a percussion hammer. It causes contraction of the gastrocnemius resulting in a brisk plantar flexion (Fig. 79).

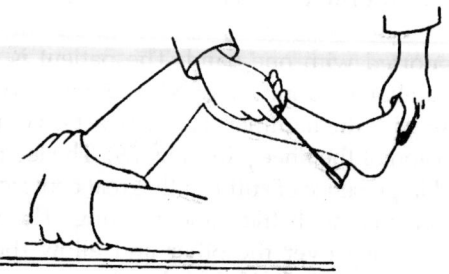

Fig. 79 Ankle jerk.

The reflex is an involuntary motor response to the stimulation of the stretch receptors in the tendon and muscle spindle. The tendon reflex is diminished or absent in any interruption of the reflex arc, either on the afferent or efferent pathways and in diseases of the anterior horn cells (diseases of the lower motor neuron). In lesions above the level of the anterior horn cells (the upper motor neuron lesions), deep reflexes are exaggerated.

In hypothyroidism, though ankle jerk shows a quick response there is a delay in its return to the resting position. In chorea the knee jerk appears sustained, and the raised leg hovers for a short while, and then falls to the resting position. The knee jerk becomes pendular in cerebellar disorders on the same side of the lesion. Ankle jerk alone is lost in lesions of conus medullaris. The lesion frequently extends into conus from higher part of the cord. In such situations there is loss of both knee and ankle jerks, and there is extensor plantar response.

Rossolimo's reflex: The ball of the foot is struck with the hammer when the patient is lying supine with leg extended and foot partially dorsiflexed. There is brisk contraction of all toes in hypertonic states. It has same significance as Hoffman's sign in the upper limb.

Clonus: When there is exaggeration of deep reflexes as a result of a pyramidal lesion, a sustained stretch of the tendon results in rhythmic contraction and relaxation of the muscles. It is referred to as clonus. It is elicited by stretching a muscle briskly, and maintaining a certain degree of stretch.

Patellar clonus: The knee is kept in extension. The patella, held at its lateral borders by the thumb and forefinger, is pushed downwards suddenly, and the pressure is maintained. The presence of clonus is revealed by repetitive jerky contractions and relaxation of the quadriceps which pull the patella upwards.

Ankle clonus: While the patient is lying supine, the hip and knee are semiflexed. The leg is held parallel to the bed, giving support to the leg with a hand in the popliteal fossa. The forepart of the foot is grasped with the other hand and is pushed suddenly backwards (dorsiflexion) and the pressure is maintained (Fig. 80). The presence of clonus is exhibited by sustained repetitive flexion and extension of the foot due to the contraction of the calf muscles. The condition is always associated with increased tendon reflexes and an extensor plantar response. As unsustained (false) clonus is noted in individuals who are very tense or anxious. The true (sustained) clonus increases by dorsiflexion of the foot and the false clonus tends to diminish and become irregular.

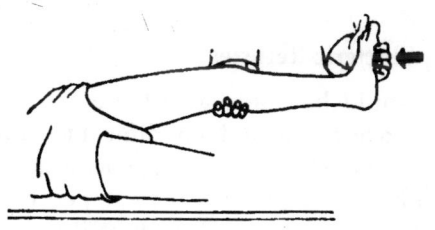

Fig. 80 Ankle clonus.

Abnormal Tendon Reflexes

The reflexes are exaggerated in the upper motor neuron lesions at all levels above the anterior horn cells. Brisk reflexes may be encountered in anxiety, following violent exercise, nervousness, thyrotoxicosis and tetanus. The exaggerated reflexes gain pathologic significance if they are asymmetrical, or if there are other signs of the upper motor neuron lesion. Cerebellar disease associated with ataxia, may exhibit an excessive swinging and oscillation in a pendular fashion, and the leg moves back and forth four or five times when the knee jerk is tested. This is due to hypotonia of the muscles.

In myxoedema, there is slow muscular contraction and delayed relaxation. Commonly delayed return of the contracted muscle to the resting phase is demonstrated when the ankle jerk, or biceps jerk is elicited (myotonic reflex).

Certain tendon reflexes may be absent in the lesions of the sensory nerve (polyneuropathy), the posterior root (tabes dorsalis), the posterior column (subacute combined degeneration of the cord), the anterior root (spinal compression), the anterior horn cells (poliomyelitis, progressive muscular atrophy), the peripheral motor nerve (trauma), terminal nerve endings (polyneuropathy) and the muscle (myopathies, periodic paralysis). The tendon reflexes may be absent temporarily in spinal shock, coma, raised intracranial tension, diabetic ketosis and uraemia. Advanced spastic paraplegia and severe extrapyramidal rigidity are associated with reduced or absent reflexes.

Grading of the Reflexes

The tendon reflexes may be graded depending on their briskness as 0 (absent), 1 (normal), 2 (brisk), 3 (very brisk), and 4 (clonus).

Organic or Sphincteric Reflexes

Enquiry should be made about the acts of swallowing, micturition and defecation, and any difficulties during these acts should be noted. The act of swallowing, micturition and defecation are a reflex phenomenon, and they depend upon complex movements of both striated and unstriated muscles excited by raised tension in the wall of the viscus concerned.

Swallowing: The patient should be asked for the presence of any difficulty in swallowing (dysphagia). This is necessary when there is a history of regurgitation of food through the nose. There is difficulty in swallowing liquids in dysphagia associated with neurologic disorders. Mechanical obstruction of the oesophagus is associated with difficulty in swallowing solids.

Micturition: Micturition is a reflex act. Normally micturition is initiated by a voluntary effort, but once started it becomes a reflex act which is then difficult to stop. The patient should be asked whether he finds any difficulty to control or initiate micturition, and whether he can appreciate bladder and urethral sensations. The reflex path is partly through the plexuses in the bladder wall, and partly through the pelvic plexuses and it has the controlling centre in the spinal cord at various levels. The innervation of these plexuses is dual from sympathetic system (L2, 3 and 4 segments) through the hypogastric nerves and from the parasympathetic system (sacral 2, 3 and 4 segments) through the pelvic nerves (*nervi erigentes*). The stimulus for micturition reflex is distension of the bladder with urine, and the stimulus passes to the spinal cord by way of the *nervi erigentes*. Evacuation of the bladder occurs by contraction of the detrusor, and relaxation of the internal sphincter under the control of *nervi erigentes*. The voluntary initiation of the act of micturition is under the influence of the motor cortex through the cerebropudendal pathway. Pudendal nerves supply external sphincter.

The complicated process of micturition may be affected by disease or injury at different levels within the central nervous system. It results in different types of neurogenic or neuropathic bladder. The former may be hyper-reflexive or areflexive. It is directly analogous to the upper or lower motor neuron lesions respectively. The lesions within the sacral segments of the spinal cord result in areflexive bladder. Bilateral lower motor neuron lesions result in a flaccid atonic bladder that overflows without warning. Hyper-reflexive bladder is noted in the lesions above that level. Bilateral upper motor neuron lesions cause frequency of micturition and incontinence. The bladder is small.

Bladder function disturbances may be in the form of urgency, hesitancy or frequency of micturition or dribbling or retention of urine.

The damage to the spinal cord (acute transverse lesions of the spinal cord) may result in retention of the urine, and the patient is unable to pass urine. The excessive retention causing distension of the bladder (atonic neurogenic distended bladder) may result in overflow (overflow incontinence) or the bladder may fill up and empty periodically by relaxation of the sphincter without the knowledge of the patient (reflex incontinence or automatic bladder). It is noted in tabes dorsalis with destruction of posterior roots. Sometimes it is seen in diabetic autonomic neuropathy.

In overflow incontinence, the distended bladder may be recognized on palpation and percussion, and pressure over the suprapubic region may result in expulsion of urine from the urethra.

Destruction of both afferent and efferent fibres of parasympathetic innervation to the sphincters of the bladder is noted in cauda equina lesion and it results in an autonomous bladder. There is loss of bladder sensation. The bladder is emptied incontinently and inefficiently from time to time due to the action of local and axonal reflexes.

In reflex neurogenic bladder the sacral bladder centre remains. intact, but there is destruction of both afferent and efferent connections with a higher centre. It is noted in paraplegia. The bladder which is devoid of sensations empties incontinently from time to time. There is usually certain amount of residual urine. Retention and incontinence of urine is also noted in situations affecting the brain. Lesions of the superior frontal and anterior cingulate gyri (stroke, tumour, hydrocephalus) cause a reduction in awareness of bladder and result in incontinence. There can be retention of urine from more posterior lesions of the frontal lobe. There is spasticity of the striated muscles of sphincters. There is no involvement of the local reflex mechanism in the spinal cord.

In slowly progressive compression of the spinal cord, there may be hesitancy (initiation of the act of micturition taking a long time) or precipitancy (inability to control the act of micturition) during the early stages. In frontal lobe tumours the bladder sensations are retained but there is loss of ability to inhibit spontaneous contractions. It results in an uninhibited neurogenic bladder. There is a disturbance of awareness of micturition resulting in frequency and urgency.

Defecation: In acute lesions of the spinal cord, particularly of the sacral segments, there is laxity of the sphincters and incontinence. The patient may be asked for any difficulty in defecation and for the presence of rectal and anal sensations. It is lost in lesions of conus medullaris. The reflex depends upon the sacral third and fourth segments. Higher spinal lesions cause contraction of the sphincters and result in constipation.

Anal reflex: The anal reflex (S3, 4) is tested by scratching the skin around the anus. It results in an immediate contraction of the voluntary anal sphincter. The anal sphincter also contracts when the patient is asked to cough. This reflex has to be tested particularly in any patient with suspected injury to the spinal cord of lumbosacral region. The anal sphincter normally contracts briskly in reflex response to a sudden cough (the 'cough reflex').

Sensory System

Modalities of Sensation

The determination of sensory loss is of great importance in conditions of paraplegia, peripheral nerve lesion and syringomyelia. However, in the absence of sensory complaints, testing only for touch sensation on all four limbs will suffice.

The modalities of sensation are as follows:

1) *Exteroceptive:* cutaneous sensations derived from sources outside the body such as pain, light touch, and temperature

2) *Proprioceptive:* deep kinaesthetic sensations such as position, passive movement, vibration and pressure derived from the body itself

3) *Stereognosis:* combined and cortical sensations such as tactile localization, two-point discrimination and graphaesthesia

4) *Interoceptive:* visceral sensation, not routinely examined at bed side

Sensory Pathways

All forms of sensations, originating from the receptors (pain, touch and temperature) after their stimulation are conveyed through a peripheral nerve and a sensory root to the spinal cord, or cranial nerves to the brain stem. A lesion located either in the nerve or root results in loss of all forms of sensation from the area that it supplied.

1) The fibres carrying sense of fine touch, position, passive movement and vibration ascend in the posterior columns of the spinal cord ipsilaterally as they enter, to the *nuclei gracilis* and *cuneatus* in the medulla. Then the fibres decussate to the opposite side and ascend in the medial laminiscus to the brain stem along the touch fibres from the face to the thalamus, and ultimately to the post-Rolandic cortex.

2) The fibres conveying the sensations of pain, temperature, and crude touch on entering the spinal cord ascend a few segments upwards on the side of entry and then cross to the opposite side to reach the anterolateral spinothalamic tract. It ascends to the

brain stem, where it lies lateral to the medial laminiscus. The quintothalamic tract joins it in the pons, and the fibres terminate in the thalamus. During the course, many fibres end in the reticular formation of the brain stem. The sensory impulses from the thalamus pass through the posterior limb of the internal capsule and the thalamoparietal radiations to the post-central gyrus in the parietal lobe (sensory cortex).

Depending on the level of the central perception and analysis the sensations are subdivided as primary (perception at the level of optic thalamus) and cortical (analysis at the sensory cortex) modalities. The latter depends on intact sensory pathways.

Arrangement of the Sensory Fibres

The fibres from the lower part of the body are displaced medially in the posterior columns. In the spinothalamic tract, fibres from the lower part of the body are displaced to lie superficially to those from the upper part of the body. In the thalamus, fibres from the lower part of the body lie laterally to those from the trunk and arms, and the fibres from the face lie more medially. In the sensory cortex, fibres from the lower limbs terminate near the superior longitudinal fissure. The lower part of the post-Rolandic gyrus contains the fibres from the face.

Some of the afferent impulses carried in the sensory nerve fibres do not reach consciousness. They convey impulses directly or indirectly to the motor neurons for spinal reflexes or to the cerebellum through anterior and posterior spinocerebellar tracts. The latter fibres convey proprioceptive impulses from muscle and tendon receptors to the cerebellum and facilitate coordinated limb movements.

Tests for Sensation

Diseases of the sensory system may present with features such as pain or parasthesia due to spontaneous activity or irritation of sensory neurons or loss of ability to appreciate some modalities of sensation and present as anaesthesia or analgesia. These symptoms occur with disorders affecting from the end organs to the thalamus. Irritative lesions above the thalamus present with parasthesia but not with anaesthesia. There is loss of sensory discrimination and of spatial and quantitative aspects of sensation.

The following tests are employed to investigate the sensory

functions: (i) Superficial sensations: light touch, pain, and temperature; (ii) Deep sensations: position, passive movement, deep pressure and vibration; and (iii) Discriminatory sensations: stereognosis (recognition of the size, shape, weight, texture and form of objects) and tactile localizations and discrimination.

Before undertaking each one of the following tests, the nature of the test has to be explained to the patient. Then the test is performed with the eyes closed. The examination of the sensory function requires maximum cooperation from the patient and it is often preferable to test the sensations before the patient is exhausted. The test should be carried out quickly without repetition. The stimulus has to be moved from a region of diminished sensitivity towards normally sensitive areas, as it is easy to appreciate increased sensation.

Sensory examination is a subjective test, often one finds difficulty to give strictly comparable stimuli. The pulp of the fingers is relatively insensitive to pin-prick, but very sensitive to touch.

Superficial Sensations

Touch sense: This is tested with a wisp of cotton. It does not cause sufficient pressure to stimulate deep sensibility, and produces sensation familiar to the patient. It is applied over the skin lightly. The patient is asked to go on counting as soon as he feels the touch. Commonly it is started on the face and proceeded down the body in dermatome areas.

While testing for superficial touch or pain, the examiner moves the wisp of cotton wool or pinpoint vertically where the dermatomes are running horizontal (on trunk and the face) and transversely where dermatomes are vertical (arm, forearm and leg), and compared.

The loss of touch sensation is referred to as anaesthesia. It is called hypoaesthesia and hyperaesthesia when the sensation is reduced or increased respectively. The areas of sensory loss have to be noted. The hairy regions are avoided while testing. The validity of the reply of the patient, is tested by asking the patient whether he feels the touch without applying the cotton. The patient may be asked to point out the spot touched. The pressure touch is tested, by touching the skin with the point of a finger or the head of a pin.

Pain sensation: The prick of a pin or pressure on the muscles can evoke pain sensation and these sensations are tested separately.

Superficial pain: It is tested, by a sharp pin with a rounded head. It is advisible to use a pin with a shaft long enough to allow the examiner's index finger and thumb to slide downwards. The tip of a pin is applied with an identical intensity over different regions of the body and compared to identical areas from the face downwards like shoulders, the inner and outer aspects of the forearms, the thumb and little finger, the upper and lower chest, and abdomen, the buttocks, the front of the thighs, the lateral and medial aspects of the legs, the dorsum of the feet, and the little toe. The prick should not be too noxious. It should be applied at the rate of 1 per second. The patient is asked to count when he feels the pain sensation. He must be able to appreciate the sharpness of the point and pain, which the prick evokes.

Pressure pain (deep sensibility) is tested, by squeezing the calf muscles or Achilles tendon. Sometimes testicular sense, is tested by applying pressure. There is tenderness in the peripheral neuropathy. The deep sensation and the testicular sensations are lost in tabes dorsalis.

Loss of pain sensation is called analgesia. Hypoalgesia refers to a decrease in pain sensation. It should be remembered that the pulp of the finger is less sensitive to pain but highly sensitive to light touch. Hyperalgesia refers to an exaggerated sensibility wherein a mild stimulus can evoke an unnatural degree of pain.

Temperature sense: Temperature sense is tested, by using test tubes filled with hot and cold water. They are applied over the skin in turn, and the patient is asked to identify whether it is hot or cold. The sensation is compared, by applying the test tubes over symmetrical areas of the skin from the face downwards. The eyes of the patient are closed while testing. The test provides no more useful information than testing pain. The loss of temperature sense is called thermanaesthesia.

Dissociated sensory loss is a condition wherein there is loss of pain and temperature sense with preservation of touch sensation and is diagnostic of syringomyelia.

Deep Sensations

Proprioception enables the individuals to detect joint motion and limb position. It has distinct sense organs and ascending pathways in the spinal cord. However it requires a healthy contralateral cerebral cortex for full perception, thus resembling the cortical sensation.

Loss of proprioception is encountered in peripheral neuropathy and diseases of spinal cord and of the cerebral hemisphere. There is disproportionate loss of vibration sense and proprioception compared with pain and temperature in diseases of the posterior columns of the spinal cord.

Joint sense (sense of passive movement): The terminal phalanx of the big toe or thumb is moved slowly up and down to about 10-15° (extension and flexion) while the proximal phalanx is fixed by holding its lateral aspects with the thumb and finger and the eyes of the patient being closed. The patient is asked for the direction of the movement of the joint as soon as he appreciates it (Fig. 81). If the patient fails to recognize the movements of the digits, the same test is carried out at the wrist, elbow or knee. The joint sense is lost in disorders of the posterior column. A patient with posterior column deficit complains of numbness in the affected limb. Objectively it is difficult to demonstrate the numbness as loss of touch, pain or temperature.

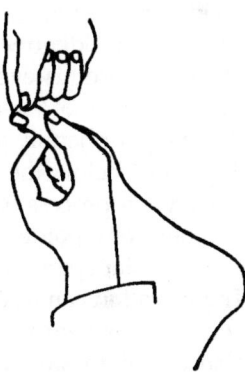

Fig. 81 Joint sense.

Position sense: One limb of the paint is kept in a particular position while the eyes are closed. The patient is then asked to keep the other limb in a similar position. If there is no paralysis of the limb the individual must be able to bring the limb to the same position as the other limb. This test is useful to demonstrate the integrity of the posterior column.

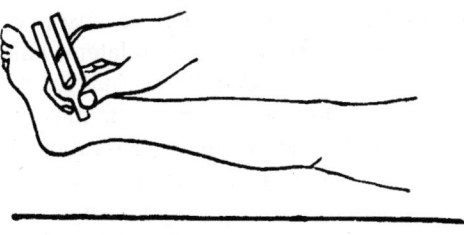

Fig. 82 Vibration.

Vibration: The vibrations are appreciated by the individual when the foot of a vibrating tuning fork is kept on the bony prominences of the body (Fig. 82). It is lost in conditions affecting the posterior column such as peripheral neuropathy, nutritional neuromyelopathy, tabes dorsalis and Friedrich's ataxia. It is the earliest sensation to be lost in diabetes mellitus and old age.

An aluminium tuning form having vibrations of 128-256 Hz per second is used for the purpose. Before the actual examination a vibrating tuning fork is placed over the sternum or clavicle to allow him to identify the vibration sensation. Then the patient is asked to close his eyes. The prongs of the fork are struck on the shoe and its foot (stem or Y junction) is placed on bony points starting peripherally at the distal phalanx of the great toe or index finger just below the nail bed, and then at the medial malleolus and styloid process of the radius. If the patient fails to appreciate it, other bony points like the tibial tuberosity, olecranon, anterior superior iliac spine, vertebral spines, ribs and sternum are selected. The vibration can also be tested in soft tissue without underlying bone. The patient is asked to say when he feels vibration. He is also asked to say when he ceases to feel it. In situations of impairment of perception of vibration, the examiner can still perceive them. Often the vibrations are stopped by touching the prongs with the hand, and its appreciation by the patient is verified. Normally a healthy adult is able to appreciate vibrations for at least 11 seconds when the stem of the vibrating tuning fork is held against lateral malleolus, and for at least 15 seconds when it is held against styloid process of the radius.

Cortical Sensations

Appreciation of the cortical senses requires their integration and processing in a healthy contralateral cerebral hemisphere. The tests are performed to assess the function of sensory cortex (parietal lobe). The sensations are from the contralateral half of the body. Cortical sensations are mediated by the parietal lobes and represent an integration of the primary sensory modalities. Testing cortical sensation is useful only if the primary sensations are intact.

Stereognosis: Normally an individual is able to recognize a familiar object by feeling its size, shape, weight, and form when kept in the hand, while the eyes are closed. It is dependent on the sense of touch, position, and movement. While testing the stereognosis, the patient is asked to close his eyes, and easily identifiable familiar objects such as a coin, a key, and a pin are put first into the hand suspected of abnormality and if the patient is not able to identify or takes a long time to decide, it should be placed in the other hand and compared for accuracy and speed of response.

Astereognosis refers to the loss of these sensations, and there is absence of normal skilled movements of exploring an unknown object. In lesions of the parietal lobe, astereognosis is evident even though the superficial sensations are normal. The sense of stereognosisis also carried through the posterior column. Astereognosis occurring with posterior column lesions is associated with abnormality of a sense of position, vibration and light touch. The patient may find it difficult to close over a small object in a partially paralysed, or oedematous or deformed hand and may give a false impression.

Sensory discrimination: Normally a person is able to discriminate between the stimulus of two blunt points of a divider or two pins when applied simultaneously over the skin while the eyes are closed. The patient is asked to say whether he is being touched with one or two points. This ability of distinguishing the stimulus of two points varies in different parts of the body. In the fingertips, it is possible to appreciate the stimulus applied 2 mm apart. Two points separated by a distance of 1 cm on the palm, 2-3 cm on the sole of the foot, and 3-5 cm on any part of the trunk can be determined normally as two points. The appreciation of this sensation depends on the integrity of the light touch sensation. The loss is evident in lesions of the parietal lobe even when the sense of touch is intact. It is also lost in the posterior column and sometimes, peripheral nerve lesions. The point of the dividers should be blunt; otherwise the pain fibres are stimulated. Calloused skin on hands and feet are to be avoided while performing the test.

Tactile localization: The skin is touched with the fingertip while the patient's eyes are closed. Then he is asked to put his finger on the same point. The patient fails to do so in loss of cortical sensation. The significance of the test is similar to that of two-point discrimination.

Graphaesthesia: Graphaesthesia refers to the ability to recognize letters or numbers written on the skin with a blunt point. The patient closes his eyes and traces the letters or numerals such as 8, 4, and 5 on the palm or forearm or leg. Absence of graphaesthesia in presence of normal peripheral sensation implies a parietal cortical sensation.

Double-simultaneous stimulation test: When two stimuli (touch or pinprick) are applied simultaneously on corresponding parts on two limbs or sides of the trunk, normally it is possible to identify them as two different points, while the eyes are closed. In parietal lobe lesions the patient fails to perceive the stimulus on the contralateral side of the damaged parietal lobe (sensory extinction).

Romberg's sign: The upright posture is dependent on cerebellar, labyrinthine and visual postural reflexes, and on the proprioceptive sensations from the muscles of the lower limbs.

Romberg's sign is a special test to demonstrate incoordination in the lower limbs, and the sign is named after Moritz Romberg, a German physician. In reality it is a test to show loss of position sense in the legs (sensory ataxia) and not a test of cerebellar disorder (motor ataxia). In conditions such as sensory polyneuropathies, subacute combined degeneration of the spinal cord, and tabes dorsalis. The patient finds unsteadiness while walking. Interruption of the pathway carrying afferent impulses from the proprioceptors of the lower limbs, affects the maintenance of posture and movement. However, ataxia is compensated by visual impulses about the position. The patient becomes unsteady on closing the eyes. Rarely Romberg's sign may be present in patients with laryrinthine or cerebellar disease in which ocular impressions may partially compensate for the disorder of balance.

The test is performed, by asking the patient to stand with eyes open and then to bring the heels as closely together as possible without losing the balance. Then he is asked to close his eyes. The patient begins to oscillate and stagger to an extent of falling if unsupported. If there is ataxia, Romberg's sign is positive. In cerebellar ataxia, and in severe vestibular disorders, the patient is unable to stand steady even when the eyes are open. The examiner has to extend his arms at the sides of the patient to prevent him from falling if he loses his balance.

The loss of position sense in the upper limbs can be demonstrated by asking the patient to outstretch his upper limbs though ataxia is absent when the eyes are open, the limbs begin to swing in different directions as soon as the eyes are closed.

Determination of Sensory Level

After noting the areas of sensory loss, it is necessary to determine the level of the lesion (Fig. 83). Spinal cord is organized in segments, from each of which a pair of anterior (motor) and posterior (sensory) nerve roots arise. The spinal segments do not correspond to the vertebrae bearing the same number. In the highest cervical region they do correspond. C_1 does not supply the skin. In lower cervical segments there is one segment difference. C_8 spinal segment is opposite C_7 vertebra. The spinal segments till the mid-thoracic region correspond to a vertebra lower than their number. The difference is of two segments in the lower thoracic region. The lumbar and sacral segments are located opposite T_{11} to L_1 vertebrae.

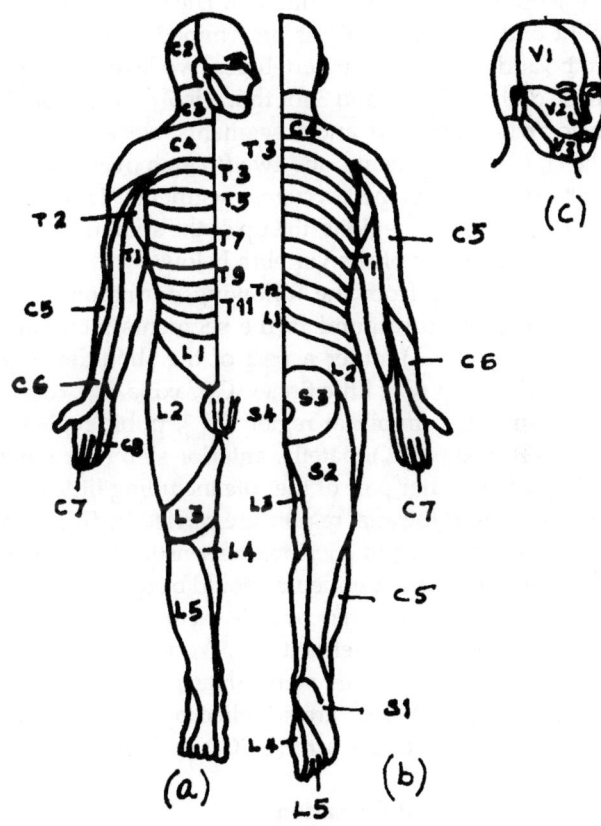

Fig. 83 Sensory dermatomes
(a) front, (b) back, (c) trigeminal nerve.

C_4 lesions are associated with loss of sensations above the clavicle and T_2 lesions are associated with loss of sensations below the clavicle. The sensation of deltoid region are carried by C_5. The sensory loss due to lesions of C_6 and C_8 extend to the forearm on its dorsal and ventral surfaces. The median nerve lesion in the arm results in sensory loss predominantly in the palmar surface of the thumb, index, middle and radial half of the ring finger, whereas the lesion of ulnar nerve above the elbow results in loss of sensation over the palmar and dorsal surface of the little and ulnar half of the ring finger.

The spinal segments till the mid-thoracic region correspond to a vertebra lower than their number. The relation between spinal segment and vertebral body is determined as follows: one level has to be added for cervical vertebrae. Two levels are to be added for those of thoracic 1–6 and 3 for thoracic 7–9 vertebrae. The tenth thoracic arch overlies L1 and 2 segments; eleventh thoracic arch overlies L3 and 4 segments, and twelfth arch overlies L5. The first lumbar arch overlies the coccygeal segments. It must be noted that in lower thoracic regions, the tip of the spinous process marks the level of the body of the vertebra below.

The sensations from the following dermatomes located in different regions correspond to the segments mentioned in the brackets: occiput (C_2), outer aspect of the shoulder (C_5), thumb (C_6), middle finger (C_7), little finger (C_8), axilla (T_3), costal margin, xiphisternum (T_8), umbilical region (T_{10}), pubic region, inguinal ligament (T_{12}), knee (L_3), patella, anterior shin (L_4), inner part of the sole (L_5) and outer part of the sole including little toe (S_1). The sensations around the anal region, are carried by S_{3-5} segments. In a situation of cauda equina lesion, the sensory loss in the 'saddle' area of the buttocks and perineum should be specifically examined.

In cord lesions, there may be a clear-cut upper level of sensory abnormality. Often it is defined by a zone of hyperaesthesia. It must be noted that there are some areas over the chest, arm and thigh where adjacent areas are supplied by a much higher spinal segment (chest T_3 and C_4), arm (T_2–C_5) and thigh (S_2–L_2).

Patterns of Abnormal Sensation

There are some common patterns of sensory abnormalities that range from total loss to very slight reduction, or even hypersensitivity.

Site & extent of the lesion	sensory abnormality
1. Thalamus & Parietal cortex	unilateral loss of position sense and cortical sensation with disturbances of light touch and quality of pain
2. Thalamus	
a) total	unilateral loss of all sensation with gross disability
b) partial	unilateral loss of all exteroceptive or proprioceptive sensation with motor impairment, cranial nerve palsies, tremors or gross disability
3. Medulla	loss of pain and temperature on one side of the face and the opposite side of the body
4. Spinal cord	
a) gross	bilateral loss of all forms of sensation below a definite level
b) partial unilateral	unilateral loss of pain and temperature sensation below a definite level
c) intrinsic central	impairment of pain and temperature sensation over several segments with normal sensation above and below
5. Cauda equina/conus	'saddle' type of loss of sensation over the lowest sacral medullaris segments
6. Sensory root/Peripheral nerve	loss of all forms of sensation over a well defined area in one part of the body

Cerebellar Function

While testing the functions of the cerebellum, the tone of the muscles, and coordination of movements and the ability to perform rapid alternating movements are looked for. The condition is associated with hypotonia. Routinely, the coordination is tested while testing the motor system by performing the finger-to-nose test in the upper extremity and heel-to-shin test in the lower extremity.

Normally, alternating movements can be performed rapidly and regularly (diadocokinesia). The condition is called dysdiadocokinesia when there is an inability to perform rapid repeated movements. This is an important sign of cerebellar ataxia.

The patient is asked to rotate the hands rapidly at the wrists with arms flexed at the elbow, and with the forearms vertical and palms facing medial wards as done during a *pooja*.

In cerebellar disease, the movements are coarse, irregular and slow. The hand is dorsiflexed and the fingers extended. The result is shaking of the palm instead of rotation of the wrist. It can also be tested by asking the patient to tap the back of the hand rapidly with the fingers of the other hand, or by pronation and supination of the forearm rapidly on each side. In testing the lower extremities, the patient is asked to touch the finger of the examiner held near the lower limbs with the big toe, or tap the foot against the bed in quick succession.

The patient may be asked to thread a needle, or to do finger counting or buttoning and unbuttoning. The incordination is exemplified in these acts.

Dysmetria is an inability to stop movements at an appropriate time. It results in overshooting or undershooting. It is demonstrated by performing the finger-to-nose test.

Signs of Cerebellar Lesion.

Cerebellar ataxia
Hypotonia
Dysdiadocokinesia
Dysmetria
Past pointing
Nystagmus
Intention tremor
Scanning speech
Pendular knee jerk

Past pointing sign (described by Robert Barany, an Austrian physician in Sweden who got Nobel prize in 1914): The patient is asked to bring forward horizontally his arm and touch with the fingers, those of the examiner, who has placed his arm similarly outstretched. The patient is asked to lower the arm and bring it back to the original position with his eyes open, and later with his eyes closed. The test is repeated. In unilateral cerebellar disorders, the arm on the side of the lesion deviates away from the original position towards the side of the lesion instead of accurately regaining its original position.

The other important cerebellar signs are:

1) *Gait:* The patient finds it difficult to walk along a straight line and the gait is irregular and staggering. There is a tendency to fall to one side, usually to the side of the lesion due to the loss of muscle tone on that side.

2) *Nystagmus:* There is presence of regular horizontal jerky nystagmus. In unilateral cerebellar disease, the nystagmus is slower, and the range of nystagmus widens when the eyes are moved towards the side of the lesion, than when moved to the

unaffected side. Rarely, there may be a skew deviation with one eye being turned upwards and outwards, and the other downwards ad inwards.

3) *Scanning speech:* Pronouncing each syllable in a word slowly without any appropriate accent (see page 218).

4) *Hypotonia:* The limbs are flaccid and hypotonia is marked in acute cerebellar lesion.

5) *Intention tremor* (see page 277).

6) *Pendular knee jerk:* A swinging character of the jerk is due to hypotonia. It is elicited in a patient seated with the testing limb crossed over the other with the leg hanging freely.

Signs of Meningeal Irritation

Meninges: The meninges cover the entire brain as a continuous membrane, that extend down to cover the spinal cord. The pia and arachnoid are in close contact in most places except in the 'cisterns'. Cerebrospinal fluid circulates between these two membranes.

The following important signs involving the stretching of the spinal roots are looked for in cases of meningeal irritation.

Neck stiffness (rigidity): Neck rigidity occurs early and later changes to definite head retraction in meningeal irritation. It is demonstrated by placing a hand behind the occipital region of the patient, and then flexing the neck to allow the chin to touch the chest. Normally it does not cause pain. In meningeal irritation, neck flexion causes pain, and the act encounters resistance from the spasm in the extensor muscles of the neck. The stretching of the spinal nerve roots causes a reflex muscular spasm. The head gets retracted when there is marked degree of neck stiffness. Neck stiffness is noted in conditions associated with meningeal irritation (meningitis, meningism, subarachnoid haemorrhage), posterior fossa tumours, lateral sinus thrombosis, Parkinsonism, increased intracranial tension impending cerebellar tonsillar herniation at foramen magnum, diseases of the cervical spine (cervical spondylosis, cervical fusion, infection or destructive diseases of cervical spine) and in generalized muscular spasm (tetanus).

Kernig's sign: Normally the knee of a supine person can be extended passively on a hip flexed to 90°. The extended knee produces an angle of 135° between the posterior surface of the thigh and the leg. It does not produce any pain. In conditions of meningeal irritation involving the lower part of the subarachnoid

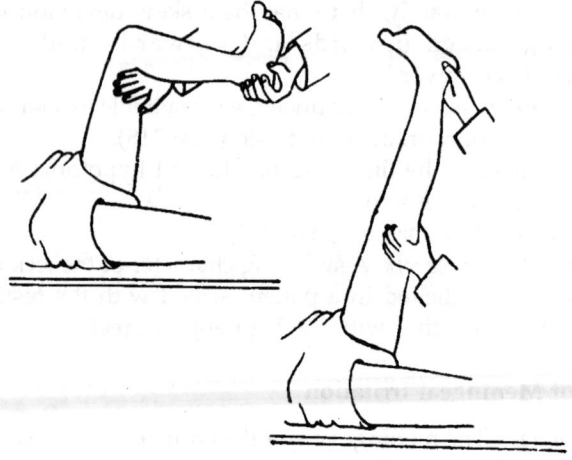

Fig. 84 Kernig's sign.

space, the passive extension of the knee causes pain. The leg can not be extended to more than a right angle when the thigh is fully flexed on the abdomen. The restriction is due to the spasm of the hamstring muscles. It is referred to as a positive Kernig's sign (named after, Vladimir Kernig, a Russian neurologist) (Fig. 84). It is due to the stretching of the spinal nerve roots of the lower limbs and inflamed meninges. Spinal meningeal irritation is associated with positive Kernig's sign in the absence of neck stiffness. Kernig's sign is also positive in prolapsed disc, and in cauda equina tumour irritating the $L_5 S_1$ roots.

Brudzinski' sign: The sign named after Jozef Brudzinski, a Polish physician, is often present in meningitis. It is due to presence of inflammatory exudates in the lumbar theca. The sign is valuable if it is suspected that head retraction is partly voluntary. It has two components: the neck sign and the leg sign. In the former, there is flexion of the knees and hips on flexing the neck. In the latter, the passive flexion of one leg produces a similar flexion of the opposite leg as a contralateral reflex.

Straight leg raising test (Lasegue's test): In conditions like sciatica, attempts by the patient to raise his extended leg are restricted by pain. The extended leg can't be elevated passively with the examiner's hand. This is due to the entrapment of spinal roots $(L_5 S_1)$ in protrusion of a low lumbosacral disc. The test is named after Ernest Lasegue, a French physician.

Gait

Act of walking involves a variety of interrelated movements of different parts of the body. It is influenced by reflexes such as postural reflex, labyrinthine reflex, righting reflex besides integrity of different arts of the nervous system.

There can be an alteration in the position of the patient during walking (gait) following neurologic disorders affecting the cerebrum, extrapyramidal system, cerebellum, spinal cord, posterior roots, and peripheral nerves, disorders of muscles, bony deformities and hysteria. To study the gait, the patient is asked to walk in a straight line for at least 9 meters, with legs uncovered, then turn and return back to the starting point. However, the best time to observe the stance and gait is when the patient has no idea that he is being observed especially during entering and leaving the examination room.

Some of the gaits observed commonly are as follows:

1) Spastic gait: In the spastic gait seen in paraplegia in extension involving the pyramidal tracts (spinal) bilaterally, the legs are stiff and are advanced slowly on a narrow base by dragging the feet. There is difficulty in flexing the knees. The foot is raised from the ground by tilting the pelvis. Then the leg is swung forwards. The foot makes an arc and the toes scrape the ground.

2) Scissor's gait: In bilateral pyramidal lesion (cerebral), there is excessive spasm or contracture of the adductor muscles of the thigh. It results in medial rotation of the legs which cross each other while walking. The patient exhibits jerky movements of the trunk and upper limbs while walking. This is seen in cerebral diplegia, and lathyrism.

3) Hemiplegic gait: Hemiplegic gait is a spastic gait wherein the abnormality involves one side only. The patient who has residual hemiplegia, or hemiparesis due to a lesion in the pyramidal tract shows the limb to be stiff on the affected side. The foot is plantar flexed. The leg is dragged forward in a semicircle, first away from, and then towards the body (circumduction) slowly, while the outer side of the foot is scraping the floor. The arm is adducted at the shoulder, flexed at the elbow,

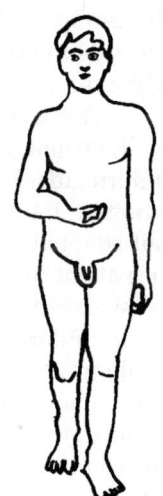

Fig. 85 Hemiplegic gait.

and pronated and flexed at the wrist. The arm swing is diminished. The patient leans to the opposite healthy side while walking (Fig. 85)

4) *Shuffling (festinant) gait:* In Parkinsonism, the patient walks in a stooped position with the head and the body bent forward. The hips and knees are slightly flexed. The gait is slow. The patient walks with a series of small, flat-footed shuffles, giving an impression of trying to catch up with the centre of gravity. There is reduction or absence of normal swinging movements of the arms. The patient, if pushed forwards (populsion), backwards (retropulsion) or sidewards (lateropulsion), is unable to stop himself and tends to fall. There is a tendency to speed up the walking (festination). Sudden changes of direction can't be made. When the patient is asked to turn around while walking, the patient takes a turn in three to four steps instead of making a swing of the body.

In diffuse cerebrovascular disease from multi-infarcts or in normal or low pressure hydrocephalus, the gait can be small-stepped shuffle. It is irregular and hesitant. The patient may lean backwards rather than forwards.

Marche a petipas, a gait named after a Russian ballet master shows rapid, short tapping gait, resembling the rapid steps of a ballet-dancer on points. It is seen bilateral lesions in the deep frontal white matter.

5. *Ataxic gait:*

i) Reeling gait of cerebellar ataxi: The patient walks on a broad and irregular base, keeping the feet widely apart (broad base) and swinging the legs unnecessarily and irregularly. It simulates the gait adapted by a drunken person. In unilateral cerebellar lesion, the patient swings to-and-fro and shows a tendency to fall towards the side of the lesion due to the loss of muscle tone on that side.

In midline posterior fossa lesions, there is ataxia of the trunk resulting in instability. The trunk becomes unsteady. The patient reels in any direction, and there is a tendency to fall backwards (truncal ataxia). Often it may be mistaken to be of hysterical origin. The condition is also seen in tumours of the vermis and foramen magnum anomalies with descent of the cerebellar tonsils. Unlike sensory ataxia, the cerebellar ataxia persists whether the eyes are open or closed.

ii) Stamping gait of sensory ataxia: This is encountered in posterior column lesions such as tabes dorsalis, nutritional neuromyelopathy and carcinomatous neuropathy. There is loss of the sense of position resulting in loss of appreciation of the position of the feet. The patient walks by placing his feet wide apart. He moves slowly lifting the thigh, high, bringing the legs forwards. The foot is brought down suddenly with the heel slamming the floor. The patient exhibits reeling from side to side while walking. The patient can be steady if he concentrates on the ground while walking. The ataxia increases when the eyes are closed, or when the patient walks in the dark.

In loss of position sense, a similar high-steppage gait may be seen as the patient is not aware of the position of his feet. The heel tends to strike the floor first. The gait is irregular and ill-controlled. The leg moves in all directions and the patient reels from side-to-side on a broad base.

Differentiation of Ataxia.

	Sensory	cerebellar
Muscle		
Power	diminished	normal
Tone	markedly diminished	diminished
Nutrition	may be slightly affected	maintained
Reflexes	absent	pendular
Signs of lesion of		
Posterior column	present	absent
Cerebellum	absent	present
Gait	stamping	reeling
Romberg's sign	positive	negative

6) *High-steppage gait:* In polyneuropathy, cauda equina lesions and peroneal muscular dystrophy, the patient raises the foot high to overcome the foot drop and brings down with toes hitting the ground first. The patient is not ataxic. The patient has to flex the limb at hip and knee so that the foot clears the ground. There is weakness of the dorsiflexors of the feet. Such a gait may be seen unilaterally in anterior tibial muscle paralysis.

7) *Waddling gait:* In conditions of congenital dislocation of the hip, pseudohypertrophic muscular dystrophy, advanced pregnancy and osteomalacia, the body oscillates from side-to-side with each step. The weakness of muscles of the pelvic girdle results in abnormal rotation of the pelvis through an abnormally large arc. There is marked compensatory lordosis as the body is tilted backwards like the gait of a duck. The feet are placed widely apart.

The heels and toes are brought down simultaneously. As the abdomen is brought forward the shoulders are thrown back.

In pseudohypertrophic muscular dystrophy, the patient has to climb upon his own legs, when he is asked to get up from the recumbent posture. This is due to the weakness of the extensors of the spine and knees. The patient turns

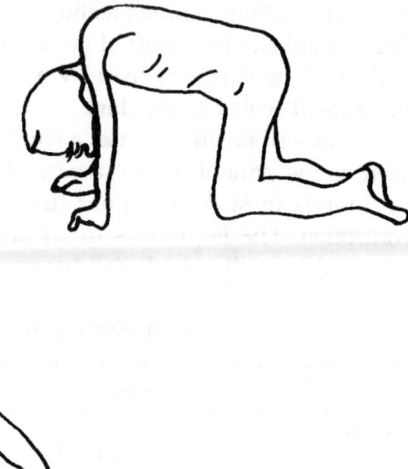

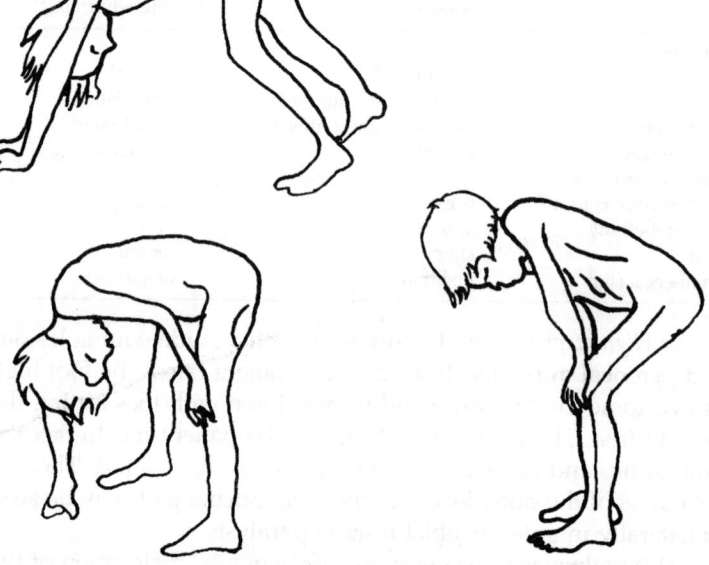

Fig. 86. Gower's sign: Patient with pseudohypertrophic muscular dystrophy climbing up the legs.

over on his abdomen, then raises the body on his hands and knees, following that he clasps the legs, knees and thighs with the hands and stands up (climbing up the legs or Gower's sign) (Fig. 86)

8) *Hysterical gait:* This is an irregular, bizarre type of gait and it alters from moment to moment and from examination to examination. It is exaggerated when the patient is being watched. It does not follow any set pattern.

9) *Dancing gait:* In chorea, the jerky involuntary movements which exaggerate during walking throw the limbs far apart. The patient walks on a wide base, and the steps are kept in an irregular fashion.

10) *Apraxia of gait:* There is disturbance in the central organization of walking due to the disorders of frontal lobe such as tumours, hydrocephalus or infarction. Though the patient is able to move his legs while sitting or lying he fails to walk in an organized way.

Autonomic Nervous System

The autonomic nervous system consists of sympathetic and parasympathetic nerve components, and it is concerned with modulation of functions in the cardiovascular and gastrointestinal systems, temperature regulation, bladder and bowel activity, sexual reflexes, papillary and respiratory reflex control.

The Clinical Presentation is Varied and the Autonomic Abnormalities are as follows.

Inability to maintain blood pressure in erect posture (orthostatic hypotension)
Resting tachycardia
Inability to slow the pulse with deep breath
Pupillary immobility
Dry skin with impaired sweating
Poor urine stream from detrusor failure
Retention or incontinence of urine
Constipation and fecal incontinence
Impotence

Interpretation of Neurologic Signs

Upper motor neuron lesion

Clasp-knife spasticity, loss of voluntary power, the presence of associated movements (for example, while yawning, the paralysed limb may be suddenly drawn up, or while trying to get up, the paralysed limb moves higher than the normal limb), no wasting except from disuse, exaggerated deep reflexes, loss of superficial reflexes, extensor response on the opposite side of the lesion.

Lower motor neuron lesion

Flaccidity, wasting and paralysis of the muscles, loss of deep reflexes, unaltered superficial reflexes, flexor plantar response, no associated movements.

Extrapyramidal lesion (Parkinson's syndrome)

Lead pipe or cog-wheel rigidity, no loss of power except poverty of movments from rigidity, presence of involuntary movements, absence of emotional movements and normal reflexes.

Cerebellar lesion

Hypotonia, lack of coordination (adiadocokinesis), nystagmus, slurring speech, intention tremors, and pendular knee jerk. Diseases affecting one cerebellar hemisphere produce signs on the side of the lesion.

Localisation of Sensory Disturbances

The sensory loss may occur from the lesion of the peripheral nerve, posterior root, posterior column, spinal cord, thalamus and parietal lobes.

Peripheral nerve

1) *Individual nerves:* Ulnar nerve (claw hand), radial nerve (wrist drop), median nerve (ape hand), anterior tibial nerve (foot drop), lateral cutaneous nerve of the thigh (meralgia parasthetica).

2) *Symmetrical polyneuropathy:* Glove and stocking anaesthesia with loss of all sensations over the distal parts of the extremities (hands and feet), symmetric distal weakness and wasting, for example peripheral neuropathy, and loss of deep reflexes.

3) *Cauda equina lesion* (involvement of all lower lumber and sacral roots): gradual onset, saddle shaped anaesthesia over the skin of perineal region, thigh and legs which may be unilateral or asymmetrical, severe root pains, wasting of the muscles and asymmetric weakness, loss of ankle jerk with retention of knee jerk, bladder disturbances late and less marked.

4) *Conus medullaris lesion* (lower sacral segments of the cord):

sudden and bilateral, symmetric dissociated saddle shaped sensory loss, root pains not common but may be severe and unilateral, wasting of muscles rare, absent ankle jerk extensor plantars early and loss of bladder and rectal control.

Posterior Root

Zone of hyperaesthesia at the level of the lesion, root pains, loss of all sensations below the lesion, loss of deep reflexes (tabes dorsalis).

Posterior Column

Loss of deep sensations below the lesion (subacute combined degeneration).

Cord type: Transverse lesion—loss of all modalities of sensation below the lesion with a definite upper level.

Partial lesion—a picture of Brown-Sequard syndrome, impaired light touch and vibration sense and corticospinal tract signs below the level of the lesion and impaired sensation and impaired temperature sense contralateral to the lesion and at the level of lesion ipsilaterally segmental zone of hyperpathia and spontaneous pain from irritation of the compressed segment. Spinal canal-dissociated anaesthesia—loss of pain and temperature sense with preservation of touch and pressure sensation (syringomyelia, intramedullary tumours).

Intrinsic spinal cord disease (intramedullary tumour, syringomyelia): dissociated anaesthesia-loss of pain and temperature sense with preservation of touch and pressure sensation, bilateral corticospinal signs, paralysis and sensory level, urge incontinence/retention of urine.

Extrinsic disease (compression of the cord from outside): progressive asymmetric paraparesis, paralysis with sensory level, Brown-Sequard syndrome (named after Charles Edouard Brown Sequard, a French physiologist, whose names bears the names of his father and mother), root pain, worsened by movement, incontinenece/retention of urine and faeces.

Localisation of Lesion in the Spinal Cord

The localisation of the lesion in the spinal cord is made on the presence of some of the following features:

	At the level of lesion	Below the level of lesion
Motor	lower motor neuron type with wasting.	upper motor neuron type of paralysis.
Sensory modalities	zone of hyperaesthesia, root pains whenever roots are compressed.	loss of all modalities of sensations below the level of the lesion with a definite upper border.
reflexes	loss of reflex.	exaggeration of all deep reflexes, extensor plantars, loss of visceral reflexes.

Spinal Cord Compression

a) *Intramedullary compression:* Absent root pains, ill-defined, delayed sensory disturbances (parasthesia) below the site of lesion which may be bilateral from the beginning, weakness and widespread wasting of muscles and features of lower motor neuron lesions, presence of fasiculations, dissociated sensory loss with sacral sparing, early bladder symptoms, absence of spinal tenderness, late appearance of upper motor neuron lesions, frequent trophic disturbances.

b) *Extramedullar compression:* Root pains may be present, well-defined parasthesia below the lesion early—unilateral to begin with, symmetric wasting of muscles and weakness, lower motor neuron lesion often absent, absence of fasiculations, loss of all sensations predominantly over caudal region, bladder involvement is late, spinal tenderness may be present, early appearance of upper motor neuron lesions, trophic disturbances uncommon.

Thalamus

Contralateral hemianaesthesia, excessive sensibility to painful stimuli. There may be ataxia and choreiform movements.

Parietal lobe lesion

Loss of cortical sense-two point discrimination, tactile localization, stereognosis, and parietal extinction.

Localisation of the Lesion Producing Hemiplegia

The site of the lesion in hemiplegia may be in the cerebral cortex. Internal capsule, midbrain, brain stem or spinal cord. The localisation of the lesions of corticospinal tract can be made by the following associated neurologic findings.

Cerebral cortex: Monoplegia (hemiplegia unlikely) on the contralateral side, with or without involvement of the face, motor aphasia in the affection of the cortex on the left side, or cortical loss of sensation in involvement of the parietal lobe, epileptic fits of Jacksonian type is frequent.

Internal capsule: Complete hemiplegia on the contralateral side with paralysis of the lower half of the face (supranuclear facial palsy). Spread of the lesion backwards is associated with sensory changes (hemianalgesia and thermanaesthesia) and sometimes homonymous hemianopia on the side of paralysis.

Midbrain: a) Base: Contralateral paralysis of face, arm and leg with ipsilateral lower motor neuron oculomotor nerve paralysis (Weber's syndrome). b) Tegmentum: In addition to the above features there is evidence of contralateral cerebellar ataxia, and tremors due to involvement of brachium conjunctivum and red nucleus (Benedikt's syndrome, named after Moritz Benedikt, an Austrian physician).

Pons: Contralateral hemiplegia with convergent squint from ipsilateral lateral rectus palsy (Foville syndrome, named after Francois Foville, a French neurologist). In addition there can be ipsilateral infranuclear facial palsy (Millard-Gubler syndrome, named after Auguste Millard, and Adolphe Marie Gubler, French physicians). The condition occurs from lesion in pons due to thrombosis of pontine branches of basilar artery.

Medulla (Tegmentum): Contralateral hemiplegia without involvement of the face with paralysis of the soft palate and vocal cord, on the side of the lesion from involvement of the Xth nerve (Avellis's syndrome). The condition may coexist with ipsilateral tongue paralysis from involvement of the XIIth nerve (Jackson's syndrome, named after John Hughlings Jockson, an English neurologist).

Lateral part of tegmentum: Ipsilateral paralysis of V, IX, X and XIth cranial nerves, Horner's syndrome, cerebellar ataxia and contralateral loss of pain and temperature (Wallenberg's or lateral medullary syndrome, named after Adolf Wallenberg, a German physician) from insufficiency of posterior inferior cerebellar artery.

Medial part of tegmentum: Paralysis of ipsilateral half of the tongue with contralateral paralysis of leg and arm and impaired sensation (medial medullary syndrome).

Upper cervical portion of the spinal cord: Hemiplegia on the side of the lesion with Brown-Sequard's syndrome. The cranial nerves are not involved.

NINE

LOCOMOTOR SYSTEM

> *"As to my health, thanks be to God, as long as I sit still without any pain, but if I do but walk a little I have pains in my legs, but that is, I think, caused by former colds and because they have carried my body so long".*
>
> *Anton van Leeuwenhock (1632-1723)*

The examination of the musculoskeletal system (muscles, cartilages, bones, joints, and soft tissues such as tendons and ligaments) is considered under the locomotor system. The skeletal system gives strength to support the body and protective covering to vital organs. It provides flexibility to perform a wide range of movements at the joints of the vertebrae and limbs. The muscles are examined under the nervous system (see page 259). Muscle weakness should be characterized as proximal or distal. Muscle wasting may occur due to polymyositis, or disuse from a painful joint.

A general examination provides information on stance, gait, posture and skeletal proportions. It is followed by examination of the bones (skull, jaw, thoracic cage, vertebral column, pelvis and limbs) and the joints. The examination involves inspection, palpation and different specific physical manoeuvres to elicit diagnostic signs.

Bones and Vertebral Column

Bones: The bones of the skull (see page 34) and of the extremities are examined for their shape, swelling, irregularity, fractures and tenderness. Deformities are referred as valgus (pointing outwards) or varus (pointing inwards).

Deformities: The knees may be separated and appear bowed (*genu varum*) in rickets, osteitis deformans, flurosis, and achondroplasia. Instead, the knees may touch each other with a separation of the legs apart (*genu valgum*). There may be bowing of the legs forwards (saber shin). The big toe may be turned outwards (*hallux valgus*). The foot may be flat (*pes planus*) or high-arched with a hollow below (*pes cavus*). There may be equinovarus deformity of the foot with the patient standing on its outer margin.

The wrists and ankles may be swollen from enlarged epiphyses in rickets. There is swelling of the costochondral junctions, and is described as *rickety rosary*. Hypertrophic osteoarthropathy shows swelling around the wrists and ankles from periosteal thickening. The bones appear irregular. In osteitis deformans (Paget's disease, named after Sir James Paget, a British surgeon) there is bowing of the tibia and femur, bony enlargement and increased local temperature. The bones appear greatly deformed in osteitis deformans and osteogenesis imperfecta. Localized bony swellings may develop from infections, cysts and tumours.

Spontaneous fractures may be noted in malignant metastatic deposits in bone, hyperparathyroidism (osteitis fibrosa cystica), osteogenesis imperfecta or multiple myeloma. Tenderness is elicited on application of pressure in chronic myeloid leukaemia (especially over the sternum), multiple myeloma, osteomalacia, generalized osteitis fibrosa and carcinomatosis of bones.

Vertebral column: Normally the spine exhibits a mild degree of kyphosis (posterior flexion) in the upper thoracic region, and slight lordosis (anterior extension) in the cervical and lumbar region. These features may be exaggerated to a marked degree.

Lordosis is present in pseudohypertrophic muscular dystrophy. A generalized kyphosis may occur in senile osteoporosis and rheumatoid spondylitis. A localized angular deformity (*gibbus*) may be caused by a fracture or by spinal tuberculosis (Pott's disease). The spine may exhibit lateral curvature (scoliosis) and it may be towards either side. There is rotation of the vertebral bodies making the spines to point towards the concavity of the curvature. Scoliosis disappears on flexion (muscle spasm) and on sitting (unequal length of legs). Often kyphosis and scoliosis exist together (kyphoscoliosis).

The vertebral column is felt with the hand from above downwards for the presence of any tenderness, and it is ascertained further by thumping the spine with the fist. There may be presence of a spina bifida (failure of closure of the spinal canal in the lumbosacral region) with depression, pigmentation or hair.

Movements: The range of movements of the cervical, thoracic and lumbar spines, is tested by asking the patient to bend forwards (flexion), backwards (extension) and sidewards (lateral bending). In addition rotation is possible in the cervical and thoracic spine. The pelvis should be fixed while testing the movements of the thoracic and lumbar spine. Spinal movements are painful and restricted in cervical and lumbar spondylosis. The spine gets fixed in ankylosing spondylitis. Elicitation of range of movements is forbidden in cases of cervical injury.

Straight leg raising test: When the patient is lying on his back with extended lower limbs, the examiner has to place the hand beneath the heel and passively raise the extended leg. Normally 90° of flexion at the hip should be possible. When the fifth lumbar or first sacral root is stretched as in a lumbo-sacral disc prolapse, the same amount of straight leg raising will not be possible (Lasegue's sign, after Ernest Lesegue, a French Physician). When the limit of straight leg raising has been achieved further tension on the root by dorsiflexion of the ankle causes compression of ultimate component of sciatic nerve, the posterior tibial nerve and aggravates the pain (Bragard sign, named after Karl Bragard, a German orthopaedist). Such an abnormality is not noted in tight hamstring muscles, or in a lesion in the hip.

Joints

The methods of inspection, palpation and range of movements around the joints ('look, feel and move') are adapted while examining the joints. The joints are examined in a systematic way in the following order: temporomandibular, sternoclavicular, shoulder, elbow, wrist, metacarpophalangeal and interphalangeal joints of the hands, hip, knee, ankle, metatarsophalangeal and interphalangeal joints of the feet, spine and sacroiliac joints. While examining the joints they are compared with the corresponding joints on the opposite side.

The following features are looked for while making the examination: shape of the joints, signs of inflammation (redness, tenderness, warmth and swelling), dryness (gout), or moistness (rheumatic fever, septic arthritis) of the skin overlying the joint, deformities, displacement, wasting of the muscles around the joint and range of movements.

Temperature: The raised temperature over the joint or the bone is detected by placing the back of the fingers on it as they are most sensitive compared to the palmar surface. Raised temperature may be as a result of increased blood flow (Paget's disease) or inflammation (rheumatoid arthritis, rheumatic fever, septic arthritis).

Pain: Distension of articular capsule causes pain and the patient tries to minimize the pain by keeping the joint particularly flexed. Such a position causes least intraarticular pressure and greatest volume. Inflammatory effusion is associated with flexion contractures. The abnormality is determined as a swelling and flexion deformity, and diminished range of movement especially on extension. Tenderness is noted by observing the patient's reaction on pressing the joint between the finger and thumb. It is graded as grade 1 when the patient complains of pain in the joint. When there is marked tenderness, the patient winces (grade 2) and withdraws the affected part (grade 3). The patient does not allow touching the joint in grade 4 tenderness as in rheumatic fever, septic arthritis and crystal arthritis. In fibromyalgia, there is no inflammation even though there is diffuse muscle and joint tenderness.

Involvement of joints: The joints that are most commonly involved in different arthritis are as follows:

Arthritis	commonly affected joints
rheumatic fever	large joints (flitting)
rheumatoid arthritis	small, peripheral (metacarpo/tarsophalangeal and interphalangeal)
osteoarthritis	weight-bearing large joints, terminal interphalangeal
ankylosing spondylitis	sacroiliac, vertebral
infective arthritis	large (monoarticular)
gout	small peripheral-first metatarsophalangeal

Swelling: When there is swelling of the joint, it obliterates the normal contour of the joint. The swelling may be due to synovial effusion (collection of synovial fluid in the joint space), or proliferation of the synovial membrane and periarticular tissue (rheumatoid arthritis), or enlargement of the ends of the bones particularly the radius and ulna (osteoarthropathy). The periarticular swelling usually extends beyond the normal joint margins or full extension of the synovial space. Synovial effusion can be distinguished from synovial hypertrophy or bony hypertrophy by palpation. Rheumatoid arthritis may be associated with fusiform enlargement of proximal interphalangeal joints,

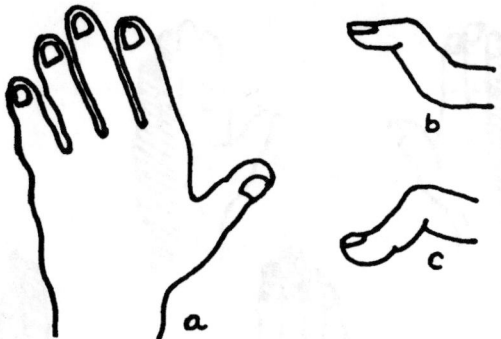

Fig. 87 Deformities of hand in rheumatoid arthritis
(a) ulnar deviation of fingers (b) swan-neck deformity (c) hyper extension of
proximal and flexion of distal interphalangeal joint.

'swan-neck' deformities of fingers and hyperextension of proximal,
and flexion of distal interphalangeal joints, ulnar deviation of the
fingers and subluxation of metacarpophalangeal joints (Fig. 87).
In psoriatic arthritis, terminal interphalangeal joints show swelling.
The joint involvement is symmetrical in rheumatoid arthritis, and
asymmetrical in psoriatic arthropthy and gout. In neuropathic
arthropathy (Charcot's joints, after Jean Martin Charcot, French
Physician who gave the first description of the condition), the joint
appears grossly distorted, and painless. It must be remembered
that muscle wasting can give a false impression of joint enlargement.

Nerve paralysis: Nerve lesions are associated with hand
deformities. Ulnar nerve paralysis causes slight hyperextension
of the metacarpophalangeal joints with slight flexion of the
interphalangeal joints (claw hand deformity). It is associated with
wasting of the small muscles of hypothenar eminence and loss of
sensation of the palmar and dorsal surface of the little finger and
of the ulnar half of the ring finger. The thumb falls into the flat,
ape—like or Simian deformity. Median nerve paralysis causes
wasting of thenar eminence (abductor pollicis brevis) and loss of
sensation on the palmar aspect of the thumb, index, middle and
radial half of the ring fingers. Damage to the radial nerve results
in a 'drop wrist' deformity (Fig. 88).

Fluid collection: Small or moderate knee effusion may be
recognised by the 'bulge sign'. The collection of fluid within the
knee joint or adjoining bursae, can be demonstrated by eliciting

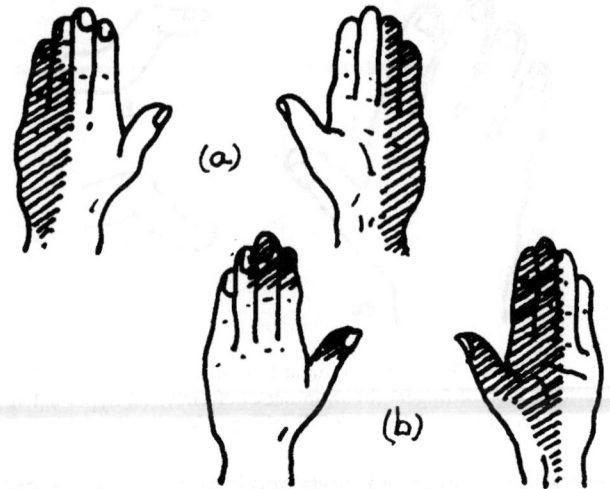

Fig. 88 Loss of sensations following lesions of
(a) ulnar nerve (b) median nerve.

fluctuation and a patellar tap. To elicit these signs the knee is kept
in extension, and the suprapatellar pouch is squeezed with left
hand towards the knee joint and kept pressed.

Fluctuation: The sides of the joint are held between the thumb
and the index finger of the right hand. When they are pressed
firmly, an impulse is felt by the left hand in the presence of fluid.
A firm non-fluctuant swelling is characteristic of synovial
thickening.

Bursal effusions (effusions of the olecranon or prepatellar
bursa) overlie the bony prominences and are fluctuant with sharply
defined borders.

Patella tap: When the patella is pushed back it causes
displacement of the fluid and of patella knocking against the lower
end of the femur ('ballotment of the patella').

Crepitus: A grating sensation is felt by the hand, placed on the
knee joint while it is moved passively. It is encountered in
osteoarthropathy, wherein the articular surfaces of the joint are
roughened. Tendon sheath creptitus may be felt in tenosynovitis
of long flexor tendons in the palm. It is associated with the trigger
phenomenon, wherein the finger is caught in flexion and it has to
be pulled back into extension.

Muscle wasting: The wasting of the muscles is recognized, by making a comparison of two sides of the body. In asymmetrical wasting, muscles appear smaller, and the limb presents a smaller girth. The circumference of the limbs kept in a symmetrical position can be compared at the same levels. Generally, a fixed bony point is taken to select the level (malleoli, tibial tuberosity, anterior iliac spine, styloid process of the radius and medial condyle of the humerus). The level at an identical distance is to be marked with a skin pencil, and the circumference of the limb should be measured at that level with a measuring tape.

Range of movements: Movement of joints is described as flexion, extension, abduction, adduction and rotation. The movements tested are active and passive. The range of movement is to be tested in all joints such as temporomandibular, cervical spine, shoulder girdle and upper limb, thorax and lumbar spine (see page 264), pelvic girdle and lower limb joints. The patient is asked to move the joint in various directions. The range of the movement, the ease of its performance and the presence of pain are ascertained. Active and passive range of movements of joints should be assessed in all planes and compared with contralateral joints. Each joint should be passively manipulated through its full range of movements. The movements are limited by effusion, pain, deformity and contractures. A periarticular process such as tendon rupture, or myopathy should be considered when the passive movement exceeds active movement.

The power of joint action is determined by the active movements and is recorded in a simple 5-point scale as recommended by the British Medical Research Council (see page 265). In neuropathic joints, a wide range of movements is possible without any pain. The movements are tested passively by moving the joints gently with one hand, while feeling the joint by the other hand. The degree of limitation of the movements is compared with that of the normal side.

The movement in a joint may be limited due to pain, muscle spasm, inflammation, contracture, effusion into the joint space, bony overgrowths and ankylosis. Diseases affecting the bone, cartilage or synovial membrane cause limitation of movements in all directions and are associated with generalized tenderness. However movements towards the affected structure such as damaged ligament or capsule is associated with relief from pain. Knee joint may be locked from material present within (meniscus or a cartilaginous loose body) in such a way as to interrupt further extension, although flexion is possible. Joint movement is not possible in injury or acute inflammation due to pain. There is lack of movement in ankylosis or arthrodesis; however it is painless. Excessive laxity of ligaments results in hypermobility of the joints in inherited connective tissue disorders such as Marfan's syndrome or Ehler-Danlos syndrome. Unusual mobility of the joint is observed in Charcot's knee joints.

INDEX